Praise

"This is a guide book for a new generation. Sure, older generations might tell young men today to man up, shrug it off, or toughen up and they are not wrong to say these things, but that advice comes off as simplistic and accusatory, so it doesn't resonate. Meanwhile, rates of depression and anxiety are skyrocketing among the young. Justin Stenstrom does speak to this generation with detailed, thoughtful and personal advice in *Elite Mind*. It's an important book. I know several young men I am going to gift *Elite Mind* to this winter season."
— Frank Miniter, a New York Times best-selling author whose latest book is *The Ultimate Man's Survival Guide to the Workplace*

"*Elite Mind* is incredibly powerful. If you have anxiety or depression this book will absolutely change your life. Get it today."
— Craig Ballantyne, author of *The Perfect Day Formula*, and the new Wall Street Journal best-selling book, *Unstoppable*

"In an ocean of voices there are few who manage to cut through the BS as effectively as Justin."
— Gary John Bishop, New York Times best-selling author of *Unfu*k Yourself*

"We all have a story and often our greatest strength comes from the challenges we face. Justin is a force for good in the fight against anxiety and depression. His story is a testament that you too can fight and grow through your pain. Thank you Justin for not only your words but the tools to strengthen our mental health."
— Ben Newman, international speaker, best-selling author, and world-class performance coach to Fortune 500 companies, business executives, and professional athletes in the NFL, NBA, MLB, UFC, PGA, and NCAA

"Unfortunately, depression is an experiential condition and until you have it, you can never truly understand the reality of the unbearable pain — the extreme heaviness in the chest, the deep sense of existential angst, the wanting to end it all. I forced myself to try any solution, from drugs, to supplements, to food, to major lifestyle changes like meditating and prioritizing sleep, to not giving a f*ck about things not worth a f*ck. Fortunately, Justin has organized all of these solutions in a try-able whole from his personal experience with anxiety and depression, and from his success with each of them. I never expected a book on depression to be uplifting, but this one is. If you have anxiety or depression, or support one who is, or simply want to finally "get" what it is like, or just feel like reading a book with a happy ending, then this book is for you. I wish I had this book when I was 16 and a college junior, when I first tried to end my own life. Give this book a flying f*ck!"
— Dr. Ted Achacoso, Founding Pioneer of Health Optimization Medicine and Practice (HOMe/HOPe), polymath, and one of only five people in the world who possesses an IQ of 200

"Hard times, anxiety, and depression are oftentimes not a choice, Justin Stenstrom proves that the path to recovery can be."
— Andrew Marr, U.S. Army Special Forces Green Beret, Co-Founder of Warrior Angels Foundation

"This book is a powerful testimonial to the power of the mind. Justin's personal journey is just as inspiring as it is heart wrenching and gives the reader a step-by-step guide to taking charge of their own life."
— Dr. Pankaj Vij, board-certified internal medicine doctor, international speaker, author of *Turbo Metabolism*

ELITE MIND

ELITE MIND

A REAL-WORLD GUIDE TO OVERCOMING ANXIETY, CONQUERING DEPRESSION, AND UNLEASHING YOUR INNER CONFIDENCE

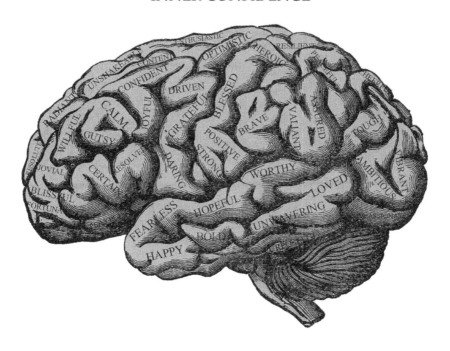

BY

JUSTIN STENSTROM

For more content, bonus material, and further elite mind training go to:

EliteMindBook.com

Copyright © 2020 by Justin Stenstrom

All rights reserved.

ISBN: 978-1-7343323-0-8

OFFICIAL DISCLAIMER

While the author has made every effort to provide accurate information with regard to references, resources, website links, scientific articles, and other citations throughout the book, neither the publisher nor the author assumes responsibility for errors or changes that may take place after this book's publication.

The author does not dispense medical or professional advice throughout this book but rather general information for entertainment purposes only. He does not recommend the use of any technique as a means of diagnosing or treating any physical, emotional, or medical condition. The information, techniques, and suggestions in this book are not a substitute for medical supervision. All matters regarding your health require medical supervision. Neither the author nor the publisher shall be liable or responsible for any loss, damage, or consequence allegedly arising from any information, technique, or suggestion in this book.

DEDICATION

I would like to dedicate this book to my father, the man who gave me life, inspired me to write, and then saved my life during a time I considered ending it. Thank you for being there for me and for blessing me with so much. I can never repay you but I will continue to thank you every day for imparting your wisdom, toughness, resilience, and sick sense of humor on me. If it were not for your foresight and outside-the-box thinking I probably wouldn't be alive today to write this book, and if it were not for your perverse style of comedy this book would undoubtedly suck ass. Haha, thank you for everything, I truly appreciate it and love you.

CONTENTS

Prelude 1

How to Read This Book 12

PART I: My Story **15**

    Chapter One: Introduction 17

    Chapter Two: My Life Now 23

    Chapter Three: My Suicidal Depression 29

    Chapter Four: Smoking Myself Crazy 37

    Chapter Five: My First Panic Attack 47

    Chapter Six: Meeting Doctor Empathy 53

    Chapter Seven: My Life-Changing Decision 59

    Chapter Eight: I Know How You Feel 65

PART II: Anxiety **71**

    Chapter Nine: My Shrink and Me 73

    Chapter Ten: Mindfully Meditating 83

    Chapter Eleven: Living in the Moment 93

    Chapter Twelve: Taking a Key Mineral 109

    Chapter Thirteen: Sleeping Away My Worries 135

    Chapter Fourteen: My Last Panic Attack 163

    Chapter Fifteen: Facing My Biggest Fear 179

    Chapter Sixteen: Taming the Beast 193

PART III: Depression **199**

    Chapter Seventeen: Cultivating Gratitude 201

Chapter Eighteen: Hypnotizing Your Depression 221

Chapter Nineteen: Working out Your Blues 239

Chapter Twenty: Supplements for Depression 255

Chapter Twenty-One: The Antidepressant Diet..........................269

Chapter Twenty-Two: The Power of Community 283

Chapter Twenty-Three: Having a Purpose 291

Chapter Twenty-Four: Loving Yourself 309

PART IV: Confidence 319

Chapter Twenty-Five: Your Untapped Confidence......................321

Chapter Twenty-Six: Pretend to Be Great 329

Chapter Twenty-Seven: A Powerful Confidence Tool 341

Chapter Twenty-Eight: Shattering Your Comfort Zone...............355

Chapter Twenty-Nine: Improving Your Self-Image......................367

Chapter Thirty: Averaging Your Way to Greatness 389

Chapter Thirty-One: It Takes Work...403

Last Words 415

Epilogue...423

REFERENCES 435

ACKNOWLEDGMENTS 461

RESOURCES 462

ABOUT THE AUTHOR 463

ELITE MIND

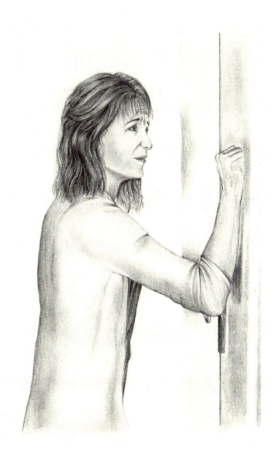

Prelude

John Smith was a typical American teenager: a fair-skinned young man with brown hair, brown eyes, a splattering of freckles around his nose, and a nice warm smile that evoked nothing but joy for those fortunate enough to see it. He was handsome in the eyes of most, had a frame that affirmed a natural predisposition for athletics, and bore a mind that revealed his greatest innate blessing of all, a profound intellect that destined his future to be one that just about ~ would envy. Yes, John's occupational trajectory wo·¹ ˙ include that of a doctor, lawyer, physicist prestigious. It wasn't a matter of *if*, but *what* he would choose to impart his brilliance upon.

He excelled in academics and sports for as long as anyone could remember, from Little League where he was a perennial All-Star, to the classroom where he was a regular honor-roll student. He made friends with ease and had many during his younger years. Sports teams, backyard ballgames, birthday parties, straight-A grades, and a close circle of loving family and friends encompassed all the years of young John's adolescence. He led a fine life by all accounts and was lucky and fortunate to have all he did.

John was blessed with much, and certainly thanked his lucky stars from time to time like any good young boy would do. He was happy and life was good.

But like all things in life, change occurred.

It didn't happen overnight, but slowly, a gradual shift began to take place in John's world.

As puberty set in, John, like many his age, became a bit insecure with his transforming body. Overzealous facial acne, frequent recalcitrant fluctuations in voice, unwanted facial, armpit, and pubic hair growth, and uncontrollable spikes of sexual desire in the form of embarrassing pant bulges in the midst of any given school-day lesson, all accompanied his development.

The once confident and self-assured John began to take a step back and become a bit more reserved to cope with the unpredictable changes with which his maturing body might betray him. He stopped raising his hand to answer questions in class; he stopped having his friends come over for backyard games and birthday parties; he withdrew a little from his family and even his really close

Prelude

friends; and he began to focus more on himself in an unconscious effort to reassert control over his physiological chrysalis.

As high school commenced, John only drew deeper into his emotional shell and further from the young, happy boy he'd formerly personified.

He lost touch with his old friends, stopped caring about sports, refrained from trying much (if at all) in school, and exhibited a loss of performance in nearly all areas of life. He didn't mean for things to spiral downward, but they did, and by that point he didn't know how to stop them. On the outside, of course, he played it cool and pretended he was fine, but on the inside, he was really struggling.

The once friendly, lovable, gifted John Smith was now becoming a withdrawn, quiet, troubled young man. Sure people still knew John, and most people still liked him, but nobody really seemed to care anymore. No old friends seemed to want to hang out with him, no new classmates seemed to want to make his acquaintance, and the love and passion he had for sports and for being active drifted away with his childhood innocence, leaving him resigned to spending his days at home, in a self-imposed isolation.

And so continued his downward descent. Only now the pace was picking up.

Desperate for change, John began acting erratically. He got into trouble at school, began hanging out with the wrong crowd, and started experimenting with drugs and alcohol. He was still a good person, but his misguided efforts to ease his omnipresent emotional woes took control of his rational, otherwise well-intentioned young mind, and led him into exacerbating his problems with even deeper anguish.

A few nearly failed classes, several suspensions, and many experiments with alcohol, marijuana, and even some pills later on, and John was completely lost. The nice young boy was all but gone from the nearly grown but disturbed young man. And the pain John so desperately tried to cover up for some time, had only gotten worse, and was about to hit its peak.

The loneliness that had been his closest friend for the past few years began to take over. It grew like an uncontrollable tumor and festered into a crippling depression he couldn't shake. Day after day he'd wake up with the feeling that he would never get over it. That he would never have real friends again. That he would never be an A-student again. That he would never get a girlfriend, even though girls had used to really like him and tell him he was cute when he was younger . . . He must not have been . . . or at least that's what he thought.

He dwelled on everything that wasn't going his way in life and began to believe that everything he thought he'd once known was really all wrong the whole time. He didn't know anything anymore and had even lost the drive to try to figure things out. None of it made any sense. The only thing he really knew was that life wasn't fair. It sucked. It never gave him any breaks and always seemed to work out well for all the jerks. But good guys like him always got screwed over.

Yes, he knew this, and only this, to be true. And he didn't want any part of it anymore.

And this was when his anxiety kicked in. A habitual feeling of uncontrollable nerves and wild thoughts, that would surge through his mind and body and leave him feeling utterly terrified, soon got mixed into his cacophony. He had no idea what this was at first, but soon began taking medication after getting the diagnosis from a family doctor a short time later.

Along with antidepressants, he thought he'd found a solution to his problems, but quickly realized the transient hope was nothing more than wishful thinking. The pills didn't necessarily inflame his condition, but they certainly did nothing to alleviate it. And after a few more days, John was back at it, having panic attacks, and feeling more hopeless than ever.

He held out for a few months, fighting off the emotional torment, for no other reason than to make his parents think things were okay and that the meds were working. But deep down he knew he'd never get over those feelings.

The loneliness that gripped him at every moment. The anxiety that became a constant companion. The panic attacks he was forced to withstand, sometimes multiple times in a single day. The sleep he'd rarely get. And the depression. The depression that made him sink into the lowest strata of his soul and make him feel like he was, and never would be, anything. The depression that made him want to end it all. The depression that kept calling after him, edging him, tempting him, enticing him with the only solution to his perpetual suffering.

And one day this allurement proved to be too much.

WHERE'S JOHN?

John's mother, Mary, called for John to come down for dinner.

At first she thought nothing of his unanswered response, chalking it up to a typical habit whenever she wanted to get his attention. As a mother in her mid-forties and understanding how young boys are, she chose her battles carefully. Things like this didn't really bother her.

After half an hour or so, when she and her husband Jim had finished their meals, she gave another call to Jonathan, just to remind him that his plate would probably need to be microwaved now. Still she heard nothing back, but again, this was all too common.

Perhaps an hour later, after watching one of her favorite shows with Jim, she noticed the plate still out on the counter, and Jonathan still nowhere to be seen. Now she was a little worried. "He definitely should've come down by now," she thought, and gave another call up to Jonathan, this time with a touch of admonishment and a hint of worry in her voice.

After not even a full minute of silence she decided she'd had enough, and despite Jim's assurance that everything was fine, she left the sofa and marched up the stairs, hoping from the bottom of her heart that this was just something stupid, a foolish mother's over-worrying and nothing more.

But she had an intuitive dread that something was amiss.

By the time she reached the top step her heart was pounding. She didn't know why, but she knew something wasn't right. She stormed over to John's door and knocked three times with a banging that could conceal her desperation no more.

"Jonathan?" she asked after the trio of knocks.

"Jonathan, are you in there?" she repeated, her composure fading, as she prayed for nothing more than to hear her son's sweet voice.

"Jonathan, open the door right now or I'm coming in," she announced one last time in defiance, after another set of unanswered frantic calls.

Prelude

She couldn't take it anymore. She turned the doorknob, but was surprised to see it wouldn't fully rotate. It was locked.

She frenetically called out for Jim, and even he now seemed truly worried after rushing up the stairs. Both Jim and Mary instinctively knew in that moment that something was terribly wrong.

Jim didn't even wait for his wife to say anything else. In one powerful thrust of his aged but burly left shoulder he broke the door open and burst in.

The lights were off, so immediately Jim flipped on the room's switch as Mary entered too, fervently pushing past Jim's frame to get a better look at what lay before them both.

For a split second both parents noticed absolutely nothing.

Jonathan was nowhere to be found.

"Jonathan!" Jim called out in a booming voice. "Where are you so—" "Oh my God!" Mary cried out, her heart dropping, as Jim followed her gaze, and instantly realized his worst fears had come true.

In the nook on the far side of Jonathan's room where Jonathan's closet was situated stood an image that would forever haunt both Mary and Jim for the rest of their lives.

John Smith, their kind, brilliant, and beloved boy, was dangling just inches off the ground from a rope whose noose wrapped around his neck and whose other end was tied tightly around a screwed-in metal bar, one which many years back had been installed by Jim to support a toy basketball hoop for young Jonathan.

Jim instinctively ran over and lifted Jonathan up onto his shoulders, in a futile attempt to give his boy another breath. But it was far too late. Jonathan had been there for hours now, his blue face revealing this unfortunate reality.

Mary, following suit, immediately reached up and ripped off the knot from the bar, her desperation giving her more strength than usual, but even in doing so, she knew deep inside that it was over.

Both Mary and Jim tried everything they could think of for the next half dozen minutes, including an emergency call to 911 of course, but try as they might, Jonathan was gone. And nothing they could do would ever bring him back.

Their little boy would never breathe another breath again, would never say another word, would never bring home a girlfriend, would never graduate from college, would never have that great job, would never marry a beautiful woman, and would never bring grandkids over for them to relive the most precious moments of life with.

It was over.

THE AFTERMATH

Jim and Mary, aunts and uncles, cousins, many old friends, and a good number of classmates all came to his funeral. And the emotions ran unbearably high throughout. Not a dry eye was found amongst the crowd of family, friends, and contemporaries, and the palpability of this tragedy could be felt by all.

Nobody could discern why Jonathan had done it.

His classmates knew he'd been quiet the past few years, and maybe more so the last few months, but he'd never shown any signs of being depressed. He just seemed bored.

His old friends hadn't seen him as much to accurately make note of any emotional change, or at least that's what they said when dialogue

Prelude

inevitably broke out on the matter. But they too, in the infrequent exchanges they'd had with Jonathan every once in a while, had distinguished no real difference in personality. To them, he seemed normal, just perhaps a little more quiet than they remembered. Even his parents, who'd seen him every single day, could not detect any significant change in his mood.

Yes, he'd gone through a lot of crap the past couple years, and especially the last few months, particularly with his anxiety and depression issues, but they knew so many other kids his age who had gone through the same. They'd chalked up his misfortunes as being part of the maturing process, and had truly felt he would grow out of it in a year or two.

Sure, the anxiety and depression had worried them at first, but the medication he'd been taking had seemed to really help and appeared to solve the problem. Never, in a million years, had they ever imagined he would do something like this.

To say they'd been completely shocked when they found him that fateful day hanging from that rope would be the biggest understatement in history. They'd been completely shocked that he'd ever even had a thought about doing this, never mind actually following through with it. Not their boy. Not the one they'd known and loved for so many years.

Jim and Mary were in denial for a long time following the funeral. It still seemed like any minute now Jonathan would come down from his room and smile his warm smile, and fill up their hearts with joy like he always did when he told a joke or acted goofy. It seemed like he was still there and that none of what had happened really happened. That it was all just a bad dream, a nightmare that would end at any moment and everything would go back to normal . . .

But unfortunately it never did.

This nightmare would never end, as it was their reality. And they had to live with it the rest of their lives. The sadness, the grief, the anguish—they would harbor these sorrows as long as they lived.

THE REFLECTION

John, or Jonathan as his parents called him for 17 years of his life, is of course a fictional character.

I crafted him from the anamnesis of my mind, as the representation of a number of people I've known well, been acquainted to, and been friends with. And as you may be able to tell, a little bit of myself can be found in John's essence.

The truth is, John is me. John is you. John is your brother. John is your son. John is your friend. John is each of us and all of us.

He's that kid you went to school with who hung himself. He's the friend you knew who intentionally took too many pills to end his suffering. He's the young man you read about in the newspaper who jumped off the town's bridge. He's the gossiped-about boy who everyone remembers through the years as the tragic, sad, misguided young man who had the world in the palm of his hand but couldn't shake his demons.

John is not an anomaly. Unfortunately this story's been told over and over again. And it's only becoming more and more common. It's shocking fewer people these days because it's becoming less of a surprise to hear, see, or read about. The regrettable truth of the matter is that suicide is becoming an epidemic, and its prevalence is spreading as fast as any disease in history.

We all know people who have killed themselves; for most of us, we know many. The heartbreaking reality is that our young men and women are dying at alarming rates because of mental disease.

Prelude

But even our older men and women, the many forgotten adults of our world, are too falling victim to this heartrending act. The true certainty of this endemic illness is that it affects everyone. Every race, creed, gender, nationality, and age is at risk for falling prey to the depredations of this truly morbid mental affliction.[1]

But it has to end.

It's killing some of our greatest minds and souls and leaving us tortured and grieving for eternity. We need a solution. And we need one now.

My hope is that in the coming pages, I can share some of the many solutions, and help put an end to this universal tragedy. My hope is to end anxiety, panic attacks, and depression, or at least drastically reduce their burden to the point where people can reasonably manage them, and in turn, wipe out the suicides that are taking out so many of our loved ones.

Hope, as you'll come to find out, is a very powerful tool, and when combined with action, can facilitate incredible change.

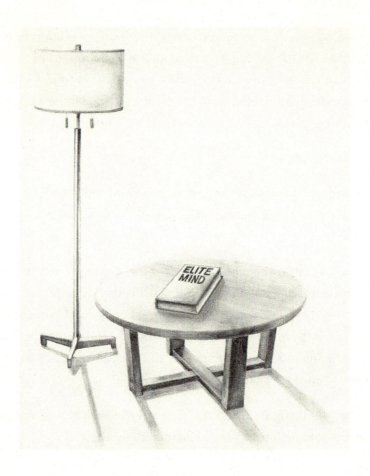

How to Read This Book

The following tale is a compendium of side-splitting anecdotes, distinctly exhilarating first-person narratives, and uproariously funny accounts of exemplary tales of mischief and adventure, designed to invoke apothegms of truth and wisdom at their conclusion. But more importantly, it's a compilation of action-packed and useful strategies for taking back control of your mind, and mastering it thereafter.

How to Read This Book

This book is essentially divided into four individual sections: The first, my captivating background story which gives you a good idea of where I come from and why I've written this book. Next is the section on anxiety, which gives you all the tools you need to get it out of your life. After this is the segment on depression, which shows you exactly how to extricate yourself from its powerful grip and reclaim your contentment in life. Finally, we have the portion covering confidence, which is reserved for teaching you the strategies for acquiring the unheralded, unbelievable, and mind-blowing self-confidence that'll propel you into living a life full of thrill-chasing and dream-catching success.[1]

You can read right through, one page at a time, which I recommend most people do. Or you can skip to the section most pertinent to the area you'd like to master right away. The choice is yours of course.

Ideally, you'll be so entrenched in the wisdom and entertainment oozing out of every page, you'll read it all from cover to cover in one sitting, and then go back and read it again many times over—but again, feel free to do as you like. This book was meant to be a guide for helping you overcome some of the toughest challenges in life. Fold over pages, highlight shit, underline words, make notes and annotations wherever you see fit, and jump back to different places to go over and really learn something again.

Skip around if you like, and use this as the guide it's meant to be: a guide to help you in your battle. I'm giving you permission to deface and defile the pages from hereafter if it helps you remember or keep your place for easy access to something later on (but only for this reason!).

Lastly, each chapter within the sections on anxiety, depression, and confidence-building offers a main action-step to implement in your life. Every single one of these action-steps taken individually has the power to change your life, but combining them with as many other action-steps from other chapters just increases your odds of unworldly triumph.

In an idyllic world you'd use all of the steps in all of the chapters. But being a human being who takes up residence on planet Earth who wasn't born yesterday, I know that some steps you'll probably use more than others, and others you might omit altogether. I'm here to remind you that's okay too. But use as much as you can, and implement as many of the strategies as possible. This is really the fastest track to seeing success.

Cultivate the elite mind housed deep within the shadowy depths of your brain, and optimize it to live the most heroically fantastic life you can imagine. Trust me, you deserve nothing less.

Now, let's begin.

PART I
My Story

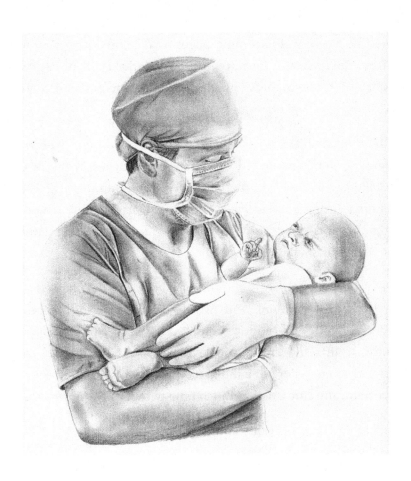

Chapter One
Introduction

About 90% of my life is spent making fun of people. The other 10% is spent wondering why I'm not making fun of people. But before you get all uppity and think I'm a complete asshole for this, let me add that even *I*, myself, am not immune to my own self-amusing expulsions of humor. You see, I don't take myself too seriously. And I especially don't take life too seriously. I take it the way I feel it was meant to be taken, in stride and with laughter, much laughter.

As you'll observe in the coming pages, I've come a long way in my life, from the lowest of lows (the deepest, darkest pits of depression and anxiety) to the highest of highs: a happy, hopeful, and confident place of earnest contentment.

But the ride wasn't easy, as you'll see, and it's still not over, not by any means. Yet I've learned over the years to cherish the ups and withstand the downs, and (perhaps even more importantly) to enjoy the entire journey in between. And so the overwhelming majority of my time now is spent doing what I love doing the most: laughing and making others laugh as well.

Whether that's in person, online, or via a book like the one before you now, I truly love playing with words and nestling others into the wonderful world of humor. There's truly something magical in comedy. It lifts the spirit, connects two individuals, and creates happiness, even if only for a moment. But that moment is special, and so I've naturally cultivated as much time with it as possible.

With that said, let's officially end the formal pleasantries.

I swear quite a bit throughout this book. If you're easily offended by a few well-placed f-bombs, s-bombs, and other curse-words of note, this is probably the wrong masterpiece for you. Do us both a favor and pick up something more suitable, like say a Mr. Roger's greatest hits DVD or something by some other wimpy asshole.

I'm honest, upfront, and genuine, and sometimes describing the true authenticity of a moment requires a pejorative term or two. Get over it. I'm not perfect and I'm not going to sugarcoat shit and pretend to be.

Also in my defense, I'm from Boston, Massachusetts, being moderately crude is kind of in my blood.[1] We Bostonians get spit out of the womb with guts and blood splattered across our naked little

Introduction

bodies and two clenched fists with middle fingers hoisted toward the obstetrician for rudely awakening us from our cozy nine-month slumber. (It's been historically proven.)

Furthermore, I make fun of various notable characters throughout the book. Again, if you continued reading after the last warning, stop now. If this is going to offend you, take your bizarrely-directed angst out on someone else. I've already told you to find something else to tickle your fancy, perhaps *Little House on the Prairie* will do.

But seriously, what's a self-help book without some cleverly placed comedic descriptions of fucked-up people here and there?

In addition, as you can probably tell by now, I don't really give a shit whether you like how I talk or not. I'm here to help you and deliver my profound message, in the only way I really know how: by sharing with you techniques that actually work, and making you laugh so you remember them thereafter.

It's really the best approach for getting someone to recall what they've been taught, and it also happens to be far more entertaining to me to write this way.

So, let me apologize in advance to anyone I may offend in the upcoming chapters. Again, not that I really give a shit, but do remember that if I say something that offends you or some crippled person you know, it's only said to help you (and the crippled fucker you know), and to make you laugh. I don't take myself seriously and neither should you. You can make fun of me all you want, and call me any name in the book. I'll just laugh and talk shit right back to you, it's called having thick skin—and having a sense of humor. And yes, this is something our society is in desperate need of at the moment.

So stop being such a sensitive butt-licker and allow me to tell you the story of how I became such a wise, humor-filled, and confident young man (young if you're reading this within 30 years of the original publication—when I hit 57 I'll relinquish my "young" title), and how I overcame two devastating problems that leave so many disheartened and hopeless in life: anxiety and depression.

As you can probably discern by now, this isn't your prototypical self-help guide. It's not a book that talks about abstract concepts, ra-ra shit, and woo-woo philosophies designed to make you feel all warm and fuzzy for a few fleeting seconds. If you want the "You-can-do-it-Johnny" mantra you can open up the scores of other self-help books that are littered with that motivational crap, for it leads to nothing but continued frustration and unanswered questions. You won't find that disappointing dogma here. Instead, I present to you raw, honest, and unfettered truth about combating your mental struggles and cultivating a winning attitude.

It's not pretty, it's not for everyone, and it's not going to make you feel all snug and special, but it fucking works!

If you want real you've come to the right place. If you want the perfect blend of narrative allure and personal growth guidance, you've come to the right place. If you want a story that entertains you and occasionally makes you spit out your freshly-poured hot coffee amidst uncontrolled bursts of laughter, you've come to the right place. And finally, if you're sick of turning over self-help stones, one after the other, in search of the answer to your own mental health woes, look no further . . . you've also come to the right place.

Self-help books are cool, trust me, I've got a nice collection of them I use to impress girls that come over from time to time. But the staggering majority of them are as useless as a great big pile of steaming dog shit. And it's mostly because of three reasons:

Introduction

One, most of them suck balls in terms of their content, meaning the vast majority of them just don't deliver enough value aside from the "you-can-do-it" attitude.

Two, the practical takeaways for readers are either overwhelming or non-existent; the reason for you, the reader, to pick up a self-help book in the first place is because you want to change something in your life, hence the cleverly titled genre. But so many of these uncleverly written books either have far too many actionable steps to take (they tell you to do an exorbitant amount of shit, naturally leading you to do *nothing*, because you, like every other human being in existence, will get overwhelmed by such an overburdened approach) or, oddly enough, provide you with zilch to do in terms of actionable steps, which is clearly just as bad, if not worse.

And finally, the third reason most self-help books suck big hairy donkey balls is because they're written in the quintessence of a 99-year-old Catholic Church priest giving a sermon on Easter Sunday. That is to say, they're about as entertaining as watching a freshly-painted fence dry. They spit facts, how-to's, and well-meaning tips, but they can't get the reader to pay attention, because they're so goddamn boring. (Trust me, if there's one thing you will not be while reading this book, it's bored. I'll bet your depression on it.)

So strap in and enjoy the ride. Have a few laughs, keep an open mind, and most importantly, take action on the advice laden within this book. No matter how much I joke around and bust people's balls, I am truly in it to see people get better. I know just how bad life can suck when things are off for you mentally, trust me, it's the worst fucking feeling you can possibly have. I know it all too well. At the end of the day, I want you to be happy again, to have hope again, to have confidence in yourself again, and most importantly, to laugh unrelentingly at all life has to offer . . . after all, humor is truly magical.

Lastly, everything mentioned in the forthcoming pages is all either backed by science, backed by personal experience, or backed by both. Simply put: it all works. If you truly follow the steps outlined within this book you will most certainly heal your mental issues and master your mind. It's not easy and it takes a lot of work on your end but the formula for success is quite simple: Follow this book, take action, change your life.

So many others have already done just that. And yup, you can thank me later by writing me a heartfelt note I'll probably never read.

But seriously, good luck and God bless.

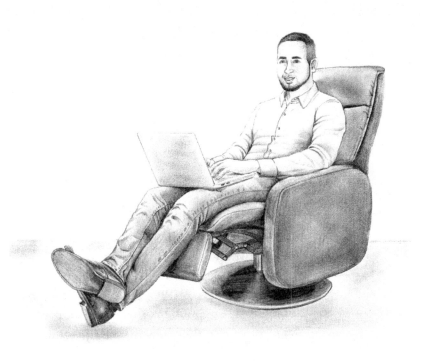

Chapter Two
My Life Now

I'm relaxing on an oversized blue La-Z-Boy writing chair that's beat up and worn down from years of use. It's got countless leather wrinkles, several prominent holes peeking out of its sides, and dozens of scratches and scrapes that memorialize the many days it's seen. But it continues to chug along, like a faithful old pup on its last leg. Yes, it's got sentimental value and I refuse to let it go. Not to mention, it's comfortable as fuck.

It's 3AM in Boston, Massachusetts. As I write these words I look over at the beautiful brown-haired naked woman lying across my bed just a few feet away. She is absolutely gorgeous and she fucks like a

Greek Goddess, though she's Puerto Rican. Puerto Rican girls are some of my favorites, and this girl in particular, is probably one of my all-time favorites. She looks stunning and her personality can be summed up in one word: *feisty*.

She's entertaining, loud, and exciting all at once, and keeps me on my toes. Exactly the formula to turn me on.

It's been about half a year since I broke up with my ex of three years, but I'm finally getting to the point of being happy and being myself again. She was a great girl, my ex, but it just wasn't meant to be at that point in time. And so even though it was the right decision to mutually end things, it still hurt. Really fucking hurt.

For someone who's faced anxiety, depression, and feelings of loneliness and abandonment throughout his life, a breakup can be crippling. It can be even more crippling when you truly love that person. But it was something that had to be done, and something that I'd slowly conditioned myself over the years to withstand.

Though clearly being a night owl is something I've not yet grown past, I grin to myself for a moment thinking of how far I've come over the years. I think to myself how fucking lucky I am to be sitting here now writing this book. How happy I am with where I am in life, both personally and professionally. I'm truly blessed and enjoying every moment of the ride.

Running a top-rated podcast for men's self-help advice and a website that accompanies it is easily one of the coolest occupations I could possibly think of having. Not to mention coaching guys into overcoming their day-to-day struggles and running live events throughout the year, which is just as much fun, if not more. I absolutely love my job and really don't even think of it as a *job* per se. It's more like a daily passion that just so happens to make me a shitload of money.

My Life Now

I regularly get to chat with some of the world's most successful entrepreneurs, authors, doctors, and high-achieving individuals (virtually any time I want to have them on the show) and pick their brains for advice that would otherwise cost tens-of-thousands of dollars to receive. I always say, interviewing some of the guests I bring on is like a free personal coaching session for *me*. I learn just as much as anyone listening.

I've had legends like Robert Greene (international best-selling author of *The 48 Laws of Power*), Kevin Harrington (billion-dollar business mogul and original shark on *Shark Tank*), Bas Rutten (UFC superstar and former heavyweight champion of the world), Grant Cardone (*New York Times* best-selling author and top business strategist), Dr. John Gray (best-selling author of the iconic book *Men Are From Mars, Women Are From Venus*), Dr. Dale Bredesen (a famous neurologist who's literally reversing Alzheimer's Disease) . . . the list goes on and on (I could also mention Dan Millman, Paige Hathaway, Dorian Yates, Dr. Bruce Lipton, Mark Manson, Gretchen Rubin, Jocko Willink, and Wim Hof, to name just a few).[1]

These names aren't listed to brag or to impress you, but to impress upon you how far I've come. I went from pushing carriages and taking shit from old ladies at my first job at 14 years old as a Market Basket bagger, to running my own business now, making my own schedule, and getting to do something I truly enjoy every day.

On top of the great fun I have in business, as I alluded to at the beginning of this chapter, my personal life is fucking kickass too. I have a handful of really close friends with whom I hang out all the time and who I love like family. We drink together, party together, sit back and shoot the shit and laugh together, brainstorm together, and share secrets and goals about our lives with each other. Most importantly, we really enjoy each other's company.

I also have a really close family who I love dearly and who I spend as much time with as possible. Dinners, football games, movie-watching, and much more is spent with the family. I've got their back and would do anything for them, and I know they have mine.

My dating life too is exceptional. I truly enjoy being single now, unlike any other time in my life. I'm content. I enjoy the peace and quiet. I crave the novelty of new women, yet I'm okay when I don't get it. I enjoy my alone time and use it productively; but I equally enjoy connecting with others and forming new bonds and relationships. It's a very interesting point in my life and one I've fully embraced, though it hasn't always been easy to do so, and certainly hasn't come naturally.

Yes, life is great at the moment. It's not perfect, nor do I imagine it will ever be, but it is really fucking good. I can only hope that my level of contentment and happiness will carry on for a hundred more years, until I'm incredibly old, feeble, grey, and too senile to know the difference.

Yes, my life as it stands right now is quite special.

But it wasn't always this great.

There was a time when all of what I have now seemed like a fairytale in somebody else's book. Having great friends, a happy family, beautiful women, a job that pays great and that I truly love doing . . . this was all completely foreign to me once. My life a decade ago was nothing like it is today. None of the positive elements of my gratitude today could be found back then. In fact, it felt like everything around me was exceptionally dreadful.

Because it was.

I was a completely different person back then. And living in a completely different world.

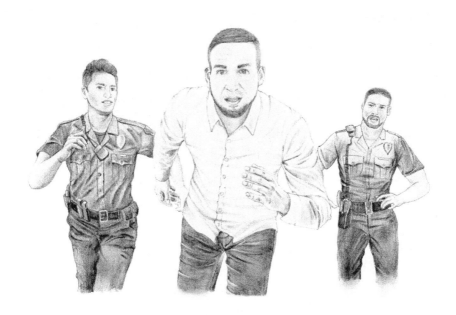

Chapter Three
My Suicidal Depression

"I could get in my white Pontiac Sunfire and drive down route 44 at a buck-twenty, cross over the median, and hit a truck head on. That would definitely work," I thought to myself. "Or, I could easily sneak into dad's gun rack and take his hunting rifle when he goes to work. That might even be easier. But I won't, WILL NOT, use a rope and hang myself like so many other kids have done! That just seems too painful and like so much work . . . but on second thought, I've heard it doesn't hurt nearly as bad as people think. And the neck is supposed to break instantly if you do it right."

These were the words I uttered to myself internally as I sat on the couch in my living room about 10 years ago. I was depressed—no, *severely* depressed—and for about a year or so (I was 17 at the time) I constantly thought about ending my life.

The stress of life had gotten to me.

The pain of being alone had crippled me for some time and ascended to a level that had become completely insufferable. I simply couldn't bear it anymore.

You see, I'd always had this feeling of loneliness, even when I was younger. I remember having friends over and every time they would have to go home I felt a fear of being by myself, and a minor feeling of gloom would creep through my body.

I think it's in my genes.

I looked it up once, and some people are just naturally predisposed to feel more aloneness than others.[1] Just as some people are inherently wired to be musicians, or write books, or build houses (or be overly-happy do-gooding assholes like Ned Flanders), some too, are innately blessed with feeling lonely. And I had this gift.

Alas, along with this celebrated endowment came another true blessing: episodic stints with a modest yet occasionally substantial depression. Not manic, or bipolar, or schizophrenic depression, like many unfortunate others have had to endure, but a periodic, shitty, down-on-yourself depression, that always seemed to show its face whenever things weren't going well in my life.

And in this particular period of time, things were going *awful*.

In fact, it had gotten so awful that I could no longer manage my low-grade melancholy like I'd been able to do for the majority of my life. At this point in time, it had taken over.

MY CHILDHOOD

Looking back at my early childhood there was always a bit of depression behind the scenes; I just didn't really notice it. Blessed in those early years with truly loving parents, incredible siblings, and great friends, the grisly features of depression were never able to showcase themselves in a conspicuous light.

The outdoors was where I lived as a kid. No matter what season it was, we Stenstrom kids always found something to do outside. The summertime was filled with wiffleball games and barbecues; the winter with snowball fights and sledding.

I always enjoyed being active and competing with other kids my age, whether that was slipping past tackles in backyard football or chasing down my enemies during nighttime contests of hide-and-seek or manhunt. The competition of just about anything fueled my joy. And this kept me content and kept the background despair at bay. In fact, it was virtually non-existent for many years, other than the intermittent periods of loneliness and the occasional nights where I couldn't sleep because of the lively nature of my mind.

But as the years progressed and the wiffleball games ended and the snow melted away, I became less active with others and delved deeper into my own head, a head that I soon realized was full of deep-seated fears, shame, anxiety, self-consciousness, and yes, dark, unwavering depression, a much darker depression than I'd previously experienced or even knew existed.

THE HIGH-SCHOOL YEARS

By the time high school rolled around I was lost.

In middle and elementary school I'd managed to be a fairly popular kid and reveled in having naturally good looks and a pretty decent charm. The girls liked me, my friends enjoyed hanging out with me, and my grades were better than those of just about any other kid in school. I was a pretty decent-sized fish in a small pond.

But when I became a freshman at Taunton High School, this all changed.

Amidst the transition into the vast sea of high-school students, I lost connection with just about every friend I'd made in my former lagoon. My claim of being a moderately cool kid was gone almost overnight.

I then hit the devastating lows of puberty, delved deeper into the pessimistic confines of my mind, and stopped caring about my grades.

Unbeknownst to me, these were the initial rumblings of a distant storm brewing on the horizon, but one that was closing in fast.

FRESHMAN YEAR

My freshman year consisted of signing up for the football team and trying fruitlessly to make the starting lineup. I was fast as hell which was great. But I was also small as hell which was really shitty. I weighed about 130 pounds soaking wet and stood maybe 5'7 on my tippy toes.

Naturally, after getting crushed in practice day in and day out for the first few weeks by kids weighing 30-60 pounds more than me, I started lifting weights to increase my frame. This was my first real foray into health and fitness, and a first step into what would become a true passion for me later on.

But I had no real idea what I was doing in the beginning. I did manage to fortuitously gain maybe 10-15 pounds or so by virtue of sheer luck, but it wasn't nearly enough to be competitive on the field. Needless to say, I sucked because I was just too small.

Strike one.

I went out for the team, like most teenage boys, to become more popular and to get girls, and I guess to have some fun playing football as well. Unfortunately though, when you get pummeled in practice and you don't play during the games, you kind of don't catch on as one of the trendy kids. Consequently, if you're using this as your main apparatus of choice in getting girls, you kind of don't get any. And, as a final obligatory cherry-on-top, when you get your ass kicked every day, don't become popular, and don't get a single girl . . . you have absolutely no fucking fun. Strike two, three, four and five.

Yeah, that pretty much sums up my first year of high school. A culture shock of ass-kickings, failures, and dejection.

SOPHOMORE YEAR

My second year in high school, things started to look up for me. Just kidding; it sucked equally bad if not worse than my freshman year. I took up boxing in the hopes of getting tougher, as by this point I'd gotten it in my head that I needed to be tough to be cool, and I needed to be cool to get girls, and football wasn't doing either for me.

Well, to make a long and excruciating story short, I was neither tough nor cool, and I still didn't get any fucking girls.

In fact, the only tangible things I received from boxing were multiple concussions and considerable brain trauma from doing it every day for four to six hours and for nearly two years (until I finally smartened up and quit). I had fully committed to learning the craft and tried with reckless abandon to get good at it. At one point I firmly believed I was going to be a professional boxer, and nobody could convince me otherwise.

But truth be told, I can't bash it completely. As much as boxing didn't come naturally, and did leave some lasting damage, it did teach me some good things. It taught me how to fight, how to not quit, and how to hang in there when you're scared shitless, all lessons I've needed to use time and again throughout my life.

As an aside, if I was smarter back then and knew what I know now, I would have approached it quite differently. I would have rested more, and taken breaks after getting many of those knocks to the head, to give myself time to recover. Oftentimes you have to take several steps back and relax, even when you want to keep pushing forward. But it's lessons like this that typically only come with time. As someone who wants to be the best and wants things right away, patience has been a virtue I've consciously needed to cultivate over the years. And it's something I must continually remind myself to embrace.

With boxing being the main focus of my second unsuccessful year in high school, the social facet of my life continued to plummet. My friends completely disappeared and the girls I tried to impress weren't impressed.

JUNIOR YEAR

My next year was where shit really hit the fan for me. I persisted with my futile attempt at becoming a professional boxer for most of the year, but also added in smoking weed, drinking alcohol, and law-breaking to this terrifically fucked-up recipe for success.

This year was essentially my troublemaking year. After a couple of years of pent-up frustration and accumulating despair, I started to lash out, at the world and at myself. I hung around with some kids who weren't really my friends, but with whom I wanted to fit in. And I did what they did, only being the high-achieving go-getter I am, I did it better than them.

I started smoking weed all the time. I started drinking alcohol. And I started committing countless amounts of crimes. (I'd like to be brutally honest here and just own up to many of these crimes, but to be even more brutally honest, I'm not entirely well-versed in the Massachusetts Statute of Limitations. There could be some fucked-up loophole somewhere that could potentially bite me in the ass. So, suffice to say, I'm not getting into specifics, but I did some pretty bad shit for a short period of my life.)

I'm not proud of this nefarious past, but like it or not, it happened. I'm also truly lucky (and blessed) I never got caught.

In fact, it took a really close call where I *was* nearly caught by the cops (for one of these aforementioned acts of criminality) before I finally smartened up and quit doing stupid shit.

But as you can see, my life was spiraling out of control.

THE REASON I DID IT

I was and have always been the same guy inside, for the most part anyway. And that is a good man, and a good person. But I think time, frustration, and hopelessness can make anyone waver in their moral convictions. And it did that to me.

Not to mention drugs and alcohol can also play a big role in this moral decision-making process (though it was not as pronounced in my case, it certainly is in many others), and stress within the brain (of which we'll certainly be expounding on soon) can also lead many to do things they otherwise never would.

So to recap, I clearly wasn't in the best state of mind.

I'd been doing drugs and drinking alcohol intermittently, taking shots to the dome from boxing, hanging out with people who were not really my friends and who had a horrible influence on my well-being, and to top it all off, I still, for the life of me, couldn't get a fucking date to save my life.

As you may be able to surmise at this point, the ingredients for something extraordinarily shitty to take place were carefully being laid out. The papers had been rolled up and spread around systematically, the kindling had been meticulously placed over them, and the freshly split logs were neatly arranged on top of it all. The only thing needed now was a match.

And a match is what I got. Literally.

I remember it like it was yesterday . . .

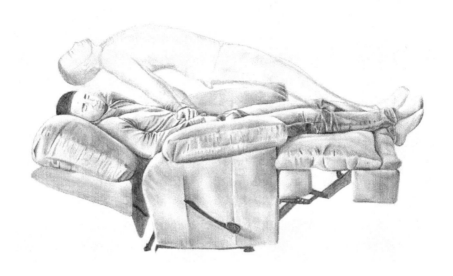

Chapter Four
Smoking Myself Crazy

We'd gotten a $20 bag of really good Haze from one of my brother's friends. It smelled phenomenal. I'd grown very fond of the smell of good weed over the last few months, and this one made me extra giddy.

I kept taking a whiff of it every few minutes and kept telling my "friend" John how fucking awesome this smoking session was going to be. We'd just skipped out on the second half of our school day, after getting the brilliant idea of snagging some weed and hanging out at my mother's wide-open house (she was a flight attendant and was away on a trip somewhere).

"I'm going to be fucked off this stuff dude! I can tell it's good. Look at how green it is and how shiny these leaves are." I waved the baggie around in front of John's face. "My boy always hooks me up. Wait 'til you try this shit, man."

About 30 minutes later we strolled into my mother's garage and turned on an old radio that had been left out there. I was never good at rolling blunts but John was. And so he took the puffy leaves and started breaking them up while I inhumanely crooned out some rap songs on the radio, in a glaring attempt to appear hip.

As sad as it was, it was times like this that I felt cool: skipping out on school, living on the edge, and hanging out with someone—ANYONE, other than myself. These were the only times when I was able to escape, if only for a few brief hours, the loneliness and depression that had built up and hit a steady crescendo over the last few years.

I knew even back then that life was shitty, that I was fucking up royally, and that I needed a big change; I just didn't know what to do. Little did I know this day would inadvertently force me into figuring that out. I didn't know it then and wouldn't fully understand it until many years later, but this day was perhaps the single most important day of my life. It changed the entire course of my life.

THREE JOHNS

"You have no idea how to hit that, man! Give me that fuckin' blunt I'll show you how to rip it right," I bragged to John.

He handed me the rolled up Black & Mild cigar and laughed. "You're a fuckin' dumbass, dude! Every time you smoke you cough. And you're not even inhaling it the right way. You gotta' really suck it in. Like a girl's tit!"

"Fuck you, watch this," I fired back. And I proceeded to take the rest of the blunt and smoke as much of it as I possibly could in the next few minutes. I must've killed half that blunt by myself, and in under two minutes. By the time I handed it back to John it was nearly gone and I was celebrating this fact.

"I told you I knew how to smoke it, you dumb mitch," I said to him. "You're takin' to the bigst webb smoker around. Nobidy smoks like meeeee."

"You are fucking stoned, bro," I remember him saying. And then I remember him laughing. A laugh just like you'd see in the movies, in some main character's nightmare. You know, where it's really vociferous and sinister and it just seems to keep going on and on and getting louder and louder? Yes, John was laughing. But I wasn't. And then it hit me.

"Why are there three Johns?" I asked myself.

I was looking at him and I could see his face and his body, but there were two more of him on either side of the John in the middle. I looked down at my left hand, and I noticed I had two extra appendages that had somehow grown out of my one left arm.

And then it *really* hit me. I was fucking hallucinating.

I started freaking the fuck out.

"What's going on man!?" I frantically tried to ask John.

But he either couldn't hear me or I wasn't actually saying anything aloud (this I'll never truly know). And like any good friend, he just laughed at me and continued to enjoy what was unfolding.

I got up and started walking upstairs. But even the elementary action of placing one foot in front of the other seemed to be too laborious a task. I kept falling down the steps, and after a number of failed attempts I eventually began crawling and literally dragging myself up the stairs like an infant child might do.

I don't know if it was the maddening hysteria of it all or the terrifying adrenaline coursing through my veins, but some internal device gave me enough strength to pull myself up those stairs, even in this catatonic state. Though admittedly, it seemed like hours before I reached the top.

When I finally got there I collapsed on my back, certain of nothing else but the fact that I'd lost my mind and was going to die.

WAKING UP

After what I can only deduce was maybe 20 minutes or so (it just as easily could've been many hours, if not days), I mustered enough energy and determination to stand up. I felt great, for a moment, but as I took a few steps I realized I was still incredibly out of it . . . and still hallucinating.

I continued seeing threes of just about everything in the room. And I was scared beyond belief.

In those moments there was nothing but pure terror surging through my veins. But I tried to remain calm. I even told myself out loud, "Everything's going to be fine. It's just a bad trip."

But it wasn't.

I went to the fridge and opened up the door to get something to drink. I found orange juice, which was a favorite of mine at the time, and managed to pour myself a glass, spilling only a bit of it on the floor and on the table.

"See," I thought to myself, "I'm already starting to come out of it."

I then picked up the glass and brought it to my mouth to take a sip of nice, cold OJ. But as I brought the glass up and was about to take a sip, I instantly realized the orange juice wasn't orange. In fact, it was red!

In a shock, I dropped the red-orange-juice glass and smashed it on the floor. I then looked back at the orange juice container that was just momentarily in my hand and realized it wasn't orange juice at all. It was a fucking ketchup bottle!

As if things weren't bad enough, another jolt of pure horror raced through my body once again. I looked at the table and then at the floor next to the broken glass, and sure enough, there was red ketchup splattered all over the place. My mother's kitchen looked like the murder scene from one of Stephen King's movies.

Blood, I mean ketchup, was doused all over the floor, table, refrigerator door, and even on the walls somehow.

"I've fucking gone crazy," I thought to myself, and collapsed onto a kitchen chair in sheer trepidation.

And then it happened.

SEEING MYSELF

I had next what could only be described as an out-of-body experience.

But it wasn't like a near-death experience, or an incident I look back on with happiness and inspiration like so many others talk about. You know, the ones where somebody nearly dies or gets in an accident and they meet God and he tells them everything is okay and that their life has meaning. No, it was not one of those at all (though I believe in that shit and do wish I had that kind instead).

My out-of-body experience was a lot different.

Mine was simply a hallucination by a misguided and stoned-off-his-ass teenager who was having one of the worst trips you could imagine. You can think of it as a mystical vision, with delirium-infused distortions of reality, by an adolescent young man who smoked a terrible batch of weed. A batch that I can only infer at this point was laced with either Angel Dust or LSD, or some variant of the two.

No, there's no happy ending bound at the conclusion of this out-of-body episode. What happened to me in those moments was even more terrifying than anything I'd already been experiencing.

Yeah, I know, as if it couldn't get any fucking worse. It did.

In my mystical haze of delusion I came out of my body and rose up off the chair, hovering maybe six or seven feet above the kitchen floor. I had no control over what I was doing and no idea of what was happening. In fact, I honestly can't remember much more than that, other than I can recall just watching myself slumped down on the chair with my head resting on the table.

I can't recollect how long I was up there watching myself, or really much else (which is probably a good thing in hindsight); I just know I was scared to death in that moment and thought I had either died, or worse, lost my mind for good.

I know this whole retrospection of events sounds bizarre, and actually, I know it's completely fucking nutty, but it's true. These things happened, and they happened to me that fateful day.

WHAT REALLY WENT DOWN

My best guess is that while under the influence of some really powerful narcotics (PCP perhaps?[1]) that had been unwittingly added to the marijuana I thought I was smoking, the neurotransmitters and signals in the brain that typically function normally had been thrown tremendously out of whack and caused me to hallucinate this entire experience.

So was I really floating six feet above the ground like some kind of inebriated angel? Probably not. But did I truly envision this happening as if it were real and as if I could actually see myself from a third-person point of view? Absolutely.

PCP and drugs related to it can make people have all sorts of fucked up hallucinations and distortions of reality. They can also cause unbelievable mental and cognitive side effects[2] after the fact, which in retrospection leads me to believe this toxic gem was in fact the true culprit.

But I digress . . .

COMING TO

After what could've been days, weeks, or even fucking years for that matter, I managed to come to. I was now on the living room couch just a few feet away from the kitchen and all the blood-smeared ketchup plastered throughout it. I cracked my eyes open a little and sat up. This time I actually felt somewhat like a human being.

My head was pounding and I got a rush of panic once more, but it was more in the anticipation of me seeing threes of things again. But to my complete and utter relief I could see normally. And I calmed down a bit.

I looked out the window and noticed it was pitch-dark outside. It was the wintertime in New England and it got dark around five or six, but we'd left school around noon. So hours, probably many, must've passed since I got here.

I walked into the kitchen with my head still throbbing, but felt relieved that I could even walk again, and began cleaning up the mess. It took me 40 minutes or so of wiping up ketchup and broken glass and other shit I'd managed to knock over or spill, before I decided the evidence of any wrongdoing had been destroyed.

I then checked my cell phone, and sure enough I had about 20 missed calls and 10 voicemails. As it turned out, it was 7:30 at night, and I hadn't been heard from by anyone (mainly my grandmother and father with whom I lived) in hours. I checked all the missed calls and listened to a few of the last voicemails really fast.

Exactly one missed call and exactly one voicemail caught my attention because they were the only ones not from my parents. They were from John.

He'd called about an hour ago and left a voicemail that I played and it sounded something like this, "Hey dipshit, I told you you didn't know how to smoke. Hahaha. I left your house earlier, my boy picked me up. See you tomorrow."

I was too hurt to be mad.

I wanted to cry. But nothing came out. I called my parents to let them know I was okay and made up a story about playing pickup basketball after school at the gym with some friends I didn't have. Then I went downstairs to the garage and cleaned up any last pieces of substantiation to my presence that day.

About five minutes later I left.

I was scared, sad, hurt, and disheartened at what I'd experienced that day. And as I drove away I told myself I would never smoke weed again for the rest of my life.

And I never did.

But unfortunately that pledge wasn't enough.

I'd hoped I'd never again have to endure any of those chilling emotions. But I had no idea this was really just the beginning. It was the start of a long, terrifying, and uncontrollable roller-coaster ride of mental health and emotional woes.

I'd only now just embarked on the true storm that lay ahead.

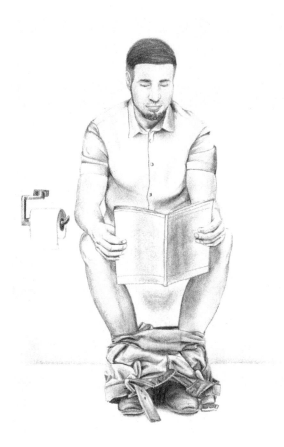

Chapter Five
My First Panic Attack

The good news is that the storm never got as bad as it did the day I hallucinated, went out of my body, and saw threes of everything in sight.

The bad news is that I had to deal with a constant blitz of emotional struggle that would never let up, a struggle that at its peak nearly led me into killing myself.

I got back home that night and went almost immediately to bed.

I took a shower, lied about playing basketball to my dad, and went to my room, where I passed out from exhaustion after just a minute of resting my head.

THE NEXT DAY

The next day I got up and went to school like any other. But I kept thinking about my horrible experience from the day before. I couldn't shake the constant thoughts of going out of my body again at any moment, or starting to see threes of things.

I was worried the entire day. And I felt sick and nauseous.

Come to think of it, I felt off for about three or four days after the delusional trip. And just to reiterate my hypothesis of the tainted marijuana being laced with PCP, it turns out PCP can stay in your system for this approximate amount of time, sometimes even up to 8 days.[1]

So while I wasn't "high" per se, these next few days my mind still wasn't its normal, albeit unhappy, self.

Not only did I feel like I was going to vomit throughout the school day, and not only did I feel anxious about getting another hallucinatory experience, but I also felt this unbelievable sense of despair. I felt like my life was absolutely meaningless, that I was a complete loser with no worth. Whether this was heightened by the drugs being in my system or just a true realization of what a fuck-up I'd been for the last few years, I'm not quite sure. But this feeling was intense, and real. That I know.

I couldn't shake it.

It was actually something I'd never felt before, something I neither quite understood nor could comprehend at the time. I chalked it up to the bad psychedelic mishap, and just kept promising myself I wouldn't smoke ever again. This gave me enough reprieve to keep going, at least for a bit.

I bumped into my incredibly compassionate and caring friend John in school later that day and he immediately started laughing when I saw him. "Dude, you were so high yesterday it was a fuckin' riot. I think you straight trashed your mom's crib too!"

"Yeah, you're an idiot! Go fuck yourself!" I walked away.

I never really talked to John after that day, and certainly never hung out with him again. I had zero interest in being around someone who could so clearly care less about my health or well-being, essentially having left me to die or lose my mind without giving a shit either way.

He tried calling a couple of times over the course of the next month or so, but after not answering any of his rings, he got the point.

Fuck him.

Looking back, this was one thing I have to give myself credit for at that time, though not much else. Cutting ties with him, and several others like him, turned out to be one small but effective step in the right direction.

THE DAYS AFTER

The ensuing days were not much better.

I kept having this weird feeling that I was going to leave my body again, or more specifically, my mind. It felt as if my mind was going to drift out of my head and be swept away by a wind. It's weird, and kind of hard to explain, but it wasn't a good feeling. And it gave me incredible anxiety.

In fact, I now incessantly had to deal with a feeling of anxiousness like I'd never experienced previously in life. Of course, we all feel stress and get a little worried about things from time to time. That's completely normal and a part of everyday life. But what I was experiencing was far different.

I was literally becoming worried every few minutes, about nothing at all. I could be sitting in class listening to a teacher lecturing about math, when all of a sudden I'd get a burst of anxiety jolting through my body about losing my mind again. Or I might just be watching TV at home, and out of the blue my heart would start pounding and my mind would start racing; I'd start thinking this was going to be the incident that would turn me batshit crazy for good.

These constant fears I had were unshakable and they were only getting worse.

MOM'S HOUSE

Several days, maybe even a full week after the initial madness at my mom's house, I was back over there as she was home from her trip. I was staying over and I remember staying up late watching sports in the living room—the same one I'd passed out in the last time I was over there.

It must've been 10 or 11 at night when I decided to go to the bathroom. By now I was the only one up and I've always liked taking a nice, peaceful shit, taking my time while leisurely reading a book or magazine on the john.

To be completely honest, I didn't even really have to go. I was kind of just bored and wanted to sit on the toilet and pass some time. I did this often back then.

So as I sat down I picked up an indiscriminate and totally arbitrary magazine that had been lying next to a couple of other random defecational compositions on the floor. I then proceeded to skim through the pages, not really interested in anything particular.

But as I was passing through the midway section of the publication something caught my eye.

It was an article about schizophrenia; I immediately narrowed my focus and began to read. I'm not really sure why this piqued my interest, but it did. It talked about what schizophrenia was, when people typically get it, and yes, all the symptoms associated with those who have it.

Now, as you can imagine at this point, this particular story doesn't end well.

Hallucinations, delusions, depression, withdrawal, irrational thinking, anxiety . . . symptom after symptom was listed, and I was checking off every single one of them to the tee.

"Yes, yes, yes . . . Oh my fucking God . . . yes," I thought frantically to myself. "I have schizophrenia!"

And this realization hit me like a ton of bricks.

The second I'd come to this irrational mental diagnosis of myself was the moment I completely lost all control. My fear, my anxiety, and my terror all reached record-shattering highs.

At that very instant my first panic attack ensued.

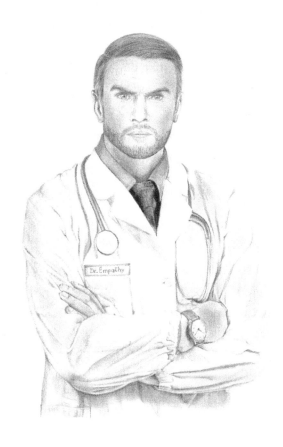

Chapter Six
Meeting Doctor Empathy

I got up with a surge of anxiety and ran for the door. I just couldn't sit there anymore, as I knew something was terribly wrong.

My heart was pounding, my palms were sweating, I was dizzy and felt light-headed as if I was going to pass out, and my thoughts? My thoughts were completely unhinged.

I kept thinking that I was crazy, that I had literally lost my mind and that I'd somehow developed this schizophrenia disease that only mental patients get. "I have it. I know I do. I should never have smoked weed in the first place. What will my parents think? What have I done? They're going to lock me up in a mental institution. Oh God, please help me! I've lost my mind!" I kept repeating these phrases in my head, over and over again, as I couldn't stop them.

And they only made things worse.

I was getting blasts of pure terror shooting through my body every minute or so and I was getting more and more dizzy and physically unsteady by the second. I felt like I was going to pass out. I felt like I was going to depart my body again. I felt like I'd never be able to go back to normal. I was petrified beyond belief.

I kept pacing around, trying to calm myself down and wanting nothing more than to be relaxed and over this devastating experience. But no matter what I did it just wouldn't let up. I even walked outside at one point, hoping that fresh air would help ease the panic levels, but it did nothing to stifle my stress.

I actually grew more anxious being outside in the middle of the night; I got really, really cold as it was the dead of winter in Taunton, Massachusetts, and I only had a tee-shirt on. Ironically enough, the frosty air seemed to stoke the flames of this wildly out-of-control inferno of emotions, adding to their intensity.

I went back inside and sat down on the couch again, trying not to think about everything that was happening. But I couldn't. I just kept thinking over and over again that this was it. That I'd really messed up this time and there was no going back.

Meeting Doctor Empathy

I got a few blankets and covered myself up trying to keep warm. But this too failed. I was shaking by then and no matter how many blankets I used I couldn't stop the bitter bite.

I debated, over 100 times throughout this episode, going to my mother's room and waking her up. I knew this would definitely be just cause to visit the ER. Honestly, I even thought of calling 911 myself several times and allowing them to take me away on the stretcher. For all I knew this was a fucking heart attack and thus a life or death situation.

But something kept stopping me from doing either of these things. It might've been shame, it might've been fear, but I just sat on the couch and continued this losing battle with anxiety.

This first panic attack lasted around 45 minutes or an hour, before it slowly faded away into a more manageable, yet still dreadful anxiety.

I sort of just slowly dozed off into sleep after a while and it all seemed to go away . . .

But it didn't.

The next morning I woke up really early, at like four or five, and immediately felt weird. Instantly I felt the anxious feeling creeping back up and felt my thoughts seemingly escape my control again. There was an incredible tightness in my chest and a feeling that I couldn't breathe. Naturally, my mind began racing wildly once more.

I was getting another panic attack. And I could not, for the life of me, stop it.

This second event lasted for another 30-40 minutes, with all the sensations of the last and all the thoughts of losing my mind, until again, after much distress and defeat, it slowly faded.

Around this time my mother woke up and came out of her room. She asked me if I wanted any breakfast and I said, "No thanks, I'm not hungry."

I couldn't work up the nerve to tell her what had just happened, what had happened last night, and what had occurred a few days prior, in this very house when she was away. So I kept quiet.

I would have carried these secrets with me to my grave if this was the last of it all. But of course, it was really only the beginning.

THE NEXT DAY

I held out for a full day and went through at least a half a dozen more panic attacks, with a dull but chilling anxiety cornering my sanity and filling in the gaps when the actual attacks took their periodic breaks.

But then I caved in. After waking up the next day and truly believing that I'd gone far beyond the crazy point, I decided to come clean.

I told my grandmother something was wrong (she'd always been the easiest to talk to about anything). She listened and calmed me down, and called my mother to come pick me up from my father's house (where I lived and stayed the majority of the time). My mother came, and listened to me and calmed me down some more, and together all three of us drove to the hospital.

On the way I came clean about everything: the weed trip, the lying, the cover-up, the anxiety, the panic attacks, the despair, the schizophrenia, the out-of-my head feelings I kept getting . . . everything.

They listened, and though I could tell they were sad, and perhaps more than a little bit disappointed, they helped. They just wanted to see me healthy and happy again. And I could sense the love they had for me. I felt good in those few minutes.

We got to the hospital and after a short while I was led in to see a doctor.

I was ready for my fate. Although terrified as ever, I just wanted to get it over with and be cured. I wanted them to give me some medication, like when you have strep throat or a fever, and I wanted this whole experience to be behind me—if that was even possible.

I was hoping against hope that it was, though. It was either this, or they were going to lock me up and ship me off to Taunton State Mental Hospital, where all the crazy fuckers got sent. Maybe I'd too become one of these poor crazy fucks . . . I kept praying this wasn't the case.

THE SORCERER

To sum up the doctor's visit that day it would have to be described in one word: dismissive.

The doc didn't seem too concerned about my story of having an out-of-body experience; he didn't seem to care that I felt like I was having a heart attack and losing my mind every few hours; he didn't really care about my belief that I'd somehow gotten schizophrenia (this I can't really bash him for now, but even still); he could really have given a shit less that I'd felt a constant feeling of dread, anxiety, and fear for the past few days; and he gave off the impression that he was needed somewhere else and couldn't be bothered much longer with his time. In fact, I should've just called him Dr. John because this guy had as much empathy and care as that asshole "friend" I used to hang out with.

But on the bright side, he did give me the "cure" I'd been looking for. After a few minutes of essentially dismissing all my symptoms, he offered up a solution to my problems and wrote up a script to end my suffering. As if some sorcerer with magical powers, he bestowed on me the note and proclaimed that I fill it at my nearest pharmacy.

"Take as directed and you'll feel better," the sorcerer decreed. "Also, here's a list of psychiatrists to meet up with to work on your dosage. Along with the Clonazepam, you're going to want to get on SSRIs[1] and they can help you with that. Good luck."

And then he waved his wand and black smoke clouded the room, and just like that he was gone . . .

Just kidding, but the hasty, old, emotionless doc did disappear faster than you can say, "Fuck."

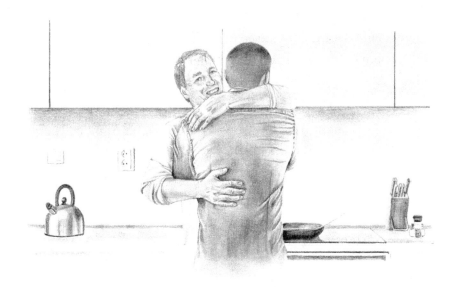

Chapter Seven
My Life-Changing Decision

Being young and dumb and desperate for a solution (like many others who fall for this trap), I immediately went home and took the Clonazepam (also known as Klonopin, or "K-Pins" by people on the street, looking to dull their brains and feel less stress) after getting a bottle from CVS.

After about an hour or so, I felt a little better after taking one pill "as directed," like the grumpy wizard had suggested. And after not sleeping particularly well for the past few nights, I went to my room for an afternoon nap, and for the first time in days had a restful slumber.

I awoke many hours later and noticed it was pitch-black outside. Maybe 9:30 or 10 in the evening. I remember getting up and walking into my kitchen to take another Klonopin pill before any more anxiety could set in, only to see my father sitting on a kitchen stool, Clonazepam bottle resting on the counter before him.

"Your mother told me everything," he said. "The whole story."

Just when I thought things were looking up, a jolt of panic coursed through my veins once more.

"I . . ." I hesitated, searching for a defense.

"Don't worry Son," my father said. "I'm not mad at you at all. I'm just happy you're okay."

Whew. What a relief, I thought to myself.

"I just wish you'd told me about this yourself," he went on. "I'm always here for you and I want you to know that. No matter how bad you fuck up, I'll always be here and I'll always love you."

I got a pit in the back of my throat in that moment. And my eyes began to water up.

My father is an old-school, Irish-Catholic from South Boston. He was raised poor, lived a hard-nosed life for many years, and then raised all his children to be tough like him. With that in mind, he'd never been the easiest to talk to. His solution to many problems was either, "Smarten the fuck up!" or "Quit being a fuckin' pussy, will ya'?" (Hence why I typically turned to my grandmother, or my mother, in times of emotional need.)

Not to say my father hadn't been there, because he always had, and I always knew it. But in terms of communicating my problems or talking about touchy things like this, it just wasn't the easiest thing to do. Men are not good at talking things out in general. My father,

My Life-Changing Decision

who'd been raised in one of the toughest neighborhoods in Boston, was even less adept at this.

But despite this, I loved the man unconditionally (and still do) and I knew he felt the same for me—even if he'd only said it once or twice in my entire life. Where my grandmother and mother had instilled love, communication, compassion, and tender qualities of the feminine nature, my father had fostered toughness, courage, determination, and resolve, a combination I look back at now and am truly grateful for. I honestly did get the best of both worlds there.

But anyway, back to the intense moment in my kitchen . . .

"I know I don't always talk about stuff with you," he continued, "but I really want you to know I'm always here if you want to talk about something. I know you're going through a tough time right now but you're going to get past it. You're a fighter Justin. You're tough and you'll get over this, trust me."

I couldn't hold back. The tears began sliding down my face. "I hope so," I said. "I just don't know how. Everything's been so off the last few days, I feel like I'm going crazy and losing my mind."

"You're not going crazy," he said. "I've gone through this exact same thing before too. Do you think you're the only one who's faced problems with anxiety, and feeling like you're going fuckin' nuts? You're not. I had the same problems too when I was your age. And I got them again many years later when your mother and I went through the divorce. Justin, it happens to everyone. Trust me, every single crazy thought that's gone through your head—EVERY, SINGLE, ONE—has gone through my head too at some point."

"I know, but it's just so scary and I have no control over it," I blurted out, through a few sobs.

"I know it is, but you WILL get over this. I know you. Your mind has the power. (He motioned to his head with his right hand and tapped it once.) It might be working against you right now, but you're going to figure out how to work with it. And I know you can do it. You're smart, you're tougher than me, and you don't give up. But this (he picked up the bottle of Clonazepam on the counter), this isn't the answer."

I was both relieved and disappointed at the same time.

I didn't trust the doc at the hospital and felt a little weird blindly taking medicine like this, but again, I knew no better. He'd given me these pills and at least it was something, where before I'd had absolutely *nothing* in terms of ideas on how to curb my rapid emotional plunge.

"A friend of mine from work went on these and some depression meds a little while back," he continued. "She was always in a great mood and really a good person to be around. I know she'd always had a little bit of an anxiety problem, but it was never really bad, as she would tell me everything. I loved chatting with her and shooting the shit. But she started taking these when her doctor recommended them, and got all sorts of crazy side effects. She tried to commit suicide a few times, had to get institutionalized for a brief period, nearly lost her job, and gained a ton of weight. She's finally off them now and on her way back to being herself, but man, it really fucked her up for a while. I was really sad to see it."

"Holy shit," I thought to myself. I would've never guessed these prescribed pills could cause such harm.

"Wow. I had no idea," I genuinely mumbled out.

My Life-Changing Decision

> **Benzodiazepines**
>
> It turns out my dad was pretty dead-on. Clonazepam and many other anti-anxiety drugs like it (Xanax, Valium) belong to a family of drugs called Benzodiazepines. Benzodiazepines, although modestly effective in short-term cases, and useful for *some* people, are vastly over-prescribed and can quickly generate a physical dependency for their use.[1] They also come with a laundry list of potential side effects: a few that my father mentioned, and many more, such as worsening anxiety, insomnia, anorexia, headaches, memory problems, mood changes, and too many others to list out completely.[2]
>
> Look, if you're taking this, or other medications like it, right now, it's okay. It's not the end of the world. But talk to your doctor and at least have the conversation about maybe weaning yourself off them at some point, and going with one of the many safer alternatives (we'll talk about these later).
>
> But please, don't do anything without having a conversation with your doctor. This is not medical advice I'm giving, just a suggestion and an observation about what's worked for me and many others in the past. Ultimately, the choice is yours. You can very well stay on prescription meds for the rest of your life and still be healthy. But you should at least know there are other options available. I'm simply here to shine the light on them.

"Yeah, they're just not as safe as some of these doctors want you to believe. And they're fuckin' addictive too. Once you start really taking them, you can't go back. You're going to need to keep taking them and be dependent on them just to function. Trust me son, you don't want to use these," he said.

"And you can beat this problem on your own," he reaffirmed. "You're a goddamn fighter, just like me."

And then he walked over to me and gave me a hug. This too, was something that he had rarely ever done in my life. So in that moment, it was truly powerful. I felt both his strength and his love right then and there, and for an instant in time all my fear went away and I felt good again.

And it was then that I decided that I wasn't going to rely on those pills sitting on the counter. I was going to beat this problem the right way. The natural way.

I still had the willpower, even during that period of total weakness and fear, to believe that I could do it. I was going to go to hell and back, searching for the true answer to my problems. And I would do anything it took to beat this, even if it killed me.

And as turns out, it almost did.

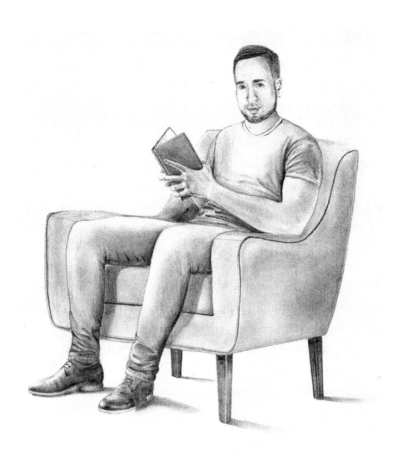

Chapter Eight
I Know How You Feel

As much as I'd like to say my life changed the minute I had that conversation with my dad in the kitchen, the truth is, it didn't.

As inspired for success as I was in that moment with my father, sadly, it didn't translate into any immediate outcome. Yes, I'd received the determination I'd needed to fight, but that didn't convert into any lasting emotional triumph, at least not right away.

He'd given me one thing that I was able to take away, however, and that was the encouragement to keep fighting and not give in. And honestly, if I hadn't had that conversation with him, there's a good chance I might not be here today.

Over the next year and a half or so, I had a lot of ups and downs. I tried just about every self-help technique I could find to combat my issues. Some of it helped (and I'll dive into that in a bit), but most of it did not. But by the end of this long, grueling stretch, I did manage to master my problems with anxiety, depression, and self-confidence, in that respective order.

But as I mentioned, this didn't happen overnight, and there were many, many pitfalls along the way. In fact, that scene I described earlier in the book? The one where I was sitting on my couch and obsessing about the various ways of killing myself? That was one of them.

WANTING TO END IT ALL

That day on the couch was several months after that talk I'd had with my father in the kitchen. I'd been trying all sorts of things for my anxiety and depression, but hadn't really made any ground.

But that particular day ended up being a turning point of sorts in my crusade for self-help.

You see, after spending hours contemplating ending it all—via car, gun, rope, or other malevolent means—I had a stark realization that things weren't okay anymore. It wasn't just a benign sense of depression or anxiety I'd been getting, but a dangerous one, one that was now posing a real threat to my life.

I'm not sure, even now, if I'd ever really have gone through with killing myself, had things continued to deteriorate. I'd like to think not. But the thought of ambiguity both then and now is what struck a true fear in me. The fact that I was even having these thoughts, coupled with the belief that they were justified, propelled me to take massive action that day. I drastically needed to find answers.

I knew in the back of my mind that the panic attacks and anxiety were what I really had to dial in on first. The suicidal ideation was dangerous, and I'd kind of been smacked in the face that day on the couch by it, but I knew deep down that the depression and suicidal thoughts were really being fueled by my inability to control my fear.

I could be unhappy. I could be a loser. I could have no friends.

If these things were true, yes, I would be depressed, and I *was* depressed, because of these circumstances. But my belief then and my belief now, at least with me (and with most people[1]) is that taking the leap from being a depressed person to a suicidal one is directly attributable to your inability to take control of your mind, especially when it's constantly dominating you in the form of anxiety or panic attacks.

Essentially, my rudimentary hypothesis, which turned out to be correct, was that if I could first take care of my anxiety and stop these unbelievably crippling panic attacks from wreaking havoc on me throughout the day, my thoughts about killing myself would go away. And then I could fight the depression I'd had for so long, and maybe, if I was lucky enough, even become a happy, confident young man.

And that's exactly what I did.

HOW THIS BOOK IS BROKEN UP

As I mentioned before, this book is divided into four sections.

The first section, which you've just read, is basically the back story of my life dealing with anxiety, depression, and confidence issues. The following segment contains my tips, strategies, and tactics for beating anxiety. The third portion discusses the techniques and game-plan used for conquering depression. And the last section talks about how to cultivate unbelievable fucking confidence in your life.

As you may notice, and as I'll be sure to point out, there is definitely some overlap between sections. For instance, some of the natural approaches I talk about for combating anxiety can, and *will*, also be effective against depression, and even for improving your confidence in some cases.

The same of course can be said of the depression and confidence chapters, respectively, in their natural overlap and applicability to other segments.

Rather than talk about the same strategies, over and over again in multiple sections, I've put each strategy in the section where it's predominantly most effective, and made note of its potential use elsewhere when appropriate.

I KNOW HOW YOU FEEL

All of the core strategies outlined in this book have been researched, tested, and applied in real life by yours truly (meaning they fucking work).

I wouldn't talk about things I didn't think could help, because I know just how devastating and crippling anxiety, panic attacks, and depression can be, and how bad it sucks not having any self-esteem or confidence.

I Know How You Feel

I also know how much it blows thinking you have something that might help, only to find out much later on that it's fucking useless. Don't worry, this book is anything but that.

By this point I hope you can understand: I've been in your shoes. I know exactly what you're going through because I've gone through it myself. As my father once said, "Every single crazy thought that's gone through your head—EVERY, SINGLE, ONE—has gone through my head too at some point. You're mind has the power. It might be working against you right now, but you're going to figure out how to work with it."

Over the years, I learned how to work with my mind and solve my problems. And now I'm going to teach you how to do the same.

Without further ado, let's commence your quest for an elite mind.

PART II
Anxiety

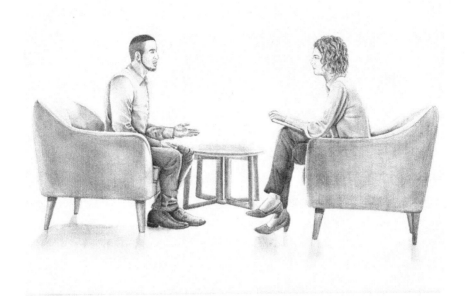

Chapter Nine
My Shrink and Me

"Oh my God, I've lost my mind and I don't know how to get it back."

Those were the words I continually thought to myself whenever I would first begin getting feelings of anxiety. The surges of fear that would accompany my every move. The unremitting sensations of butterflies swirling around in my stomach. The uneasy premonitions that something terrible was about to befall me at any moment.

I couldn't shake any of this. Not for a second.

GOING CUCKOO

I once saw a movie called *One Flew Over the Cuckoo's Nest* with Jack Nicholson playing a man who pretends to be mentally insane to avoid prison and serve his time in a mental asylum. In the film, Jack's character, Randle McMurphy, seems to think he's gotten one over on the system. But it's not long before he realizes the mental institution is a nightmare, and the head nurse is evil incarnate. She fucks with all the patients, including him, and appears to see right through his ploy.

Randle keeps his cool for some time and withstands the horrible treatment while befriending and uniting most of the other patients. But after many months of constant torment from the nurse and the rest of the staff, McMurphy snaps one day and attacks the malevolent caregiver. She survives, however, and soon after enacts her revenge on McMurphy, by having him lobotomized with the help of the other guards.

The corrupt staff then fucks with his head so badly that he actually *does* become insane. McMurphy goes from being this very sharp and witty guy throughout the movie, to being a total fucking dud by the end of it.

He's got virtually nothing going on upstairs in the form of cognitive faculties and by the film's conclusion has been transformed into a walking zombie. In an ironic twist of fate, Jack Nicholson's character becomes a true nut, but only because of the very nuthouse supposedly designed to "help" him.

MY WORST FEAR

Try as he might, time and again, there was nothing McMurphy could do once he was locked inside that asylum. Call it fate, bad luck, or destiny; he was fucked no matter what he did and doomed from the start to go crazy in there. They didn't seek to help him; they sought to make him worse.

Once you're in a place like that, there's no getting out. At least that's what I thought and it was exactly what I feared happening to me.

My biggest and worst recurring fear was ending up like poor McMurphy in *Cuckoo's Nest*. The humiliation of not being able to care for myself. The shame of not being as good as everyone else. The fear of not being able to do whatever I wanted to because I was so mentally fucked up . . . That was what really got to me.

Of course this was all in my head: a complete fabrication of reality, yet one that I was so unfortunately willing to partake in and elaborate on quite often.

The degree to which these mental contortions of actuality began to lessen, however, occurred soon after I first began visiting a shrink.

MEETING MY SHRINK

"Sit down and relax," the middle-aged, bushy-haired lady with a British accent said to me in a somewhat soothing voice. "You're safe in here."

"Okay," I meekly replied as I sat down on the couch and glanced around the room.

It was a very plain room. Professional, yes, but not really inviting or fancy, aside from all the plaques and certificates hanging on the wall behind the bushy-haired woman's desk.

I always liked observing other people's rooms. They give you a good idea of the personality of their owners. Are they serious, quirky, neat, messy, lazy, cool, eccentric, unique, ordinary, or something else entirely? This woman was unequivocally, undeniably, and ridiculously *ordinary*.

Nothing really stood out about her room or her, aside from the slight European accent which I could surmise as British.

Considering her spectacular unremarkableness, I couldn't immediately decide if I liked her or not. Usually I know one way or the other pretty quickly. But I couldn't tell with this one.

"Tell me about what's going on," she said. "I read your file and it seems like you're getting a lot of anxiety lately. Where's that coming from?"

"I'm not sure," I mumbled. "I just feel like I'm losing my mind and can't control it."

"Yeah, how so? Can you tell me what's causing you to think that and what kinds of thoughts you're having?"

"I'll be sitting around doing nothing and then all of a sudden I feel a burst of fear go through me and my mind starts racing and I keep thinking that I'm going to leave my mind and not be able to come back to it. Does that mean I'm crazy? And can you even stop this from happening? I just keep thinking I'm going to go crazy because I can't control my thoughts from giving me these crazy feelings . . ."

"Well, like I said, I reviewed your file already and I can tell you right off the bat, you are NOT going crazy," she said. "You are going through some anxiety and depression, which is actually very common, but trust me, you are not going crazy. And, just to be clear, you are not currently crazy either."

"Are you sure?" I said back, hoping to be consoled a bit more. "I've just been getting so many panic attacks lately and I feel like I just constantly have this sense of anxiety like the whole day. I can't get rid of it and I never had it before . . . How can you know for sure if I'm not crazy?"

"I know crazy," the Brit went on. "I've been doing this for over 20 years and I've seen many, many crazy people in my time: People who see things that aren't there. People who hear voices in their head that they can't explain. People who are in one moment totally happy and in a state of utter bliss, and then in the blink of an eye become unbelievably angry or depressed beyond belief. People who think they are different people at different times of the day. Do you have any one of these symptoms regularly?"

I thought long and hard for a moment and said, "I was hallucinating that time I smoked with my friend at my mom's house. Did you see that in the file?"

She nodded.

"Does that count for being crazy?" I said.

"No," she replied. "That counts for being young and dumb. That was a hallucinogenic drug you consumed that day. It would make *anyone* temporarily lose their mind. But you clearly haven't lost your mind beyond a couple of hours that day. I could tell that just by reading your file and it's even more apparent now when speaking to you." She paused before continuing, "Besides, people who are really crazy don't actually know or think they're going crazy. If you can think that thought at all, it actually means you are *not* crazy." (I found this last statement particularly interesting and very profound at the time.)

To say I was relieved would be the understatement of the year. "Okay, then I guess I don't have any of those symptoms."

"Well okay then," she laughed. "I guess you can finally believe me that you're not crazy."

And I laughed too, for the first time in a long time.

I started to like her after that moment.

I did add a question: "What happens to those people who *are* really crazy? Do they end up getting locked up in mental hospitals like in the movies?"

"No, not really. That doesn't happen the way people think it does. All of the people I mentioned to you a moment ago are people I see regularly. They make up a very small amount of my patients, but most of them are normal-functioning people. Even the *crazies* can be helped (she smiled at me). They just typically need a lot more help and almost always require several medications of some sort."

We went on, as she continued to ask me about my symptoms and I began to open up and tell her about the issues I was having.

After that first ice-breaking moment things got a lot better in the British woman's office.

I remember another key point she made that really struck home during our first day together. "I bet you would be blown away with some of the faces that come into my office and those of my colleagues in this building. Beautiful girls your age, handsome young men your age, young adults who seem to have everything you could want and seem to have the perfect life. But they don't. Nobody does. Some of the people you think have it all are those who suffer the most."

"Really?" I asked, completely shocked, just as she'd predicted I'd be. "I never knew that. I thought I was the only one going crazy here."

She laughed again. "I'm telling you. This problem, the anxiety, the depression, it's so much more common than you realize. You're not going crazy and you're not alone!"

The Numbers

It's currently estimated that 18.1% of the American adult population suffers from an anxiety disorder.[1]

That's quite staggering when you actually take into account the proportion of this figure for a second. Let me put it another way: one in every five people you come across has a clinical problem with anxiety.

That's shocking to me.

But on second thought, when I really think about it, it makes a lot of sense. There are so many people I know, both personally and professionally, who've dealt with this mental disorder, and so many more I can only imagine who are too reticent to admit it. There's an obvious negative stereotype associated with this condition, so naturally, many individuals choose not to seek help for it.

Bearing in mind this fact, anxiety (and depression for that matter) may likely be grossly underreported. But either way, the fact remains, even if we go off these numbers alone, a ton of people are suffering who shouldn't be.

Also, while we're on the subject, let's discuss some of the depression figures, because that's quite alarming too.

According to the World Health Organization, over 300 million people globally suffer from depression, and even more sadly, about 800,000 people every year are killed from suicide.[2]

Different studies claim different particular figures,[3] but depression is currently believed to affect between 7%-11% of Americans, aged 12 and older.[4] What's worse is our youth is suffering the most, having higher instances of depression, and continuing to see dramatic increases in the rates of depression.[5]

Lastly, when you look at the comprehensive list of depressive behaviors and characteristics (including anger attacks/aggression, substance abuse, and risk taking) it's believed that about 30.6% of men and 33.3% of women will experience depression at some point in their lives.[6]

> It's quite clear after examining the numbers that we have a major problem on our hands when it comes to mental illness. If we don't do something now, it will only get worse, and countless poor souls will lose their quality of life, or their lives altogether, because of the dangers of this disease.

I felt even better about myself and about her.

As we continued, I told her about my personal problems, my family, my fears of the future, my depression, and my troubles with having something to motivate me. I told her just about everything I could over the course of the next few months. And it helped.

It helped because she was one person I could count on every week, to listen to me and actually care about what I had to say.

As much as I had my parents and my family, it's different talking to someone who has no stake in the game. For whatever reason (this is really a strange but true phenomenon for the majority of human beings out there), it's typically easier to open up and share your biggest secrets and fears with a complete stranger than it is to open up to someone really close, like a family member. Perhaps it's a tribal-mentality based concept here, where we fear being vulnerable because it might damage our standing within a tribe (primordially speaking, that is), so we hold a lot of things in. Or perhaps it's something else. Whatever the case, it does seem to occur habitually.

But speaking to a shrink allows you to circumvent this problem and open the fuck up. And that's what I did. I opened up for truly the first time in my life and shared with another actual living person my greatest fears and worries. And man was this feeling fucking awesome.

I'd carried so much baggage for so many years leading up to that point it's actually quite astonishing that I wasn't batshit crazy anyway. There were the problems with my parent's divorce, with my mother always being away, with my feeling of being too short, too skinny, and too ugly compared to everyone else. And the problems with feeling like my friends had abandoned me over the years, that I couldn't make any new ones, couldn't get a girlfriend, wasn't getting good grades anymore, had no idea where I was going in life, and didn't like the person I had become. And the list went on and on.

As much as I hadn't wanted to see a shrink in the beginning, I quickly realized how invaluable our time together was.

Talking about my problems and opening up didn't change my problems or magically make them disappear, but it did allow me for the first time to really become aware of the origins of them. And in turn, this allowed me to start working on getting past them. Before, I'd basically been trying to shoot at targets in the dark. Now, the lights had at least been turned on for me.

TALKING WITH SOMEONE

Talk therapy, whether that's with a psychologist, a counselor, a friend, a family member, an acquaintance, or maybe even a complete stranger, can help you tremendously when it comes to talking about your problems. Find someone, anyone, who is willing to listen to you and hear you out. It's one of the most important things you can do.

Don't fall for the bullshit stereotypes. There's no shame in seeing a psychologist or a professional counselor of some sort. I still occasionally pop into my new therapist's office and bounce ideas off her. (I've had several different ones over the years and lost the British woman years back over an insurance policy change. Though frankly, I currently have one with whom I connect even better, and we've developed a great rapport.) Again, it's incredible to be able to open up and unpack things that you aren't able to unpack alone. Trust me, I'm not crazy because of this and you're not either for deciding to see someone. You're actually pretty fucking smart, because it works.

On a final note, I do advise you to shop around when it comes to finding a therapist. Sometimes it may take you a few tries and a few doctors before you connect with someone you really like. A rule of thumb is: if you get a bad feeling, like they're judging you or being mean or uncaring after the first session wraps up, it's time to keep looking for someone else. Good therapists are worth their weight in gold and will make you feel comfortable right away.

Embrace the process of opening up, and you can begin to take aim on the issues before you.

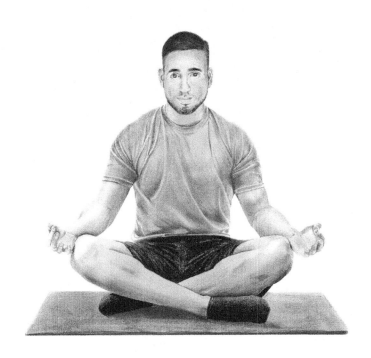

Chapter Ten
Mindfully Meditating

I sat with my legs crossed in the middle of my room like a half-assed pretzel carelessly twisted up by a teenaged Annie's Bakery employee. My legs were awkwardly positioned in ways I could not replicate again if I lived another thousand years. With my head up and my back straight I tried focusing on my breath.

The lights had been left on at first after setting everything up. Soon after though, they became too distracting so I shut them off. But then my anxiety started to creep up in the blackness so I turned my reading lamp on and positioned its head down and away, so that it let off a dim but fair balance of light and dark. *This is it. Now I can focus,* I thought to myself.

Actually, let me turn on that relaxing music CD I just got. The waves are really soothing when they crash down on the shoreline. I got up and turned on the track, using an old CD player in my room.

(Yes, we still used these ancient devices called CD players during this time period. It was just after the Paleolithic Era and right before the iPhoneithic Era. You may recall their purpose if you think long and hard, or just Google what the hell they were.)

I then sat back down and pretzeled up my legs again.

"Focus. Just focus on your breathing," I said out loud. "That's what the guy online said. Don't think about anything else but your . . . knees." *My knees? Why the fuck do they hurt so much when I cross them? . . . And my back too, now that I think of it. Why is my lower back starting to hurt?*

"Shit, just forget about it, you'll be fine," I reassured myself. "The guy in the video could hold his legs and back like this for hours. If he can do it, you can too."

I kept fighting through the uncomfortableness, determined to make it work. *10 seconds in and 10 seconds out.*

Breathing in deep breaths and letting them out, I told myself it felt good. I lied.

"Keep focusing on just your breath. Let your thoughts wander," I reminded myself, rehearsing what the mediation guru online had kept saying in his video. "You are at peace with the world," I recited. You are one with the world. Your breath *is* the world." *Wait, my breath is the world?* I was questioning my other, guru-impersonating voice. *What the fuck does that even mean? And my knees are fucking really starting to hurt now. Shit. How can I focus on my breath when my kneecaps feel like they're about to pop?*

I gave in. "Fuck this. This is stupid and it doesn't work," I said, this time extra loud for the world to hear.

And then I threw in the towel on meditating. At least for the time being.

That had been my first experience with meditation.

Needless to say it totally sucked ass. I was uncomfortable throughout and couldn't concentrate for more than a second or two on my breath. I was anxious, impatient, and completely clueless on how it all worked. I'd watched a meditation video online and figured I had it all down after that. I didn't.

My first mistake was thinking I had to contort my legs into some kind of bizarre bakery pastry. My second mistake was watching some wacko guru online and buying into his unadulterated spewing of esoteric shit.

But my biggest mistake was giving up on it so quickly.

MEDITATION WORKS

Meditation actually works. The more research that comes out on it the more it proves just how effective it can be. It helps lower stress, reduces anxiety,[1] improves mood,[2] brings your focus to the present moment, enhances executive functioning,[3] and so much more.[4] World-class athletes, high-performance coaches, Fortune 500 CEOs, incredibly successful celebrities, and so many more . . . all swear by its value.

It's really caught on the past few years and become incredibly popular, with apps like Headspace, Calm, and Insight Timer making it easy to learn how to meditate.

I'll be honest though, I didn't fully commit to meditating, in the traditional sense of the term, until after I figured out my issues with anxiety. Had I done so earlier, however, I'm fully confident in saying it would have certainly sped up the time it took for me to successfully overcome my anxiety. And this is why I'm adding it to this book.

If there's one thing I would've done differently in my crusade to recover my mind, it would've been sticking with the meditation and figuring out how it works. Because it does.

And I now meditate regularly.

I try to practice meditation a few days a week for about 10-15 minutes each time. Sometimes I'll meditate a few days in a row, sometimes I'll skip a bunch of days. I'm no longer stressed or anxious like I once was, so I don't adhere to any strict routine. If I was still anxious, like I was so many years back, I'd incorporate meditation into my life every day. But for me, right now, it's used more as a biohacking tool for optimal performance, and it does a great job at that too.

HOW TO MEDITATE

There are an infinite number of ways to meditate, everything from Mindfulness Meditation, to Metta, to Vedic, to Transcendental, to Taoist, to Qigong, to Guided, and so many others that I have absolutely zero idea (or quite frankly *interest*) in learning about.

My best advice is simple: They all work.

Whatever resonates with you on your quest to implement meditation and reap its profound benefits is the one I recommend you use. It doesn't really matter which you choose to go with, only that you take action and select something. That much I recommend.

Don't get caught up in trying to get everything down perfect in the beginning either like I did. Your feet, your legs, your back, your room lighting . . . none of that shit really matters. It's really about just trying it out and sticking with it.

That said, probably the easiest meditation to go with, and the one I inevitably settled on was Mindfulness Meditation.

This is the one I employ now as it's the one that resonated most with me.

Why?

Because it's really fucking simple to do.

Again, when I first embarked on my meditating trek I over-complicated things and couldn't get down to the brass tacks of just doing it. With Mindfulness Meditation, it cuts out all the fluff and keeps things very basic. As the great Leonardo Da Vinci once famously uttered, "Simplicity is the ultimate sophistication."

MINDFULNESS MEDITATION

In its most elementary form, Mindfulness Meditation is done by focusing your attention on a single detail for a certain period of time. This could mean fixating your concentration on a spot on your wall, on an object in your room, or on something as simple as your breath, which is usually the most recommended option and the easiest recipient of my own awareness.

ELITE MIND

Just before I start meditating, I take a deep breath or two, in and out, and then carry out a little breathing technique known as "The Relaxing Breath." This breathing exercise is great for calming you down and relaxing your mind, in and of itself, but is even more effective for getting you in the right mindset for meditation. To perform it you simply breathe in for four seconds through your nose, then hold this breath for seven seconds, and finally, breathe out through your mouth for eight seconds making a "whoosh" sound as you do. This three-part sequence is considered one full breath. You do a total of four of these breaths.

This respiratory practice relaxes you incredibly and is ideal just before meditation (and sleep as we'll cover soon). I love this technique and first heard it from Dr. Andrew Weil,[5] one of the top alternative health docs in the world.

After a minute or so of going through these specific breaths, I'll take one more deep breath in and out, and then breathe normally. From here, I'll concentrate on nothing else but my normal breathing.

My room is typically dimmed, I sit in a nice comfortable chair, and I make sure I'll be undisturbed for a predetermined amount of time.

That's it. It's really not complex at all.

No pretzel twisting, no music, no keeping my back straight as an arrow, no sitting on the floor in a Kumbaya-like attempt at reaching enlightenment . . . none of that shit.

Just me, my mind, and my breath.

The latter of which occupies all my attention.

I breathe in and I breathe out and I breathe in and I breathe out. And I repeat this over and over again, solely concentrating on these breaths for about 10-20 minutes until my alarm clock sounds and tells me it's time to wrap things up. (Or, if before sleep, until I begin to nod off, at which point I dive into my nearby bed and pass out.)

HOW I FEEL AFTER

When it's all done, I feel great. I really do.

I feel slightly energized (unless it's just before bed, in which case I feel sleepy) and more grounded and focused on what I want to get done.

I truly believe my productivity levels, on days when I meditate, skyrockets. It's like going to the gym for your mind. The neurotransmitters are firing on all cylinders, there's increased oxygen to your brain, more blood-flow throughout your body, and an enhanced sense of being in the present moment.

This is why I recommend you dive into this and hop aboard the meditation bandwagon. It's one bandwagon I don't feel ashamed in saying I'm a member of. (Sadly, there are a few others I'll omit from this volume, in hopes of preserving my good name.)

YOGA

I mentioned above a few of the different forms of meditation. I'm sure there's a million more on top of these and an infinite number of variations you could add to that as well. You could invent multifarious factions of this practice until the end of time, and I'm sure people will. All sorts of wacky, ridiculous, and downright moronic off-shoots are just waiting to be expelled from the young and dopey minds of hippies galore.

But whatever, let the hippies create. They're harmless.

Anyway, there's one subset of meditation I didn't mention and that's yoga. I left it out above because I wanted to cover it in more detail now.

To make things clear: I'm a fan.

I love yoga, and unlike my first experience with meditation, my first experience (like just about *all* my experiences with yoga from that point forward) was great.

Yoga, at least in my eyes, is essentially a stretching and moving meditation. So while it's not typically considered "meditation" in the traditional clichéd sense of the word, it actually is one of the many subtypes of the discipline, and in my view one of the best.

And just like meditation, yoga has so many fucking variants that it would be nearly impossible to list them all. Here's a short list of just a few you may have heard of: Vinyasa, Yin, Restorative, Kripalu, Hatha, Bikram, and Ashtanga.

You may have tried one of these before, or maybe you've done another type not listed; again the possibilities are endless. But as with meditation, it doesn't really matter what you settle on, as long as you enjoy it.

Personally, I like doing forms of both Vinyasa and Ashtanga Yoga (I've also tried and enjoyed Bikram, aka Hot Yoga, in the past). They're both forms of yoga where you go through a sequence of stretches (or poses) and breathe and hold the poses for a specific amount of time.

I relax, and take comfort in listening to the instructor's directions throughout the session, usually on my TV via a YouTube video, but occasionally in person. I've never done yoga without following the lead of an instructor, and probably never will. I've just never gotten good enough to do it without any guidance. Perhaps this is the one drawback to this style of meditation as opposed to something like Mindfulness Meditation, which can be easily carried out alone.

Yoga is more complex in nature, but on the plus side it's also a bit of a workout. In fact, if you do some of the moderate or challenging yoga sessions, you'll be sweating your ass off.

For me, being athletic and naturally into fitness, I initially gravitated to yoga and preferred it over plain-old meditation (now they're on the same level).

YOGA WORKED

When I started doing yoga I started very simple, as should just about every beginner out there. I popped in a yoga DVD (another technology once used in the same era as the CD) and listened to and mimicked what the young and fit yoga trainer dished out.

I moved around on my cheap green yoga mat for about 25 minutes, testing out all sorts of poses, breathing in deeply throughout the routine: Downward-Facing Dog, Cobra Pose, Warrior Pose, Child Pose, Plank Pose, Bow Pose, Cow Pose, Cat Pose, and every other animal-themed pose you could think of, I tried them all.

But unlike with meditation originally, it was much easier for me to keep my focus, and my interest for that matter, on the task at hand. Breathing in deeply, relaxing, and letting my worries dissipate for 20-30 minutes out of the day was really valuable to me in the early stages of my battle with anxiety.

So I stuck with it.

I did yoga regularly, probably three times a week for about 20 or 30 minutes each time. It helped me release my worries and de-stress. It wasn't dramatically life-changing by any means, but it truly was a good step in the right direction when it came to conquering my long-standing battle with anxiety.

I highly recommend you give it a shot. It can only help. And more often than not, it does.

WHICH ONE I USE NOW

So to wrap things up, yoga was my preferred method of anxiety release initially, but meditation, in the long-term, became more of my go-to option. For me, it's easier to set up (you don't really have to do jack-shit for setup) and can be done without the help, or in my case the *hassle*, of trying to find a yoga instructor (whether on your TV or in person) to walk you through a session.

But they both work. And they both work well in terms of helping you release stress and remove anxious feelings. My recommendation of course is to try both and go with the one you prefer more. Or, if you're like me, use both of them from time to time.

I currently do yoga periodically, to relax and unwind sometimes, but mostly if I feel like switching things up from my normal gym routine and substituting in a decent workout. I'd say I do a yoga session now maybe once or twice a month, whereas I've incorporated meditation, and more specifically the mindfulness aspect of it, into my life probably three to four times a week.

So yeah, I love them both.

Pick one or pick both. Just pick something. Trust me, they both can change your life and immediately start reducing your anxiety, improving your focus, and keeping you present and in the moment.

Which brings me to my next point . . .

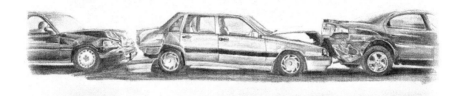

Chapter Eleven
Living in the Moment

Ever have your whole day just completely suck balls from the minute you wake up? Like for whatever reason you rolled over and woke up in Shitville?

You stub your toe on your bureau.

You accidentally drop the improperly shut and nearly full milk gallon all over the floor.

You realize only after the freezing water starts pouring down on you in the shower that you fucking forgot to pay the oil bill this month.

And to top it off, when you step outside and try to shake off the awful start to your morning, you make it but a mere three or four steps before you realize you've just planted your size 12 Oxfords in a steaming pile of freshly made dogshit—courtesy of Charlie, your neighbor's obnoxious pit bull.

As if your day couldn't get any shittier. It literally did.

Yes, quite the ironic twist indeed.

Pissed, you head back inside to clean up the messy infraction.

After about 10 minutes of wiping Charlie's half-digested meat scraps from the night before, you look up and realize you're running late.

You give it one last wipe, rinse your hands, and head out again.

Rushing now, you could use a break.

But you don't get one.

About 15 minutes later on the highway you peer up ahead only to realize there's really heavy traffic (like gridlocked traffic) about a mile up. You scream, "What the fuck!?" in utter frustration as you know this is going to cost you at least another 20 minutes that you already couldn't afford.

"What's the boss gonna' say this time?" you ask yourself. "There goes that raise I've been working up to for the last six months!"

All of your problems begin to manifest and swirl around in your mind, and you begin getting an unbelievable amount of stress and even anxiety. The anxiousness and worry seep through and dance around your body like a pissed-off bull in a china shop, touching, tagging, and knocking over just about everything it comes across.

"If I don't get this raise there's no way we can go on vacation. What're the kids going to think? What's the wife gonna' say? This is definitely going to cause another fight!" you say to yourself with aggravation.

Living in the Moment

But, just as you're pondering these troubles and gearing up for the anxiety to officially stake claim over your mind, you instinctively jam on your brakes and jerk your car to the left, and off the road.

In this haste of excitement you narrowly maneuver your car away from the SUV in front of you who unfortunately didn't have the same destiny and went barreling into the vehicle in front of him.

The same fortune befalls the truck behind you; a split-second later it comes crashing into the SUV you just avoided.

BOOM!

His airbags go off as do the guy's in the SUV, who you now realize has further jammed his front fender into the rear bumper of the vehicle in front of him. And this same domino effect seems to extend about five or six cars up.

In fact, you seem to be the only one in the immediate vicinity who didn't just get creamed. Like Vincent Vega or Jules Winnfield from *Pulp Fiction*, through some one-in-a-million stroke of luck or divine intervention, you stand alone, unscathed.

"Holy shit!" you say as you run over to check on the SUV guy who appears to be badly hurt. You help him out of his vehicle as cars behind you start to slow down and file in, and the truck guy slowly gets out as well, blood casing his forehead.

Immediately, all the problems you had a few minutes back disappear. Your focus is completely directed on the well-being of this man in the SUV and the others around you.

You call 911 after helping him off to the side. Then you ask the truck driver if he's okay and lend your shoulder for him to lean on as you assist him onto the nearby guardrail to sit down and relax. A family of four gets out of their van a few cars up, and so does the old lady next to them, everyone checking and offering a hand of help where needed.

You bring out the emergency kit in your trunk and pass out some bandages, a couple ice-packs, and a few bottles of water to those in need.

You're intuitively attending to these injured and innocent people and talking with some of them to show your support. Again, the troubled thoughts from before, all but a distant memory.

Within minutes paramedics and police arrive.

What's happened within the blink of an eye is you've changed your emotional disposition. You've gone from worrying about all your mess-ups and issues that day, to serving others and living in the present moment.

Your thoughts about fighting with your wife, losing out on that promotion, spilling milk all over the floor, and stepping in Charlie's dogshit are all gone. Not because you decided that they were unproductive thoughts, but because you were forced by unbelievable circumstance to direct your attention on the present moment.

And here's a little secret I learned many years back: Anxiety cannot live in the present moment.

ANXIETY DOESN'T EXIST IN THE NOW

It's true. Think about it for a minute.

Have you ever had anxiety whilst doing something and being *fully* present? The answer is no. You may think, "That can't be true, I got anxious when I was playing baseball when I was a kid and I loved playing ball." Or maybe, "I get anxious when I have to give a speech at my work meetings." Or perhaps you're thinking, "Justin, this can't be true. I'm fully present all the time, and even when I'm just sitting around the house doing nothing, anxiety will creep up on me. Explain *that* please!"

I will.

The answer is you're *not* fully present.

In fact, in all of these examples, nobody is fully present. You may think you are but you're really not. If you were, you'd be 100% focused on whatever it is you were doing. Thinking about absolutely nothing at all except what's in front of you. And this is quite hard for many people to do.

It's very easy to think you're being fully present and mistake this for *true* presence.

For instance, if you were thinking about giving that speech and you started getting nervous, but you kept telling yourself to calm down and that everything was going to be fine, you've already abandoned the present moment. You're playing into the anxiety of messing up, whether you mean to or not.

A better approach would be accepting, at first, that you're having the anxiety and then carrying on with what you were doing. You don't need to self-talk yourself (at least with regard to remaining present) or try to pump yourself up. If you want to be present, just be.

Focus only on what's in front of you, and when it comes time to delivering the speech, focus only on performing it to the best of your ability.

Immerse yourself in that speech, centering your mind on your words, your energy, your passion, your attunement with your audience, and your enjoyment of being there in that moment. Go right down the line with these things naturally, and don't think about anything else but delivering that speech.

Of course what would happen is you'd be fully present, and you'd fucking crush it.

Look, I'll concede that emotional reactions to physiological chemicals like adrenaline and cortisol are important and certainly serve an incredible role in our survival and safety. For instance, consider the surge of adrenaline you might face if a grizzly bear crosses your path in the woods. Your ass better have this powerful chemical to propel you to either run or fight, or you're fucking toast (though you're probably toast either way if you're up against a bear, but you get the point).

However, don't mistake these biomarkers for what we've come to call *anxiety*. Anxiety, in the generally accepted use of the term, is a negative emotional reaction to a thought process that stems from the mind projecting something negative or harmful happening in the future. Naturally, these negative emotional reactions include fear, uneasiness, worry, obsessive thinking, terror, panic, and more.

Natural jolts of adrenaline and cortisol to save our lives from wild animals or other pertinent threats is not the same. These are real threats. Anxiety is not.

When it comes to examples like the bear crossing paths with you in the woods or you nearly avoiding a car accident and instinctively tapping into your helping-others-to-safety mode, you're not thinking about anything else other than what's happening right then and there. Of course you have adrenaline coursing through you, of course you have the cortisol hormone pumping through your blood, but this isn't anxiety. This is your natural survival mechanism kicking in and keeping you alive.

Anxiety is an altogether different experience. Just to refresh your memory, anxiety was what you were feeling just before the highway pileup, when you were worrying about all your problems and projecting the imminent trouble in your converging future.

What happens when a life or death situation pops up, or something profound and unexpected, or something that really grabs hold of your attention for whatever reason, is that you are drawn into the *now*. And when you are cast into this moment, your incessant concoctions about future trouble disappears.

Depression

Depression is also an emotion that cannot live in the present moment. But it's sort of the opposite of anxiety, in that anxiety is a projection of a negative experience occurring in the *future*, whereas depression is a negative spawn of your thoughts surrounding *past* events. Essentially, it's the culmination of feelings of regret, thoughts that you missed out on something, or events that you wish had transpired differently.

But these two mental states are indeed still quite similar. Depression, like anxiety, is too caused by a thought process that takes residence away from the present moment and rubs its insidious tentacles on your current livelihood.

Consequently, the practice of living in the present moment can also be incredibly helpful for overcoming your depression and should be one of the first lines of defense in your winning battle over it. All we have is the here and now, and when you can live in this moment, both your anxiety and depression evaporate.

It's the same reason why some people get off on being adrenaline junkies and jumping out of airplanes, or doing wheelies on street bikes on the highway (or even robbing banks and committing crimes for that matter). The rush of adrenaline, the potential for death, and the attention that you're forced to have in those moments are all powerful. For some, it's the only way they know how to get rid of their anxiety. For others, they're just adrenaline-seeking nutcases (and typically very interesting people) who enjoy spending as much time being present, and feeling the thrills of life.

Living in the present moment is a powerful thing. When we allow ourselves to embrace it, life completely changes.

THE POWER OF NOW

An entire book could be written on this subject. And as it turns out, an entire book has been written on this subject, a very profound and incredibly wise book that introduced me to the whole concept of living in the moment.

It's called *The Power of Now* by a guy named Eckhart Tolle. You may have heard of it. Eckhart was all over Oprah and the news many years back and he's still quite popular today.

I'm a big fan of his.

The book is a great resource and a perfect place to start when it comes to realizing our existence is really just a series of present moments. Nothing we accomplished in the past really means anything and nothing we accomplish in the future can affect us now. All we have is the time we have right now.

You reading this book at this second in time is the present moment. And now this second in time. And now. And now. And, well . . . you get the point.

It's truly fascinating and liberating, I think. It takes the pressure off worrying about what's going to happen tomorrow while also taking focus off what we missed out on yesterday.

Look, it's good to reflect on our accomplishments from time to time and it's okay to be proud. It's also good to be motivated about our future and excited for what it holds, don't get me wrong. The problem occurs when people begin spending too much time in these places.

There's a balance here like anything.

Too much past dwelling and you have depression in your current life. Too much future projection and you get anxious right now. By seamlessly balancing the past, the present, and the future, however, you become one happy and enlightened motherfucker.

And it's pretty cool being an enlightened motherfucker. Trust me.

By the way, I love Eckhart's writing and thinking, but he's pretty dull, if not downright boring to listen to. Look him up if you think I'm kidding. The man's got a voice that would throw the worst insomniac into a Rip-Van-Winkle-like coma.

As much as I praise him for introducing me to this mind-illuminating concept, sometimes I consider whether he's spending too much time in the now and forgetting to enjoy all sides of the conscious amalgamation.

But that's not the worst problem you could have, I guess.

HOW TO LIVE IN THE PRESENT MOMENT

So how do you live in the present moment?

Well, there are many ways of gaining more presence and releasing yourself from your anxiety, or depression. But to be clear, presence isn't just something you automatically obtain once you decide you want to have it. It takes some practice being able to step into the present moment at will (unless you want to rob a bank, of course).

But assuming you're not in the business of committing felonies, here are a few ways that can help you become more present and live in the now.

MEDITATION

Meditation, as we mentioned before, is a great way to train yourself to focus on what's happening now. Through continually conditioning your mind to focus on one thing alone, like say your breath in Mindfulness Meditation, you practice the art of living in the present moment. Meditation might be the most effective of all strategies for stepping back in the moment.

DOING EXCITING THINGS

Okay, you can certainly rob a bank to become entrenched within the now if that's your thing, but I really don't recommend this—not because I'm some holier-than-thou saint with supreme moral conviction, but because you're almost positively guaranteed to get caught. And when you do you're just as prone to end up being butch Bubba's bitch in prison. (Forget living in the now, you'll be living in Bubba's sick, perverted world for years to come.)

Instead, I suggest doing new and novel things to keep your dopamine healthily active.

Drugs, alcohol, jumping out of planes, committing crimes . . . all of these work, but they're highly dangerous. A few better options would be taking a dance class, hopping on stage for a karaoke song, signing up for a fun improv class, training in a new martial art, traveling to an interesting new city, hiking through a beautiful mountain range, or learning a new skill, like say an instrument or language.

Anything that gets your blood boiling, in a good way, will have the same effect as doing dangerous things, but in a much safer and supervised environment. As human beings, we crave novelty, mainly because it brings us into the present moment.

SPENDING TIME WITH INTERESTING PEOPLE

On the same token as doing exciting things, being around exciting people will force us to live in the moment.

When we are engaged, interested, or intrigued by someone, our attention is drawn to what is going on right now. We stop thinking about our work issues, our favorite TV show that's airing later that night, or who liked our last Facebook post.

Interesting people captivate out attention like super-charged magnets, forcing us to take up residence in the moment with them. If you have friends who keep your attention, spend more time with them. If you don't, go out and start meeting new people.

Furthermore, whether you're a man or a woman, the excitement we derive when we encounter a very attractive person (whether physically, socially, or emotionally) is something special. We're intuitively ingrained with this need to connect with others, especially those we're attracted to on some level, and it has a profound effect at inducing presence. Connect more with those you're attracted to.

SPENDING TIME WITH LOVED ONES

Our family, especially our children, are great facilitators of presence. When we focus our attention on being with them and enjoying our time with them, it's easy to forget about other problems rattling around in our minds. The future anxieties we hold and the regrets of the past get lost when we share laughter, stories, jokes, and love with people we care deeply about.

Sure, families can sometimes get boring and yes, we can occasionally feel like we've had too much time with people we love and need a break from them, but all-in-all, spending meaningful time with loved ones is one of the best prescriptions for stepping into the power of now.

SEX

Sex is the ultimate form of physical connection and in my estimation the ultimate form of emotional connection. When you have sex with someone you're really into, like a wife, husband, girlfriend, boyfriend, or just somebody really fucking sexy, you're absolutely living in the present.

It's a healthy act I partake in often and one I highly recommend you start doing more of.

Who doesn't love sex?

Not only does it bring you into the now, it's also a hell of a good workout and the physiological benefits of it are amazing.[1]

DOING SOMETHING YOU'RE PASSIONATE ABOUT

Doing work that you are passionate or excited about is a very effective way to live in the moment. Think about it. How often do you daydream, contemplate what you want for dinner later, think about a beautiful woman you want to sleep with, think about a Snapchat video to post, or otherwise dabble in the nonsensical thoughts of procrastination when you're at work (assuming you don't always love your nine to five job)?

Juxtapose this illustration into a moment where you're loving what you do.

For me, it's writing about something I'm passionate about, like this book, or coaching a client into overcoming a major struggle, or giving a speech to an audience full of cheering people. In these instances, I'm fully present.

How often do you wander off when you're engaged and excited about your work? Occasionally your mind might drift, but for the most part, when you're really passionate about what you're doing, you're focused and living in the present moment. Doing something that gets you jazzed up and stimulated is an incredibly effective way of maintaining your presence.

It doesn't just have to be work of course. Having avocations, hobbies, and activities you do for fun can invoke just the same effect. But the key is that you need to have these things.

If you don't have passions, fix this immediately. Start trying, testing, and engrossing yourself in everything that seems somewhat interesting or piques even the smallest amount of curiosity in you. From here, decide what you like, what you love, and what you want to dive into even further. These things will now become your passions.

ACCEPTING THE PRESENT MOMENT

A final, straightforward tip for stepping into the now, is accepting it.

"What the fuck does that mean?" you ask.

Let me explain.

Accepting the present moment is as simple as letting go of your desire to want to control things. I know, we're all guilty of this, including me from time to time. We're all so eager to want to take charge, manipulate things in our favor, and do our best to twine things into benefiting our lives. It's quite natural to want to do this, and it has been carried on since our childhoods as a survival mechanism.

But as much as we yearn to favorably plan things out, focusing on this perpetual scheming can cause us stress. And it often does.

When we focus on the contemplative aspects of manipulation and command, we cause anxiety surrounding our success. Again, it's okay to bounce around in this place, but taking up continuous settlement is highly problematic.

But that's what so many people do. They reside in this place of constant longing for control and dwell far too long in their future projections, inevitably (and paradoxically) leading to less control and more anxiety.

Step back.

Realize you can't control most things in life.

You can only truly control YOU.

Accept that life is neither good nor bad, life just is. It doesn't discriminate when it dishes out shitstorms and it doesn't single out those bound to succeed. It just is. And whether good or bad you just are.

One of the most empowering yet often overlooked tips for getting into the present moment and finding happiness is taking responsibly over your life and accepting that good and bad things are going to happen. Some days you'll feel on top of the world. Some days you'll step in a pile of dogshit. But no matter what, you have the power to get past whatever comes your way.

And you will.

Surrendering to the now and accepting all that life has to offer is the best way to initiate your ability to live in the moment. Accept the now and enjoy life in all its wonder—both good and bad.

LAST NOTE ON THE PRESENT MOMENT

The present moment is all we truly have.

It's incredible how powerful this concept is and how powerful our reality becomes when we can live more and more in the present. Anxiety disappears, depression vanishes, contentment and happiness abounds.

Being able to step into the now is a skill. Like any skill the more you work at it the more effective you'll become at being able to use it. So practice now, using the strategies above and begin reaping the benefits of this extraordinarily beneficial practice.

And remember, the next time Charlie shits on your lawn, smile, knowing it's all a part of the ebb and flow of life. (Either that, or build a fence to keep that little fucker out.)

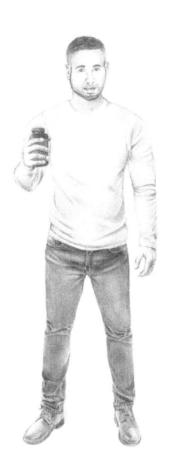

Chapter Twelve
Taking a Key Mineral

The old shop was sandwiched between a tiny little bookstore (which housed roughly the same amount of books as those collecting dust on the bookstand near my bed) and a musty-looking pizza shop whose pizzas appeared as equally appetizing as a bowlful of leather shoes.

I walked in reluctantly.

As I entered, a grey-haired lady with a blue mothball-infested sweater and a top-hat right out of the 17th century greeted me kindly enough.

"Hi, can I help you find something, young man?" she asked in a croaking voice.

"No thanks, I'm just looking around," I replied back, kindly trying to avoid eye contact and thinking to myself, *Why the hell did I come in?*

She smiled sheepishly and sat back down on her stool behind what could only have been the first cash register ever invented: a dull, simple contraption that had collected more dust than any of the books on my own shelves. This antique, like the novels next to my bed, clearly hadn't seen use in years.

Looking around, the inside was about as attractive as the pizza shop next door. The walls were decaying, the shelves were rusting, and there wasn't another human being in sight.

I felt equal parts pity and equal parts wary as I didn't know what sinister creature might be hiding in the back, ready to spring out at any moment to kidnap or kill me. After all, I hadn't told anyone I was coming here; I would've been far too embarrassed. But part of me did feel bad for the old woman who, despite looking and sounding like some character out of a Bram Stoker book, probably wasn't that bad.

The bottles of various supplements, workout powders, and healing remedies were scattered aimlessly throughout the store. I, who naturally takes ZERO pride in organization and tidiness, was disturbed by the disarray. In fact, if Detective Adrian Monk ever set foot in this boutique, he'd have a terminal heart attack on the spot. Guaranteed.

Taking a Key Mineral

I walked around for the next few minutes, trying to find what I had come there to get, while trying to appear like I hadn't come for anything specific. I didn't want the old crone hounding me or rubbing off any of her weird mothy-clothing shit or musty essence on me. I was already anxious enough; I didn't need to start worrying about contracting some weird witch-doctor disease.

After about 10 minutes of playing this disinterested game and browsing around, I finally found what I had come here for. I picked it up and looked on the back of the bottle. *Citrate, it's got to be citrate like the woman online said*, I thought to myself. *All the other forms are useless.*

"Oxide," I frustratingly read, and placed the bottle back on the shelf.

Luckily for me, there was another container next to it in a different brand.

This too had what I came here to purchase, and unlike the previous bottle it read "Citrate" on the back. *Yes, this is what I need.* I picked it up and walked over to the old lady who I knew had been watching my every move since I walked in.

"Good choice," she said, as she went to ring it up. "The magnesium citrate is one of the best products in here. It can help with all sorts of things. You must've done your homework."

"Yeah," I awkwardly replied back, not knowing how else to continue the conversation, but thinking to myself, *At least she says it's a good product too. That's a good thing, I guess.*

"Yup, it's one of my favorites," she blurted out after a few more awkward seconds ticked away.

"I've been taking it for years," she chortled out and smiled, what was most assuredly meant to be a friendly and rapport-building smile, but was sincerely taken in the only way a 17-year-old boy at the time could have taken it . . . *horrifyingly*.

The old bag had just three teeth left in her mouth, and up until this point I'd been totally oblivious to that fact. (Given the opportunity to go back in time and erase this revulsion from my memory I would leap at that salvation; unfortunately the horror of that image will live on forever, somewhere deep in my mind, as there's simply no cure for that type of mental desecration.)

With the combination of this gut-churning revelation of missing molars and the fact that she'd just unceremoniously revealed she'd been taking this mineral I was acquiring for "years," I suddenly felt sick. In my mind, whatever this disgustingly decrepit woman was consuming, I wanted no part of.

Walking out, I felt like I'd just wasted $20 on another online gimmick that wasn't going to work. *Fucking old witch*, I thought to myself. *What a fucking bit* . . . "Thank you," I somehow mustered back to her in remarkably polite fashion as she said, "Have a great day," in her crony yet gracious voice.

LATER THAT DAY

My hopes of the magnesium citrate I'd purchased earlier that day working were all but shattered by the time the sunset arrived. By the looks of the place and by the looks of its keeper, everything in that store was useless. If they worked, she wouldn't be living out of a glorified closet with dust, mold, and dilapidated furnishings everywhere. And there'd have certainly been more than just me tiptoeing around in there.

"Face it," I said to myself, holding up the bottle of citrate. "This shit isn't going to work. I gotta' keep researching stuff." I put the bottle down and went back to my laptop, continuing my quest for a *real* anxiety solution.

But as I Googled topic after topic and combed the annals of the internet's indexed pages, I kept thinking back to the magnesium. *Maybe I should give it a shot.* The thought crossed my mind, along with, *Hey, it can't hurt.* And, *That lady online did seem to make a lot of sense.*

And so after a short while, I went over to the table I'd laid the bottle down on and picked it back up.

It was 200mg of magnesium citrate. The woman online recommended taking this much in the morning and in the evening before bed. She said most people are deficient in this incredibly helpful mineral, as it's no longer found in the foods most of us eat regularly.

The Power of Magnesium

Magnesium and other minerals like it are dangerously absent from the general population's food supply because of the dramatic alterations in Western agriculture over the last few decades. Our plant-based food consumption, for the most part, is horrible. And it's only compounded by the fact that when we do eat "healthy" foods, like fruits and veggies, these healthy foods aren't as nutritionally valuable as they once were. Soil depletions from improper farming practices occur regularly in our society and this wipes out key minerals like magnesium, copper, zinc, and more.[1]

It's estimated that 80% of the population[2] is deficient in magnesium. That's a ton of fucking people. For every five people you see, four of them are not getting enough of this crucial mineral. That's why it's so important to supplement with it.

Magnesium supports your energy production, bone health, nerve function, and muscle function. It also supports relaxation, calming, and sleep, and just

> so happens to play a critical role in over 300 cellular processes. It's not just a "bone mineral," it's a whole body (and mind) mineral, and one you should definitely consider taking regularly.
>
> On a related note, you can get a great quality magnesium citrate supplement at EliteLifeNutrition.com (along with many other high-quality supplements). This is my own supplement line, and one that I've put a lot of work and dedication into ensuring is highly-respected and trusted. But of course, there are many other great options and supplement companies out there and I don't want to sound like a guy trying to pitch you shit. Trust me, I hate those assholes just as much as you do. I just wanted to let you know if you're looking for a great, trusted supplement company, we have just that. See the back "Resources" section of this book for more details if you want. If not, that's totally cool too, carry on.

So placing hesitancy aside, I popped open the bottle and dropped a pill into my right palm. Then I threw the pill in my mouth and slugged down a gulp of water from the Poland Springs bottle in my left hand.

I waited.

Not really sure what would happen next, my mind naturally began to wander.

Around this time I was still getting a fair amount of anxiety and the occasional panic attack. I'd lessened the degree of these attacks, and my overall anxiety for that matter, but it was still present, hence the decision to take the magnesium supplement in the first place (and also the fact that it was allegedly great for depression, which we'll cover in detail later on).

So mind wandering, and pill nowhere near being digested and therefore absorbed, my anxiety levels began to climb. *What if this has side effects?* I started thinking. *What if it makes me crazy? I heard these pills aren't regulated by the FDA . . . How is this different than taking the anxiety medication my father warned me about?*

Taking a Key Mineral

"What if I end up like that old lady in the store?" I cried aloud. "Oh shit, what have I done?" I shouted in terror, as another panic attack ensued.

As I paced around my room for the next 15 or 20 minutes, my anxiety level went from absolute terror for the first couple of minutes, to moderately anxious a few minutes later, to completely normal by the end of this timeframe.

I went from freaking out and having a massive panic attack to being my normal, calmed-down self in a matter of minutes. And I felt even better after about an hour, better than I'd felt in a while, at least when it came to my anxiety levels.

Looking back, the correlation between pill digestion time and my relaxation was pretty spot-on. The magnesium I so desperately lacked at that time (through poor dietary intake, and excessive stress, which depletes magnesium levels[3]) now filled a big void in that moment of need. So while I can say magnesium initially gave me anxiety (not really; I gave it to myself, but it's kind of funny to say), in the long run, it helped lessen my anxiety and keep it at a moderately low level.

SOLD ON MAGNESIUM

And so began my foray into supplementation.

I've tried and tested many products over the years, recognizing the benefits early on of what preventative medicine could offer. Mood, cognition, energy, sleep, athletic performance, immune system, anti-aging, and much more can all be positively affected with optimal nutrient supplementation.

But in the beginning, before I'd embark on my bold biohacking journey of health mastery, magnesium was all I needed.

After that first day of testing out magnesium, I was sold.

I began using it every day thereafter as an insurance policy of sorts: 200mg of magnesium in the morning with breakfast, and 200mg of magnesium with my last meal, before bed.

Overall, it had a calming effect on my nervous system throughout the day and induced a better and more restful night's sleep when I dozed off.

MY SUPPLEMENTAL REGIMEN

I've since included a few other supplements that I take daily in terms of stress relief, mood regulation, immune system function, and overall health, though I certainly don't advocate everyone take these. As I said before, I've become somewhat of a biohacking guinea pig over the years, so it's quite unnecessary to mimic my supplemental routine to the tee. Not to mention, I take these supplements for *me*, and my specific goals and needs. You, on the other hand, and everyone else for that matter, have your own precise goals and needs to adhere to, and should take the supplements that suit *you* best.

That said, just about everything I take has some merit in optimizing my health on some level. Feel free to look some of these nutrients up and see if they align with what you want too. I'm neither encouraging nor discouraging their use; I'm simply stating that they work for what I want, and only at the moment. This may change, and has changed, as I grow older, and yes, wiser. But just for shit's sake, however, because I know you're wondering, here's my supplemental regimen currently: magnesium, men's multivitamin, B-complex, NAC, resveratrol, turmeric, zinc, niacin, vitamin D, vitamin C, Ginkgo biloba, ashwagandha, and occasionally ubiquinol, grape seed extract, lemon balm, and cinnamon, to cover all the bases. I'll also sporadically sprinkle in the use of herbs like valerian root, or products such as milk thistle or melatonin, for detox support and sleep regulation, respectively. It may seem like I'm some kind of vitamin nut (and maybe I am), but the way I see it is I'd rather stay healthy and operate optimally than get sick and live a poor quality of life indefinitely.

Fuck it, I don't mind people thinking I'm weird for taking all these supplements, like I thought the old witch in the wardrobe was. If it means me being healthier and happier, I'll gladly take the baton from her feeble, froggy hand . . . just don't think I'm going to smell old and musty and have three teeth when I smile at you.

That'll never fucking happen.

Vitamin weirdo yeah, maybe. Smelly weirdo, fuck no.

THE DANGERS OF PRESCRIPTION DRUGS

With that said, it's my humble belief that we can't afford *not* to supplement, at least with a few of the essential nutrients such as magnesium.

Our food just doesn't have the nutrition it once did.

Not to mention environmental toxins found in both the air that we breathe (which has gotten worse over the years) and the diet that we consume (which has gotten way worse over the years) can wreak havoc on our health and well-being.[4] Everywhere you look there's mycotoxins, allergens, and potentially harmful bacteria or viruses looking to have a fiesta inside your body. If you're not optimizing your health and doing everything you can to stave off these assaults, you're eventually going to get sick. Whether that's a chronic disease, an infection, or just a poorer quality of life, it's worth it to pop a couple pills and keep your health at its best. At least that's how I view it.

And to answer one of the questions that popped into my head when I first took that magnesium pill, and perhaps one that's occurred to you at some point as well, "How is this different than taking prescription meds?" I say this: Popping meds can sometimes do the trick and help you overcome your problems (though even their efficacy can be debated), but they come with side effects both short and long-term (more insidious in nature than people often realize). On the other hand, vitamins and other natural compounds found in food and synthesized in the body offer comparable, and often superior benefits, without the side effects and dependency typically linked to prescription drugs.

Not to mention . . . they're so much fucking safer!

In fact, nobody in the United States has ever been verifiably killed from a vitamin.[5] There have been several alleged cases (about a dozen over the course of the last 30 years or so to be more precise), but these claims have highly conflicting evidence and their merit is dubious at best. Proven deaths, absolutely none. Contrast this with the staggering number of individuals who die each year from the result of using prescription drugs. Are you ready for this? Brace yourself. According to the Journal of the American Medical Association, every year about 106,000 people die from the direct use of prescription drugs.[6] Holy . . . fucking . . . shit!

Seriously, that's shocking.

Just looking at those numbers is sickening. Running the math real quick, that's about 290 poor souls every day dropping off, simply because they had the delusion that the medication they were advised to take would, God forbid, actually improve their lives. But no, not only does it not do this, it actually takes their lives. And our doctors are the ones who're supposed to save us? Yeah, right.

THE FLEXNER REPORT

I'm not against doctors, they certainly have their place in society; but often, far too often actually, they're not educated in aspects other than what they've been taught in school. Vitamins and natural supplements work. Unfortunately you're not going to hear about this when you go for a check-up.

This information has been largely suppressed and labeled as quackery by major government organizations in an attempt to push pharmaceutical medicine. If you don't believe me, check out the Flexner Report. This was a report commissioned in 1910 by John D. Rockefeller, the richest man in modern history, who had his pal Abraham Flexner infiltrate the American Medical Association to wipe out all competition of therapies for illness and disease.[7]

Things like homeopathy, herbal medicine, and other traditional healing modalities, which had formerly been taught and used in countless medical universities and practices, were grilled, discredited, and labeled as quackery by Flexner and his team. And after that, the rest is history.

Natural approaches to improving health were out and prescription medicine was in.

"Why?" you might ask. "Why would someone like John D. Rockefeller want to push an agenda like pharmaceutical medicine into the American landscape and remove all else?"

Simple. Profit.

There is no real money in low-cost vitamins, minerals, herbs, and supplements that can be readily picked from the ground or placed into a capsule. The money comes from the chemical concoctions of synthetic substances that cannot be easily duplicated, and more importantly, from substances that require a patent.

The patent is where the profit lies and natural supplements are not patentable.

That's why good ol' Rockefeller knew he had to do something over a century ago, and he did. And most people (including your doctor) have no idea this even happened. Or that good, natural treatments for a myriad of conditions exist.

WHY YOUR DOCTOR WON'T SAVE YOU

It's not that doctors are evil people or that they're part of some vast conspiracy theory to keep natural approaches to better health suppressed (though many of them have egos the size of Rosie O'Donnell's ever-expanding ass); they simply aren't trained in alternative therapies. (They're not even properly trained in *nutrition* of all things.) In fact, of all the courses and schooling doctors have to endure, nutritional courses account for only a few hours throughout their entire medical degree.

Let me rephrase that, just so you understand the gravity of that last sentence: Doctors spend years upon years learning so much about drug therapy, working with patients, and integrating the latest "research" into the health of their future patients, but of all this training, they spend only 23.9 contact hours[8] learning about possibly the most critical component of your health, nutrition.

And just for further reference on the term "contact hour," a normal three-credit standard college class that runs approximately three times a week for 50 minutes over the course of 14 weeks, totals 42 contact hours (each 50-minute class being equal to one contact hour). That would mean doctors, in all their sage medical training, take the equivalent of—not a myriad of classes, not a modest amount of classes, not a few classes, not even one full fucking class! In all their years of study, they actually only take just a smidge over ONE HALF of a *single* fucking class!

Yeah, pretty fucking ridiculous indeed.

But the worst part of it all might be the grip the pharmaceutical industry has over the medical schools. If it wasn't bad enough that medical schools don't teach much, if any, about natural treatments to sickness, it gets worse. Pharmaceutical companies *en masse* regularly fund many of the top medical schools in the country.[9]

They essentially give money to schools to "test" their drugs and do clinical research on their products, while also effectively altering the courses being taken by these students. Not to mention, the results are then naturally skewed in favor of many of these drugs, because who in the right mind is going to bite the hand that feeds them?

And it's not just some concocted, far-out tale you'd hear from some wacky conspiracy theorist, like those hillbilly farmers who talk about being anally probed by little green Martians all the time; unfortunately, it's real, and in America, this is the norm. The pharmaceutical industry has taken over and all but monopolized conventional Western medicine.

The good news is, however, if you're interested in finding a doctor who does know about nutrition and who's studied alternative therapies, they are out there. They're not as easy to locate as the traditional American doctor is, but they do exist.

They're called naturopathic, integrative, and functional doctors, and you can search online to find one in your area. These doctors typically know a lot more than any traditional doctor would with regard to nutrition and optimizing your health in a safe and holistic manner.

SUPPLEMENTAL THERAPY

And now, I want to talk about supplements that actually work—the meat of this entire chapter.

The following supplements I've either tried, have researched heavily, or know trusted colleagues and friends who have used them to good effect.

My recommendation is to take the safest supplements first (listed under "THE RIDICULOUSLY SAFE" heading), as they are beneficial to many aspects of your health, and come with virtually no true side effects when taken in the correct dosages (warning: anything taken in exorbitant doses can kill you—even water or air!). Just follow the label's directions (or mine) to ensure this. Then, if you so desire, try some of the other supplements below these (listed under "THE VERY SAFE" and "THE SAFE" headings, respectively), but even then try them one at a time.

You don't need to throw a bunch of random, and potentially potent, mixtures of substances into your body. Test them each individually, and see how you feel after a few weeks. Some people will do great with the first supplement they add, and that's all they need. Others will have to try a few before they find something that works.

And one last reminder (to preserve myself from any wrongdoing, and safeguard against some asshole trying to sue me for fucking up and taking the wrong dosage or getting a bellyache or having some fucking peculiar allergic reaction): All of these supplement recommendations, and all the recommendations throughout this book for that matter, are for entertainment purposes only. Yes, they work, but I'm not a doctor and I'm not pretending to be.

Consult a qualified doctor before use of these or any nutritional or supplement recommendation by me, or by anyone. Don't be stupid about this stuff; be smart and take your own well-being seriously.

Okay, enough with the legal shit. Here's the goods:

SUPPLEMENTS FOR ANXIETY

THE RIDICULOUSLY SAFE

Magnesium

Magnesium might be my all-time favorite supplement. It's safe, it's simple, and it's effective. Magnesium binds to GABA receptors in the brain[10] and stimulates their functionality. GABA (technically called gamma-aminobutyric acid by science nerds), is the neurotransmitter that allows your brain to relax and essentially put the brakes on all the activity going on (i.e. racing minds). It also lowers the release of stress hormones in the body like cortisol which can ramp up your anxiety levels fast.

My Recommendation: Take magnesium (citrate or glycinate; avoid oxide at all costs!) twice a day at 200mg or 250mg dosages. (You can certainly take more as needed too just try not to take more than 250mg in one serving.) Also, make sure the final dose comes before bed, as it's very helpful for sleep optimization.

B-Complex

The B-vitamins—B1, B2, B3 (niacin), B5, B6, B7, B9 (folate), and B12—work directly to optimize brain function, and they serve as a precursor to many important neurotransmitters (regulators of mood) like serotonin and GABA. Studies have consistently shown the benefits of B-complex supplementation and its support with both anxiety and depression because of its many important functions in the body and brain.[11]

My Recommendation: Take a high-quality B-complex supplement every day. Usually a B-50 complex (most of the Bs will be in the 50mg dosage form, except for a few such as B12 which adhere to different dosage protocols) once or twice a day will do just fine. I take a B-50 complex once a day with my first meal and seem to enjoy it just fine. Also, make sure the Bs are in their activated forms for optimal absorption and efficacy.

Niacin

Niacin is a wonder-vitamin for most people, and deserves to be singled out from the B-complex vitamins because of this. It's one of Dr. Andrew Saul's (The MegaVitamin Man) favorite vitamins and one he uses every day to lower his stress and anxiety levels. It's often recommended to take between 1,500–3,000mg in one day, but the safe upper limit is actually in the 6,000–9,000mg range. It's a remarkably safe supplement.

A man by the name of Dr. Abram Hoffer did great work on niacin and its many benefits, and helped a guy by the name of Bill Wilson (co-founder of Alcoholics Anonymous) eliminate his lifelong anxiety and depression by taking approximately 3,000mg of niacin a day. Bill W. (as many know him) also went on to duplicate the effect on many of his early AA members, helping them alleviate their own anxiety and depression as well.[12]

Niacin increases the production of nitric oxide which relaxes blood vessels in your brain, acts as a precursor to NAD and NADH[13] which directly contributes to your cell's energy production, and it also boosts your serotonin levels, making you feel calm and relaxed.

My Recommendation: Take 250–500mg one to four times a day, depending on how you feel. Some people notice a great improvement in mood relatively quickly, for others it's less dramatic. But either way niacin should be added to your diet for general health. I currently take 500mg twice a day for broad-spectrum wellness. You can go higher or lower than this; it's up to you. (Also, I prefer using niacinamide, the non-flush form of niacin.)

Ashwagandha

Ashwagandha (*Withania somnifera*) is an adaptogenic herb that's been used in Ayurvedic medicine for thousands of years. It's great at combating stress and preventing the release of excess cortisol.[14]

In one very impressive, double-blind, placebo-controlled study, 88.2% of all participants who took a form of the ashwagandha herb saw a marked improvement in their anxiety levels[15] after two and six weeks, the predetermined follow-up times of observance. In another study, it performed comparably to both the anxiolytic drug Lorazepam and the antidepressant drug Imipramine, without the side effects that usually accompany the two.[16]

With virtually no side effects accompanying this adaptogen, it's a pretty solid addition to any supplement regimen if desired.

My Recommendation: I'd recommend taking ashwagandha at a dosage of between 600–1200mg one to two times per day and seeing how you feel. It's very safe to take and I wouldn't really worry about overdoing it with this herb. In fact the safe upper limit has been reported at levels of 6,000mg (taken in divided doses of up to 2,000mg each throughout the day).

Also, when looking for this particular herb, try to get the "root extract" form of the ashwagandha and find one that's standardized in the 2.5% or 5% range of its core ingredient (withanolides). Lastly, it's a plus if your supplement contains 2.5, or even 5mg of BioPerine, or a black pepper extract. BioPerine and black pepper extract both greatly increase the bioavailability and absorption of herbs like ashwagandha.

THE VERY SAFE

Theanine

The amino acid theanine has a number of key functions and works primarily by inhibiting glutamate[17] (an excitatory neurotransmitter) in the brain. It thus allows a calming of the mind, while also stimulating the brain's alpha waves (*alpha* being the preferred brain wave state for deep relaxation). And, if that's not incredible enough, theanine also increases dopamine and GABA levels in the brain, and can also boost your serotonin levels as well.

There was a double-blind study done in 2004 by researchers comparing theanine to Xanax (one of the most popular prescription medicines for anxiety) for those suffering from anxiety. They measured participants' scores in those taking 1mg of Alprazolam (Xanax), those taking 200mg of theanine, and those taking a placebo. What they found was stunning. The placebo group saw no noticeable improvement. The Xanax group saw no noticeable improvement. But the theanine group had a significant improvement in their general anxiety, suggesting to researchers that it might be a superior alternative to one of the most common anti-anxiety meds[18] out there.

My Recommendation: Take theanine at 100 or 200mg dosages, once or twice a day. (I've never tried this personally, as I've never needed it, but the research and safety records for this supplement are incredible. It works, and it's not going to harm you like prescription medicines can.) Theanine is incredibly safe and effective.

Taurine

Taurine is another amino acid that can work wonders in your brain for anxiety. It too plays many roles, but chief among them is its ability to activate strychnine-sensitive (inhibitory) glycine receptors in the brain.[19] These inhibitory glycine receptors function similarly to that of GABA, in that they're sedative and calming in nature.

Taurine also just so happens to be one of the precursors to GABA, which means you also end up producing more GABA when you take taurine. It's the perfect double-whammy. And to top things off, taurine has been shown in many studies to be great at balancing the amount of glutamate in your brain, making sure it stays at a reasonable level. Glutamate plays a major role in sending nerve signals throughout the body.[20] However, when there's too much of it (or not enough, for that matter[21]) anxiety can proliferate.

My Recommendation: Take 500–1000mg of taurine one to three times per day. I'd suggest starting at the minimum dose for this (and any supplement for that matter), so I'd personally start at 500mg and see how I felt with that. Taurine is not an amino acid I take now, but again, one that's safe and one I recommend as it seems to be effective for many. The most you'd want to sensibly take in one day is 3,000mg, but you may be okay with taking just 500mg a day, or somewhere in between.

Valerian Root

Valerian root (the *Valeriana officinalis* type) is one of the most commonly used herbal remedies for anxiety, stress, and sleep. It functions primarily as a GABA producer, and though its exact mechanisms are not entirely clear, its effects can be tremendous.[22] It can outperform benzodiazepines like Xanax, without the side effects attributed to these sedatives. It can also be a great sleep aid (more on this later).

Valerian root sometimes takes a few weeks to kick in and notice benefit from, so if you do opt to use this herb, be patient. Also, the doses for sleep are generally higher, as a higher dosage produces a sedating effect. So keep in mind if you want to use this herb, you're going to want to use smaller doses throughout the day, to tame your anxiety, but not to tame your mind so much that you turn into a zombie.

Also, although the research thus far has been optimistic, I'd be happy to see more studies on both anxiety use and sleep use going further. Its long-term use is generally recognized as safe, but no major research has really been done on this substance yet.

My Recommendation: Valerian root is a safe alternative to anti-anxiety meds like benzodiazepines. I've taken valerian root periodically over the years to help with sleep. I haven't needed to use it for anxiety, but for anxiety purposes specifically, I'd recommend taking 100–300mg one to three times a day. Again, start off at the lower dosage and see how you feel with that.

Lithium Orotate

Lithium is a mineral found in trace amounts in various foods and water supplies globally. In fact, it's so trace that almost everyone doesn't get enough of it. Dr. John Gray, health pioneer and author of the classic book *Men Are from Mars, Women Are from Venus*, regularly talks about the incredible benefits of taking this metal. He's been taking it himself, to great effect, for many years.

There's a misconception about lithium, as doctors in the past (in all their brilliant wisdom) have prescribed the wrong doses of lithium for mental health. Using lithium carbonate (an incredibly inferior form of lithium), they would tell their patients to take lithium in the 150–300mg range, multiple times a day. This doesn't sound like much, until you realize that lithium orotate (the right form of lithium) is needed at only a 5mg dose to generate a positive mental health effect, as it readily crosses the blood-brain barrier. Yes, I repeat: five fucking mgs is all it takes! These dummies have been overprescribing this otherwise harmless and incredibly helpful periodic element in the 30 to 60 times higher dosage range, numerous times a day. So, along with the overdosing, comes terrible side effects (as with anything when you take too much of it), and thus the stigma of inefficacy and danger concerns.

But when taken in normal doses (5mgs, one to five times a day, for most people), this mineral is incredibly advantageous. Not only is it great for anxiety, but it's also been used to treat bipolar disorder, manic depression, and schizophrenia. Lithium works in a number of ways in the brain; however, its primary actions are increasing serotonin levels[23] and limiting the use of norepinephrine.

My Recommendation: I've never personally used lithium (though this may change as my biohacking nature finds great allure in this mineral) as again, I've never had to. But looking at the research and listening to doctors I trust (like John Gray), I can safely advocate for its use. It seems to work great across the board and is very safe when taken in the proper dosages. If you do choose to use this supplement, I recommend taking 5mg of lithium orotate, one to three times a day, or as needed. (I'd personally feel comfortable, after looking at the literature on this, with taking up to 25mg a day of lithium orotate.)

CBD

CBD (cannabidiol) is a non-psychotomimetic constituent of the *Cannabis sativa* plant that's been used to help treat everything from chronic pain to diabetes, insomnia, dementia, depression, neuroinflammation, epilepsy, oxidative injury, nausea, anxiety, and schizophrenia,[24] to name just a few.

Cannabidiol works in a number of ways throughout the body, but one of its key functions is its almost immediate balancing out of the neurotransmitters glutamate and GABA.

Along those same lines, it works on the autonomic nervous system by balancing out the sympathetic and parasympathetic nervous systems found within the autonomic system's umbrella. Going back to Physiology 101, the sympathetic nervous system is the fight-or-flight process that gets activated when you need excitement, anxiety, vigilance, or a get-shit-done attitude. The parasympathetic system is the relax and digest mode, that has more of a resting, repairing, and calming-you-down approach. In anxious individuals, these two systems are way out of whack, with typically far too much fight-or-flight activation and far too little rest-and-repair.

I asked my friend Dr. Christopher Shade, one of the top experts in the world on detoxification and neurological health, his thoughts on CBD supplementation and he said this: "CBD stabilizes the glutamate receptors. It balances that sympathetic to parasympathetic tone. CBD comes in there and it just magically balances those two."

He then went on to add this about CBD, "I think this is one of the most important tools for functional medicine in the last 30 years.[25]"

My Recommendation: For dosage of CBD I'd recommend taking between 25mg–75mg one to three times per day. As always, start at the lower end and work your way up, but again, CBD is incredibly safe, so you shouldn't have any issues going to the higher end of things. In some of the studies on CBD, the dosages were in the several-hundred-mg range, which reiterates just how safe it can be. Furthermore, if you're taking a legitimate liposomal-enhanced CBD product, these can offer five to six times higher absorption, so you wouldn't need as much. About 5mg to 12mg would do the trick on these, one to three times a day.

Look for the product you're choosing to say the words "Phytocannabinoid Diols," "Active Diols," or "Phytocannabinoid Hemp Oil" (or "Phytocannabinoids" or of course "Cannabidiol") next to that 25mg–75mg (or 5mg–12mg) recommended dose. All of these terms describe the active amount of CBD in the product (here in the U.S. you can't just say "CBD oil," you've got to use this other nomenclature per FDA compliance). If these words are not on the product's label, don't get it. Oftentimes companies can mislead the buyer into thinking there's a lot more CBD in their product, when instead it's just hemp oil or hemp extract without the CBD part you want.

Lastly, CBD products typically contain about 0.3% THC, not nearly enough to enact any psychoactive effects in the brain (most marijuana these days contain about 15–20% THC in them). And, as it turns out, CBD itself negates any psychoactive/negative effects that even that minimal amount of THC could potentially bring, by counteracting its effects on the CB1 receptor in the brain. In short, there's absolutely nothing to worry about as far as "getting high" from taking a CBD supplement. (Believe me, I've looked into this at length because of my personal experience in the matter.)

A FEW MORE RECOMMENDATIONS

At this point I could probably rattle off literally dozens upon dozens of other incredible supplements that have been used over the years to help treat anxiety naturally and effectively. But I think the list above is a very solid one, and just picking a couple from this list to try should be more than enough.

But finally, I couldn't resist. Here are a few more (of the many) supplements that have been shown to alleviate anxiety.

THE SAFE

5-HTP

As perhaps the most potent serotonin precursor[26] around, 5-HTP is a great supplement for helping you feel better and more content with life. (We'll cover this more in the depression section as well, as it's typically used more often for depression.)

Rhodiola

Rhodiola rosea is another one of God's great adaptogenic blessings. This herb works wonders on the brain, and has been shown to decrease sympathetic nervous system activity and also boost serotonin levels in the body. It's also great for energy and focus, but just make sure you don't overdo it, as it can have an opposite effect on some who overdose, causing hyperactivity.[27] (Also, interestingly enough, this herb has been used by many as an effective treatment for ADD.)

Lemon Balm

Lemon balm, scientifically referred to as *Melissa officinalis*, is an herb of the mint family, that's been used for centuries to ameliorate stress levels, sleep, and yes, anxiety. A 2004 double-blind, placebo-controlled study demonstrated the increases in alpha waves (the brain waves attributed to relaxation) in the brains of all the study's participants.[28]

Passion Flower

Passion flower (*Passiflora incarnate*) is a plant that's been used traditionally in the Americas (finally something we've been doing right over here), by Native Americans for many years. It works by boosting GABA levels in the brain and seems to have a profound effect on reducing anxiety in a lot of people.[29]

Inositol

Inositol is a chemical compound produced by the body (sometimes considered one of the B-vitamins, though it's technically not), and is a crucial co-factor in cellular signaling, especially among neurotransmitters. At high doses (up to 18 grams a day) it can work as a quality anxiolytic and has demonstrated to be as equally effective as Fluvoxamine (a common antidepressant and panic-attack drug) in alleviating the symptoms of anxiety and panic.[30] For some people, however, an upset stomach or nausea can occur, and seems to be more common than other supplements (perhaps because of the high dosage needed).

PUTTING THIS ALL TOGETHER

General well-being supplements (multivitamins, vitamin D, NAC, zinc, etc.) are all great supplements to add into your daily routine, as I do. They won't directly affect your anxiety levels (though they will indirectly improve them to some degree), but they are an overall recommendation for good, balanced health and brain function, and as we'll discuss later, can play a big role in depression.

Also, it's important to note that a lack of any essential vitamin or mineral, even an amino acid, can cause all sorts of problems, including anxiety. Therefore, it's imperative to get your blood tested annually to ensure your nutrition levels are optimal.

Furthermore, I'd like to make a special note on some of the amino acids listed above. It's important, when supplementing with anything, but especially when taking amino acids individually, as in the case of say 5-HTP (more on this specifically in the depression section), to make sure you consider any potential competing effects that may occur because of the "positive" reaction you intend on producing in the brain. For amino acids, this can typically occur with competing neurotransmitters that use the same receptors and fight for receptor dominance. By boosting one neurotransmitter, you may be inadvertently depleting another because of this.

Lastly, if you are currently taking anti-anxiety medication, make sure you work with your doctor in easing or weaning yourself off of it, if applicable. The last thing I recommend doing is going cold turkey on any prescription med, as this can have serious side effects. (Work with your doctor if considering going off your medications. Please, if you take nothing else from this section, listen to me here.)

But yeah, as you can see, there are many, many natural options for anxiety available. The ones above are just a few of those. Prescription medicine, in my view, just doesn't cut it when there are safer and oftentimes *better* approaches. Do meds have a place? Absolutely. But they're way down the list, and certainly *last*, in my analysis, when compared to the nutrients I listed above.

Good luck and be wise.

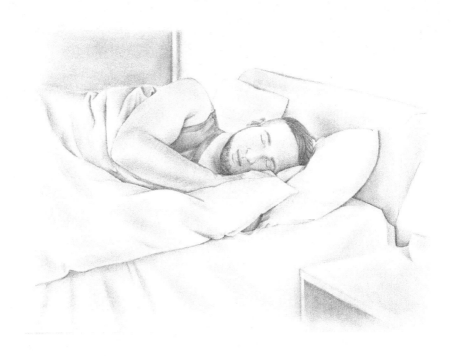

Chapter Thirteen
Sleeping Away My Worries

I rolled onto my left side for the 574-thousandth time that night, and then two minutes later rolled back onto my right side for the 575-thousandth time. "What the fuck?" I uttered aloud to myself in complete frustration. "Why can't I just fucking sleep?" *This sucks*, I thought. *What a complete waste of time. I took this night off from doing work and sleeping in my own, infinitely-more comfortable bed to come here and roll around like an asshole all night. Not to mention these wires are uncomfortable as hell, and my legs make me look like I have fucking leprosy* ... "What the fuck?" I reiterated in aggravation.

Unfortunately this declaration of contempt didn't lead to any change, and I continued to toss and turn for countless hours. Finally, as is always the case, I awoke a certain time later to the alarm that I'd wishfully set for noon, nine hours before, when I was being suited up with all of these technological gadgets affixed to my frame. I reached for my phone to shut off the unreasonably annoying monotonous jingle that so often started my days, and as I did so, a knock rapped on the room's only door.

"Can I come in?" a woman's voice asked.

"Yeah, that's okay," I sounded back.

A second or two later a short, 40-something, bushy brown-haired woman with thick black spectacles came walking in. She smiled. "Good afternoon, I'm just going to help you get all this stuff off and then you're free to go."

"Okay, thank you," I responded, happy to be able to get out of this place, and also happy I'd been able to sleep, even if only for a couple hours at most. I'd been very reluctant to even come to this place to begin with. Not because I didn't need to come here, but because I knew it was going to be really tough to sleep. I knew I'd probably be rolling around for a while and I knew there was a great chance I might not sleep at all. This after all, was my second time being here.

The location in question was a sleep study facility just outside my hometown of Taunton, MA. A tiny little structure, it was very discreet and could be driven past a thousand times without so much as a single person taking notice of its presence. That's actually what I did for many years. I'd driven right by this sleep-study place almost every day for years and years, and it wasn't until I first got referred to do an overnight study there that I even knew it existed.

But exist it did. And visit I did.

MY FIRST VISIT

The first time, a couple years earlier, I'd been recommended for an overnight stay there to monitor my occasional insomnia, rare times of quality sleep, and lack of daytime energy, which my primary doctor suspected might be caused by sleep apnea.

Long story short, I didn't have sleep apnea.

And I didn't want the sleep medicine my lazy doc wished to prescribe me. Even before all my anxiety and depression problems had grown dire, and even before I had embarked on my natural approach crusade to fix my mental health, taking pills to sleep just intuitively seemed like a bad idea. So I didn't.

Thankfully, I managed to sleep a little better for a few years, or at least managed to get by without really dwelling on my slumber habits. It sort of got put on the back burner and I didn't think much about it—until I was forced to, that is.

This time, I was hoping my doctors could shed some light on a weird sleep phenomenon that'd been occurring regularly during this period in my life. I was hoping they could pinpoint why I'd been having these strange occurrences when I dozed off; so I agreed to partake in the sleep exam again.

By the way, this was all right around the same time I'd been overcoming my anxiety issues, and starting to see some improvement in my mental health. Things were beginning to look better for me, but one day I went to sleep and when I woke up, something wasn't right . . .

A VERY STRANGE SLEEP

It was pitch-black and I could hear this weird buzzing sound emanating from an untraceable source. At first I thought it was the fan, but then I remembered we were still in the tail end of winter, and the fan hadn't been turned on in many months.

Coming to a bit, I thought it might've been the heater acting up, and maybe I needed to get up and turn it off, or at least see if I could fix its obvious malfunction. Realizing it was probably this, I reached my right arm up to pull off my blanket comforter, but was shocked to find the arm wouldn't perform this simple act. Instantly bewildered but determined still, I reached my left arm up to defy the laziness of my opposite appendage, but was met with the same puzzling result.

I couldn't move.

Immediately my steadfast resolve transformed into pure terror as I recognized the true gravity of this unprecedented situation. Trying to keep calm but fearing the worst, I tried to move my legs. To my utter disappointment and dread, I could not move either of these limbs as well. And that eerie foreign buzzing sound was becoming increasingly louder and more disturbing with each passing moment.

And then, out of nowhere, it hit me and I was able to identify its true source: It was coming from within my own head!

WHAT I HAD

As I found out later, I had sleep paralysis, a bizarre condition that befalls those unfortunate few who go to bed normally, but then wake up sometime during the night and can't move. These people can open their eyes and see, but they can't move their bodies or limbs, and are literally paralyzed. This phenomenon will typically last just a few minutes or so, but for those experiencing it, it can seem like hours. (There's a time distortion effect that takes place.)

Also, to top it off, many who have this odd experience can also hear weird noises: buzzing sounds, loud bangs, strange hummings, and more. Even more frightening, sleep paralysis sufferers may occasionally hallucinate and see demons, ghosts, aliens, and other equally terrifying visions[1] while enduring their paralysis (it's linked to a REM sleep-phase disorder, the part of sleep where you dream). Thankfully I've yet to see any ghouls of this sort, but I have had a variety of strange sounds and peculiar aberrations of feeling myself falling out of bed (or "into" my bed, like the teenage boy in *A Nightmare On Elm Street*). To say this is scary is the biggest euphemism of the decade. It's fucking petrifying!

BACK AT THE STUDY

Anyway, as the bushy brown-haired lady undid the bazillion wires leading from several complex technological apparatuses and into a vast number of areas throughout my body, I was pleased. I hadn't had any episodes of sleep paralysis that particular night, but I knew for sure that with the number of high-tech gadgets keeping track of my every move, these doctors would certainly be able to detect what was causing my sleep woes, and they'd be able to craft an admirable solution. When she wrapped up her duty and sent me on my way I was truly relieved.

Needless to say, the medical establishment would let me down once again.

A few weeks later when the test results came in, I got nothing out of them. Although I hadn't experienced the paralysis sensation that night, they still believed I had it. Which I guess was somewhat reassuring. But the truth is, they knew what they were going to do whether they saw me experiencing this bizarre sleep phenomenon or not. Their ultimate recommendation was going to be the same no matter what.

Not only could they not determine the source of the chronic sleep paralysis I'd been enduring, they didn't care to find out. They simply advised me to take a powerful sleep medication, in the hope it would somehow knock my body out and discourage it from waking up throughout the night. This they said would help, or their other suggestion: for me to take tricyclic antidepressants or SSRIs; perhaps these medications could suppress the duration of my REM sleep, or better yet, eliminate it altogether.

I once again declined their generous offer.

I'd already turned down their recommendation for anti-anxiety meds and antidepressants before, and I seemed to be getting better on both of those fronts without their help. Saying "No" again just seemed like the obvious choice.

And I'm so happy I did.

EMBARKING ON ANOTHER (MINI) QUEST

For a few months thereafter, I did my own research into sleep paralysis. Although the exact cause of this anomaly is still a mystery to many researchers around the world, several truths seem to be evident: One, it's heavily linked to an irregular sleep schedule or a disruptive sleep pattern.[2] Two, it seems to be most prevalent in shift workers or those who work overnight or have an abnormal sleep time.[3] Three, it happens more often to those who sleep in a supine position (on their backs) as opposed to on their sides or bellies.[4] Four, anxiety and stress seem to play a role, and those with anxiety disorders (like me at the time) tend to have much higher instances of sleep paralysis, compared to the general population.[5]

After learning these truths, I quickly adopted a better sleeping approach.

My irregular sleeping patterns—staying up all night and sleeping all day, or not taking sleep too seriously and only getting a couple hours of shut-eye—ended.

As much as sleep had always been an embattled foe, coming and going as it pleased and taking no direction at all from me, I began to consciously make a habit of falling asleep at a regular time, and forcibly took back some control. I compelled myself to not stay up all night, doing mindless shit like playing video games or watching movies, and slowly started conditioning myself to sleeping at around the same hours.

Following the first truth, regarding irregular sleeping patterns, I knew this was crucial. Being a lifelong night owl, however, and regularly staying up until six, seven or even eight in the morning at times, I settled on having a normalized bedtime of about 3AM. Certainly not the most ideal approach, but one I could adhere to nonetheless.

By this same token, I sort of fulfilled the second truth of improving my graveyard-shift sleep pattern in hopes of lessening my sleep paralysis. Of course, going to bed before midnight (or preferably even earlier than that) would be ideal; for me, a four or five-hour cutback from my previous slumber times was sufficient during this phase.

As far as sleeping in the supine position, this was easiest to correct. I was never too fond of sleeping on my back anyway, but I'd noticed that almost every time I'd gotten sleep paralysis, I'd coincidentally passed out in this pose. To remedy this, I simply turned to one side (some days my left, some my right), and got really comfortable lying in bed and drifting off. These side positions became my go-to postures for sleep.

Finally, for the last truth, I continued to work on my anxiety levels. Using the techniques described in this book, I immersed myself in the fight against this beast. I doubled down in my clash, and pushed even harder in my attempts to rid myself of all anxious thought.

As I implemented these strategies, my sleep paralysis slowly became less and less frequent over time. Consequently, my sleep became more restful, and my anxiety and depression improved because of it. This sleep and anxiety cycle, once vicious, was actually now working in my favor.

REM Behavioral Disorder (RBD)

I later discovered a link between sleep paralysis and neurotransmitters like GABA and Glycine, the inhibitory brain chemicals that naturally get activated during normal sleep. For those who suffer from sleep paralysis,[6] there appears to be a dysregulation in the production of these, and most likely several other neurotransmitters, during sleep.

It's believed that this imbalance causes a misfiring of information within the brain and leads to strange experiences like sleep paralysis and others like REM Behavioral Disorder (RBD), where some, rather than waking up to paralyzed bodies, actually do the opposite and act out their dreams, most commonly in violent manners, like punching, kicking, or hitting themselves (or their partners).[7]

Common (and incredibly safe) supplements like magnesium, niacin, melatonin, and various other vitamins, minerals, amino acids, or herbs can all be effective methods for naturally balancing your neurotransmitters and thus eliminating, or drastically reducing, sleep paralysis (or RBD) symptoms. (Ironically enough, once I learned of the benefits of magnesium (for anxiety), and started supplementing with it regularly, my sleep paralysis all but disappeared—a much obliged side effect of this powerful metal.)

IMPORTANCE OF SLEEP

Sleep is paramount for mental function and optimal health. There's a reason why we're genetically required to spend about a third of our lives dwelling in this state.

Sleep offers our bodies, and especially our brains, an invaluable opportunity to relax, recharge, and rest up, so that it can function optimally in perpetuity. But even when our brains do "relax," they're still hard at work, regulating our hormones, repairing neurons, flushing out damaging proteins, cleaning away harmful toxins and chemicals, and neuroplastically cultivating our circuits for growth and stability. In fact, our brains never really shut down and take a break completely (unless we die); they simply take a temporary hiatus from doing the conscious, wakeful-hour tasks we so desperately rely on them to execute, and instead do the other things we typically never give them credit for.

But it's important to recognize the powerful role our brains undertake during sleep and just how impactful it can be on our health, especially when it comes to anxiety and depression. People who don't sleep at least seven to eight hours each night are more likely to have depressive and anxious feelings. Also, according to the National Sleep Foundation, those who suffer from regular insomnia are 10 times more likely to have clinical depression and 17 times more likely to have clinical anxiety than the average population.[8]

The effects of poor, or an altogether lack of sleep, often lead to an erratically operating mind, and can cause a cascade of deleterious effects in the brain. One of these effects undoubtedly includes the excessive increase in inflammation that occurs when we don't sleep. One recent study conducted in 2015 on 2,570 men in Finland found elevated levels of the C-reactive protein (one of the best biomarkers of inflammation) in men who slept less than six hours a night on average.⁹ Inflammation of course has a strong link to anxiety, and mental malfunctioning of the brain, and is thought to be one of the true drivers of depression.¹⁰

It should be noted as well, however, that too much sleep can be just as unhealthy for you. The men in this same study who slept *more* than 10 hours (which many depressive individuals will often choose to do) had just as much C-reactive protein as those who underslept.

Another pernicious result of deprived sleep, which certainly plays a role in mental maladies, is the hormone imbalance caused from it. When we don't sleep, our cortisol (stress hormone) levels shoot up,¹¹ and our growth hormone levels come crashing down. And other hormones (like catecholamines, insulin, prolactin, and thyroid hormones) also all get thrown out of balance, leading to increased stress and numerous ravaging effects on the body and brain.¹² Naturally, chronic distortions of proper hormonal balance will certainly lead to anxious and depressive symptoms in just about everyone.

A third, and unfortunately profound consequence of this bereavement of sleep, is without a doubt the neurotransmitter imbalance that ensues. As we know, neurotransmitters are critical when it comes to the brain's functioning, especially when it comes to positive feelings and emotions.

Deficiencies in neurotransmitters like dopamine, serotonin, norepinephrine, and GABA are heavily associated with depression and anxiety in humans. We rely on these powerful brain chemicals to keep our minds sharp, focused, and happy, and when they get out of whack, serious problems arise. Sleep, as it turns out, is essential for maintaining proper levels of these chemicals, so when you don't get enough of it, you run the genuine risk of being anxious, depressed, or both.¹³

Sleeping Away My Worries

As my friend Dr. Frank Lipman, a pioneer in integrative and functional medicine, so eloquently puts it: "During the day your body makes these toxins, and these proteins, and these breakdown products. And at night is when your body cleans your brain and gets rid of them. It's like having a party one night and you get up in the morning and you don't clean up, and you have another party the next night, and you get up in the morning and you don't clean up. That's what happening to your brain if you're not sleeping. Your garbage collection is not happening, and your garbage collects in your brain.[14]"

WHAT TO DO

Look, you're not going to die if you don't go to bed at eight o'clock every night and wake up at five the next morning for a perfect nine hours of shut-eye. Trust me, I can't remember the last time I did that. (Actually, I don't think I've ever actually fucking done that.)

However, the closer you can get to maximizing your sleep each night, the better off you're going to be. In a moment I'm going to share a number of rapid-fire tips for improving your sleep. Most of them you should adhere to, some you can skip, and some won't really apply to you. Just know this: When it comes to the Big Three of eating, sleeping, and exercising, sleep is probably the most important for your mental health.

That's right. You could skip a couple of days from the gym and be fine. You could actually fast a few days without food, and still be healthy (probably even healthier). But if you skip a few days of sleep (I've done this, though not by choice, and it was possibly the worst three days of my life!), you're going to really be hurting. They say after about 48–72 hours of sleep deprivation, you can start to hallucinate and feel like you're going crazy. (My guess is any longer and you might actually.) But don't worry, the remedy for this is to sleep. And I've got some pretty damn good tips to help you do just that.

TIPS FOR OPTIMIZING YOUR SLEEP

<u>Sleep At A Normal Hour</u>

This, believe it or not, has been the biggest challenge of all my sleep struggles for years. As it turns out, I have one copy of a gene known as the Circadian Locomotor Output Cycles Kaput gene (or CLOCK gene), and this makes me inherently susceptible to a disturbed circadian rhythm. Ever since I can remember I've accommodated this propensity. I'm a night owl and always have been, but now I do my best to keep it from getting too crazy.

I mentioned before that there were times I'd go to bed at six, seven, even eight in the morning, and wake up late in the afternoon, but these days are all but gone. I typically fall asleep now by two or 3AM, still very late by most measures, but not so late that I'm completely fucking myself and turning into a vampire. (I've certainly dialed back my early-morning forays into the abyss of consciousness, but still have a ways to go before I'm where I want to be.)

Hey, I'm not perfect, and I still have many areas I could improve in. This is one of them. But who knows, maybe one day I'll stop using my genetic susceptibility to being a night owl as an excuse to stay up all night, and actually start sleeping normally like the rest of the world. Anything is possible.

But yes, if you can, try to base your sleep as close to the way Mother Nature intended it.[15] That means mimicking the sun's schedule as best you can. This helps regulate the production of powerful hormones like cortisol and melatonin, which are intended to peak and drop as the sun goes up and down, antagonistically. People with fucked-up sleeping times like myself risk having imbalances in these critical hormones and thus experiencing poorer quality of sleep.

You can get around this by using some of the other techniques we'll talk about in a minute (like I've been able to do for years), but at the end of the day, it's still best to copy nature's playbook.

Sleep 7–9 Hours

Study after study indicates our need to sleep about seven to nine hours each night.[16] The exact amount will vary from person to person, but the consensus is that within this range, humans profit most from their slumber. Remember those who sleep too little (six hours or less) and those who sleep too much (10 hours or more) are at a much higher risk for having clinical depression and anxiety. Find your sweet spot, whether that's seven, eight, or nine hours, or somewhere in between these times, and stick to it. Religiously.

Of course, you can screw this up from time to time and you'll be alright, but seriously, routinely getting seven to nine hours of sleep is a must and will absolutely improve your mental health.

I might sleep late, but I always make sure I get my seven hours of sleep every night.

Have A Normal Routine

I don't care if you work the graveyard shift, the second shift, the first shift, or some made up in-between shift, you should have a regular routine that you adhere to when it comes to your sleep. Sleeping irregularly, as the scientific studies confirm, messes with your biochemistry and sleep quality,[17] and can lead to really bizarre and downright terrifying conditions like sleep paralysis.

But even on a less extreme level, having different sleeping patterns interferes with your body's ability to follow regularly-scheduled functions. It's like having a great, on-top-of-his-shit manager running a thriving warehouse, setting up all the processes and directing all the workers to stay on task and operate efficiently; only to have a drunken owner, who's never around and out of the know, come in one day out of the blue and start aimlessly ordering everyone around and telling them to do moronic things. The inebriated proprietor is not only revealing to his employees what a complete loser and asshole he is, but more importantly, he's fucking everything up and throwing off the smooth harmony of the work environment for all.

Our bodies are the same way. We like order and hate people (whether drunken assholes or anyone for that matter) coming in and messing things up. Human beings are rhythmic animals and as much as our current society is speeding things up and distorting the natural flow of how we're designed to live, it's imperative that we try our best to maintain some semblance within the 21st century technological chaos that surrounds us.

Work with your body and assist it by upholding order and routine. It will reward you by giving you a more restful and nourishing sleep.

Go to bed at the same time every night and wake up at the same time every morning.

<u>Take An Hour Or Two To Unwind</u>

This is really a major part of the sleep process in my view. Having a designated time to set aside to get you prepared to fall asleep is almost as critical as the actual sleep itself. People who jump right into bed or who go directly from playing video games, watching an engaging movie, or messing around on their cell phones, are not giving their minds the time it needs to unwind.

It takes a certain amount of time for your brain to adjust to radically different conscious conditions. Successful transition, from alert and stimulated (robbing and shooting a bunch of people in *Grand Theft Auto*) to shutting down and turning off your excitatory brain waves is not that easy. Your brain needs time to adjust to these polar opposite mental states.

Going from being mentally aroused to jumping right into bed is the perfect recipe for rolling around for the next few hours and wondering why you can't sleep. Instead, stop the video games, movies, and cell phones an hour or two earlier, and have a relaxing routine before nodding off. Reading a book, having sex, and meditating, are some of the best ways to unwind.

Avoid Blue Light

Different colors of light do different things to the body and brain. By housing particular forms of varying wavelengths of light, certain colors can penetrate through our cells and enact radically different change to the body's systems. One of these such colors is blue light.

Blue lights have been studied by researchers and have been shown to elicit a sense of alertness and wakefulness in humans.[18] There effects have actually been compared to those of caffeine in many ways. This is great if you need to rev up your cognition to perform better during the day, but at night, just before bed, it's the last thing you want to do.

Avoiding your cell phones and laptops, and minimizing television viewing before going to bed, is highly recommended. I know it can be tough, but give yourself a break from electronics just before sleep. When you're trying to wind down and release the right neurochemicals (melatonin, serotonin, GABA, glycine, etc.) to do their job, the last thing you want to do is spend time in front of blue lights that shunt their discharge and actually increase the release of excitatory neuros.

Avoid Caffeine In The Evening

Coffee can be a Godsend to many people. It's one of the most popular beverages in the world and a necessary facilitator to the day of many. Its main ingredient, caffeine of course, being the reason why. Caffeine works by blocking one of the body's key sleep-inducing molecules, a neurotransmitter called adenosine.[19]

Adenosine is a byproduct of ATP (one of the main energy sources for your body's cells) and builds up over the course of the day in your brain as you stay awake. Adenosine functions as an inhibitory neurotransmitter and depresses the nervous system to calm you down and get you tired. When the molecules in caffeine bind to the same receptors in the brain that adenosine uses, they overthrow the function of adenosine to get you sleepy, and are able to help keep your mind awake.

Caffeine to start your day in the morning is typically fine, and can actually have some beneficial effects on the brain and body (for one, it can actually support the function of dopamine). But caffeine typically has a half-life of 4-6 hours for most people. Coffee bean lovers and tea-baggers far and wide, beware: If you're thinking of consuming caffeine a couple of hours before bed, don't. It will almost certainly disrupt your sleep.

Make Room Temperature Ideal

When your room is too cold, you can't relax; you shiver and constantly tug down on your blankets to gain more heat. But try as you might, you can't get comfy. When it's too hot, you sweat, fidget, toss, turn, and kick your legs around in fruitless attempts to find the cooler, unheated areas of your sheets, but this never helps. In both cases, the temperature works against you and sabotages the quality of your sleep. We've known this for years, but sometimes it slips our minds and we forget.

The effects of temperature on sleep have been studied in recent years and researchers are essentially confirming what many of us intuitively knew: both the heat and cold can negatively affect your sleep.[20] Thus it's imperative to set your room temp at a comfortable setting every night. This will vary from person to person, but in general, a good sleeping temperature is between 60–70 degrees Fahrenheit. Find yours and marry it.

Make The Room As Dark As Possible

We are designed to sleep in the dark. Our ancient ancestors didn't have cell phones, televisions, computers, or even light bulbs. When the day went dark, they didn't have the option of channel surfing or watching porn on their favorite website; they pretty much had one option: go to sleep, and wait for the sun to come back up to get shit done.

As it turns out, we're all still wired this way. As much as we may not like it, our brains are still geared to being in sync with the sun's light. Hundreds of thousands of years of evolution can't be erased by just a couple hundred years of artificial light. Although we may be adapting to a life where artificial light takes over, we've still yet to cross that threshold internally, and therefore must still adhere to the rules of Mother Earth—or, at the very least, compensate for not.

Ideally, as I mentioned before, it would be best to have a normal sleep schedule. Having one that closely follows that of the sun, waking up and going to sleep when it's naturally light and dark, is truly best. But if you can't manage this, or are innately nocturnally predisposed like me, make your room as dark as possible.

That means getting true blackout curtains that block out the sun in the morning when you're sleeping (or when you're going to sleep) and keeping your room dark throughout the entirety of your rest. Having just a speck of brightness in your room can mess with your melatonin and cortisol release, and critically impair your sleep. I may be bad with going to bed late, but I've been absolutely dogged in maintaining an exceptionally darkened room during sleep. This allows me to mimic nature's will pretty damn well. It's not ideal, but it is effective.

One recent scientific retroactive analysis concluded that 99% of people exposed to room light just before bed have a suppression of melatonin, a delayed release of melatonin, and a shortening (by 90 minutes) of its duration, compared to those exposed to dim or no light. Also, the study found that in 85% of the trials conducted on melatonin expression, exposure to room light *during* sleep inhibited melatonin synthesis by 50 percent.[21] Pretty shocking.

A good indicator of whether or not your room is dark enough is whether or not you can see your hand. If you can in fact see your hand, by waving it in front of your face, your room is not dark enough. Get some more curtains, or darker, thicker ones, or try another technique for blackening out your windows. But do something. You don't want to see anything when you go to sleep. (Except maybe some naked women, or men if that's your preference, in your dreams.)

Exercise

Exercising during the day is a safe and effective method for improving sleep at night. This is one of the simplest yet most supportive solutions for insomnia.

Many years back, when I'd get periodic bouts of insomnia for a night or two, my grandmother would always say something to the effect of, "Go run in the back yard for a few hours! You're just being a lazy bum! You need to do more! Run!" (And yeah, that's no typographical error you just read, my grandmother was a yeller. She was one of those crazy old ladies who always shouted to emphasize her words and swung a wooden spatula around to get her point across, even when she wasn't mad—which she never really was, though you'd never guess if you'd read a screenplay of any arbitrary day in her life. Looking back now, it's actually rather comical. Back then though, it was quite compelling.)

But as it turns out, she was right. Taking her advice, I'd often exercise for an hour or so, maybe run several miles, or go to the gym and do a nice, hard lifting session, and lo and behold, later that night, I'd sleep like a baby.

My wise little old granny knew instinctively what scientists and researchers are discovering more and more in recent studies: that moving, exercising, and breaking a sweat, favorably improves the biochemistry throughout the body and brain.[22] Critical players like hormones, neurotransmitters, proteins, and other key atomic substances all seem to sway the pendulum back in favor of improved slumber.

We'll cover exercise in depth in the depression section but remember this: If you exercise during the day, you're almost certainly going to have a better sleep when night falls.

Condition Your Bed For Sleep (And Sex) Only

Pop quiz. What do the following things all have in common: Doing late night work for tomorrow's big meeting; binge-watching your favorite Netflix series; watching fetish porn on your laptop; and swiping right for fat chicks on Tinder?

Any ideas?

No? Okay, I'll tell you. They're all things that should never be done on your bed before sleep (or ever as far as Tinder is concerned—and yeah, moderate the fetish porn if you must watch it; too much can mess with your sexual performance.[23]).

These stimulatory actions are designed to keep your mind engaged and working hard, the last things you want before nodding off. Remember, you want an unwinding routine before bed, and anything that's going to inspire the beta brainwaves is not something you want to undertake. Beta brainwaves are for being conscious and alert, the complete opposite of our intended goal.

Instead, you want to switch to having alpha and theta brainwaves, the ones closely associated with deep relaxation, meditation, and light sleep (and eventually delta waves for a deeper sleep).

Having a rule of only using your bed for sleep or sex is a great idea. Sex of course is a naturally healthy and downright amazing activity, and as such, cannot be eliminated from your bedtime routine. (If anything, you should make a habit of adding more of it.) But everything else should go. Condition your mind to recognize your bed as a sanctuary for rest.

Every time you lie down on your bed, you should either be having unworldly sex (with a drop-dead gorgeous supermodel from Russia) or sleeping (and dreaming about having sex with a Russian supermodel—or, I suppose, even sex with a modestly attractive, non-fat chick from Tinder is still acceptable.) Everything else is pure blasphemy.

Make Your Room As Quiet As Possible (Consider A White-Noise Machine)

Just as your room should be as dark as possible to align with the universal laws of nature, so too should your room be quiet. At night, activity has historically quieted down, if not ceased entirely, and so we've been conditioned to sleep in environments with little to no noise.

For hundreds of thousands of years, unexpected sounds or noises in the night would naturally arouse our conscious minds and affect our sleep, since unanticipated sounds in the night meant something bad: an animal predator approaching near; a dangerous thunderstorm; a potential foe from a nearby tribe . . . anything that could cause our primordial ancestors harm would undoubtedly alarm them and affect their rest.

We may not live in a world as dangerous as that of our prehistoric forbearers, but we're still largely wired in the same capacity. Sounds and noises, especially of the unanticipated variety, very much affect and even ruin our sleep. Again, ideally it would be best to sleep at a "normal" time; this way you could synchronize your sleep with that of most your neighbors and have as few interruptions of commotion as possible. But for some, including me, using a white-noise machine has been a solid alternative.

White-noise machines are great for keeping your mind distracted from many of the background sounds that inevitably creep up throughout the night: A dog barking down the street (even for just a few minutes); a roaring motorcycle riding by; an argument between a couple walking past your home . . . all of these sounds, which would wake most people up from their beauty sleep, would most likely go unnoticed if a white-noise machine (or two like I use) was being utilized during your slumber.

They're not going to block out every sound, and they certainly aren't foolproof, but for most sounds, they do an exceptional job of masking their presence.

One model you might consider grabbing is the Marpac Dohm white-noise machine. I've tried a few white-noise machines over the years and to be completely honest, they all kind of sucked balls. This one, however, does not. On the contrary, it works quite well, so well, in fact, I ordered a second one for travel, or for those nights when I've admittedly slipped back into my nocturnal roots and stayed up far later than I intended. For both these occasions it's worked admirably.

(By the way, I have absolutely *zero* financial connection to this company; I just like their product and know it works magnificently. Go with whoever you want though, I could truly not care less. I'm sure there are some formidable competitors out there. I've just not come across them myself.)

Finally, silencing your phones, laptop, TV, and anything else that might make a noise during the night is a given. (Ideally, you'd remove them from your room altogether, but I understand if this is too much to give up. I certainly won't hold this against you if you don't. Keeping them off or on silent, however, is a must.)

Consider Meditation

Meditation, which we spoke about at length a few chapters back, is one of the best natural remedies for insomnia. Try it right before bed. Also, just before you start meditating, try the breathing technique called "The Relaxing Breath" that I described in that very chapter.

Get Comfortable Gear

Get a comfortable bed . . . a nice pillow . . . cool but cozy sheets and blankets . . . and everything else you either put on or lie on when you go to sleep. Being at your utmost level of coziness when you rest is a necessity. Don't overlook this simple but profound step. You should feel as though you're lying bare, atop a million Hungarian goose down feathers, marinating in your own liberating comfort, and basking in all your naked glory.

If your bed is old and shitty, and squeaks incessantly each time you roll onto a different side, it's time for a new one. If your pillow has a million stains on it and needs to be folded over for actual neck support, toss it out and get a new one. If your blankets have holes and rips and really aren't (and never really were) all that comfortable, get some fucking new ones.

Sleep is one of the few things in life you really shouldn't take lightly. Even if it means spending a few extra bucks to improve it by getting nicer shit, do it.

Take Magnesium Daily

We covered magnesium extensively in the supplement section for anxiety and we'll cover it again for depression because it's so effective and healthy for both. And, as it turns out, it's also just as beneficial for sleep.[24]

It works in a number of ways, but it's probably most prominent with regard to sleep in its ability to balance out the neurotransmitters, especially serotonin and dopamine, and allow GABA, the brain's most prominent relaxing chemical, to increase functionality. (If you want to supplement with this, take 200-250mg of magnesium citrate or glycinate just before bed.)

Consider Melatonin Supplementation

Melatonin is a hormone that your body produces at night. When the evening comes, the darkness triggers your pineal gland to start producing this chemical to signal to the rest of your body to start shutting down the system soon.

Melatonin also plays a number of key roles within the brain including moderating neuronal firing,[25] balancing serotonin and dopamine levels, regulating body temperature while sleeping, and working in conjunction with a number of other important hormones.

People like me, who may operate on later time schedules, often have a flawed production of this hormone. But following some of the other sleeping tips, like using blackout curtains and avoiding blue lights (or regular bright lights), can help to get you back in the melatonin-producing swing.

If all else fails, you can supplement with melatonin, as it's generally very safe. In terms of dosage, I'd suggest somewhere between 3–10mg a night, right before you head to bed. And maybe, if you really feel so inclined, go up to 20mg. But try not to exceed this (20mg is the most I would ever do personally). Too much melatonin can have side effects, and can actually harm your sleep. If you feel like you have to keep upping your dosage for the melatonin to work, try something else. It's not your melatonin level that's the problem, it's something else.

Consider Valerian Root

Valerian root, also discussed expansively in the supplement section, can be an effective herb to take before bed for occasional sleeplessness.

Valerian appears to have a number of relaxing modalities, but its most prominent is its ability to produce more GABA in the brain. It's very effective at doing this and thus is truly great at shutting down an excitable mind. Numerous studies have shown its ability to improve sleep,[26] especially its onset, when taken just before bed.

The dosage for sleep is typically between 400mg–900mg just before bed. As always, start at the lowest dose and see how you feel.

Turn Off Wi-Fi (EMFs)

This is a developing field of study on our health, but the effects of electromagnetic fields (EMFs), also called electromagnetic radiation, is beginning to be more and more recognized. And it doesn't look good. EMFs are invisible electrically charged physical fields produced by electrical appliances and wireless devices like cell phones, laptops, and now, even many TV sets.

As the term electromagnetic radiation suggests, the effects of these electrical fields can cause damage to our bodies in myriad ways. Again, the damage is still being assessed, but many believe it alters brain function, affects our immune systems, and causes direct damage to our cells. Several recent studies found that the cortical area of the brain is excited when around EMFs and thus researchers drew the natural link to sleep disruption.[27] After all, being excited and falling asleep don't really go together.

The research is still being carried out, but right now it seems best to minimize your exposure to EMFs when you can; especially when it comes to your sleep. Turn off your Wi-Fi at night, put your phone on airplane mode, shutdown your laptop, and keep all electrical devices away from your bed. You don't want these hidden but quite evidently dangerous electrical fields unknowingly sabotaging your slumber and wreaking insidious havoc on your health. I think the coming years will reveal a lot more about the true dangers of unchecked EMFs, but until then I think it's certainly wise to play it safe and be proactive.

Just remember, it wasn't too long ago that people thought smoking cigarettes was perfectly safe too.

Avoid Alcohol

Alcohol is thought to be great for sleep. It's not. It might do the trick of knocking you out when you consume too much of it, but it turns out that the sleep you get from your alcohol-infused brain is not restful and not of quality. You don't need to completely eliminate alcohol (in moderation it can actually have some positive health effects), but if your goal is to improve your sleep, you want to minimize it, especially in the hours leading up to your bedtime.

Alcohol messes with the body's natural production of that key hormone I've referred to many times already, melatonin. It actually decreases it.[28] It also affects the natural sleep-wake cycle of the body and throws the manufacture of adenosine out of balance. Finally, although it may induce sleep faster, the sleep you undergo while under the influence of alcohol tends to be a non-restorative sleep.

Frequent wake-ups, restlessness, and irregular amounts of time spent in your otherwise normal sleep stages occur. And oftentimes, after the alcohol is metabolized by the liver, a rebound-like effect occurs where instead of your system being depressed (relaxed and shut down), it awakens and becomes alert, leaving you with just a few hours of sleep, and a bizarre influx of unwanted energy.

I'm not the prohibition police. I'm not going to tell you to stop drinking. That would just be foolish and downright profane. I love drinking a few beers or a few mixed drinks from time to time. But if sleep is paramount for you, as it is for me, and you want to improve your mental function, minimize your alcohol intake. A few drinks once a week should be fine, but try not to do much more than this.

Consider A Mental Mantra

Have you ever tried counting sheep to herd away your unrelenting insomnia?

If you've got a pulse, the answer is yes. And if your blood is still vibrantly pumping about after answering that mind-melting inquiry, you can also recall just how shitty this technique actually works. In fact, it doesn't. In all my life I've likely participated in this sheep-counting sham a dozen or so times. And not one single fucking time has it ever worked.

That said, there is a technique very vaguely related to the sheep-tallying scheme that actually does work. I found it several years back in a random YouTube search after an arbitrarily shitty night's rest where I tossed and turned for the majority of it.

The practice is rather simple and the video I saw was created by a guy named David Mark who runs a company called 10MinuteZen.[29] Normally, I would've skipped over the video and cast it into the wacky-as-fuck category, but I was feeling rather curious that day and figured I donate the three minutes of my life to seeing what it was all about.

I'm glad I did.

To perform this technique you simply breathe in and out, either solely through your nose as normal, or with both your nose and mouth, breathing in through your nose and out your mouth. (I prefer just the nose, but you can do both if you'd like, as either way works.) Whilst breathing in and out, however, you're going to add in two sounds. The first sound, when you breathe in, is "SAAAAA." And the second sound, when you breathe out, is "Ooooom."

You'll make these two sounds, in your head, every time you breathe in and out, respectively, and you'll want to keep a consistent rhythm. Each full breath, in and out, will look like this:

SAAAA, OOOOOOm . . . SAAAA, OOOOOOm . . . SAAAA, OOOOOOm . . . SAAAA, OOOOOOm

And you'll repeat this over and over again, until the next thing you know, the sun is shining on your face and you're waking up. You don't have to keep track of how many chants you do, or how long you do it for; in fact, you don't want to, as it will mess you up. Simply use this technique over and over again, relax your mind, and let the power of this calming act whisk you away into a peaceful slumber.

By the way, these two sounds, just to reiterate, are both expressed only in your mind. You don't actually utter them out loud. Just use your inner mental voice and say them inside your head. It makes it easier to do, less distracting, and more effective.

This odd but effective little routine works because saying the "SAAAA" and "OOOOOOm" sounds in your head, over and over again, creates a white-noise pattern in your brain. It's a natural way to calm the mind and facilitate sleep.[30] Try it sometime, it works.

FINAL THOUGHTS ON SLEEP

Sleeping is critical for your health, especially your mental health. Anxiety can be ameliorated with proper sleep and can be significantly exacerbated without it. Use the tips I've shared to optimize this infinitely important part of your day. Your anxiety will convalesce, your depression will improve, and your happiness will flourish.

Sleep may seem like a passive act, a trivial part of the day that warrants no extra attention. But this couldn't be further from the truth. It's one of the most important parts of your day, and needs to be undertaken with proper consideration. A few minutes of daily sleep prep can literally change your life.

Sleep long, sleep well, and fantasize of all the wonders of the world. With proper rest they may very well come true.

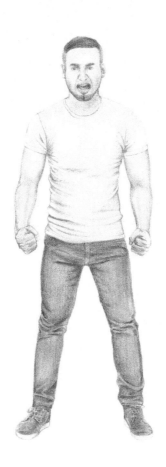

Chapter Fourteen
My Last Panic Attack

The frequency had slowed down. I wasn't getting them as often anymore. But when they came, they came with a vengeance.

Over the previous few months, I'd slowly learned how to temper my anxiety, using many of the techniques I've talked about. Overall, I was doing really well with my stress and fears, but I still couldn't shake the panic attacks completely. They hid in my shadows, lurking, watching, ready to pounce on my psyche the instant they sensed any opening.

Yeah, things were finally looking up, but the battle was far from over. My panic attacks still held profound dominion over me.

That is, until one fateful day.

In the midst of my frantic search to find my anxiety and depression cures, I'd stumbled across a million different things. Some (like those I mentioned earlier for anxiety, and those I'll bring up soon for depression) had been incredibly helpful and made a tangible impact in my life. Others I'd tried out, however, worked about as comparably well as the first straw-fortified house had for the first fat little pig who'd precariously pieced it together. In other words, they totally blew ass.

Whether they didn't work for me specifically, or not at all, I'll never know; but given my swift pace to find answers, I honestly didn't care (nor do I really care now, as I have all the answers I need, presented right here in these pages).

I bring this up, however, because during my divine crusade, I did come across something (among many things to be candid) that I'd discarded altogether, before even trying: Alternative approaches to either anxiety or depression that to me just seemed so off the deep end that they could not possibly work. (I'm a pretty open-minded guy, mind you, but some of these things were just so utterly batshit crazy, or at least they appeared to be . . .)

One technique in particular had stuck out as perhaps the most batshit crazy of them all, and I had quickly dismissed it, and probably even audibly laughed aloud at its ridiculousness. In fact, it was so fucking stupid it actually made me question the sanctity of my quest for a few brief moments. Ultimately, I carried on, of course.

But I'm getting ahead of myself, for now anyway . . .

STORY TIME

I'm sitting in my room one day watching porn.

Like any testosterone-fueled teenager at the time I get off watching all sorts of random and perverted shit. I'm addicted to it in a sense and dedicate at least a couple of hours out of the day to enjoying the craft.

(At this juncture, as I mentioned a moment ago, I'd been getting better with my anxiety. But I still wasn't nearly as "cured" as I'd hoped to be. There was still a lot, no actually a FUCKING MASSIVE amount, of work to do.)

So as I'm sitting in my room, tugging away my misery and hoping to get a quick relief from the day-to-day depression and feelings of inferiority and hopelessness, I randomly start to think about my life. I start to consider why I'm not pleased, and why I'm wasting away in my room like some kind of reject who can't get a date (I couldn't buy a date back then), and who can't be happy. I start to contemplate my existence, and ponder my true purpose and reflect on the absolute meaning of my life . . . and I don't like it.

No, as I mull over the entire philosophical gravity of everything surrounding my reality, I don't like it at all.

(Okay, actually, I'll be honest: in complete transparency this self-assessment and deep-dive into the meaning of life came after I'd sprayed semen all over my bed and lap in a short-lived climax of right-handed passion. But moving on . . .)

With seminal fluid varnishing everything important in sight, I begin feeling like a complete loser, and start thinking about how all I do is sit around jerking off in my room all day long (which was actually rather true). I continue this pessimistic opining, and quickly my feelings of worthlessness compound.

They start to fester, one insidious thought after the next, until soon I give myself anxiety. And this anxiety just adds more gasoline to the already-stoked flames. After a few more minutes of this, I find myself on the precipice of yet another panic attack. Fucking great.

My technique of late, during this precise stage in time, was to try to distract myself. I'd immediately try thinking of other things, more pleasant things—like unicorns and rainbows for instance—to alter my thoughts. If this didn't work (it never did), I'd turn on the TV and try watching *SportsCenter* or maybe some type of news show. Inevitably, when this failed, I'd get up and move around, hoping by now the panic would've had enough fun beating my ass for the day, and would kindly move on to some other future date.

Sometimes I was lucky and by this last step it would sort of fade away, like a bully who gets winded from pounding your face in for 15 minutes and decides to get off you, not because he's suddenly hit with an emotional stroke of empathy, but because he doesn't want his hands to start hurting from clubbing your face in for such an extended period of time.

Most times, though, the bully would stay longer, unmercifully hammering away, one terrifying blow after the next. And it was really up to him when he decided to leave, and come back for that matter.

So I'm in my room, freaking the fuck out, after coming to the realization that I have jack-shit going on in my life and that I literally waste a good portion of my day, every day, playing with myself. The incredibly powerful, soul-sucking feelings I begin perceiving only get exacerbated by my thoughts of getting another uncontrollable panic attack.

And then I get another uncontrollable panic attack.

My heart is racing, my palms are sweating, I feel the butterflies doing backflips in my stomach, and my thoughts are firing frantically in all directions. "Oh my god," I say. "Why can't I stop this panic? I feel like I'm going crazy again!"

"Think good thoughts! Just change your focus and you'll calm down," I hysterically blurt aloud. "You can do this man, just RELAX!" I am desperate to console myself.

It doesn't work.

The thoughts race faster and faster, and my sense of control is all but a distant memory. The bully is back and he's beating the ever-living shit out of me. Tenacious, ferocious, unrelenting . . .

After a few more boundless minutes of intolerable agony, a random thought pops into my head. It's one I've never truly considered up until this point, aside from a fleeting moment of unadulterated ridicule months back.

I don't know why, but it seems to offer some bizarre shred of hope. And right now, with the bully on top and pounding away, it's all I've got.

I latch onto it in complete desperation.

THE GAME-CHANGING THOUGHT

Months earlier, as I alluded to at the beginning of this chapter, I came across a number of ridiculous and seemingly batshit-level-crazy ideas for thwarting anxiety and depression. But one of these ideas was unequivocally head and shoulders above all others, and took the cake for being the wackiest of all, or so I thought.

This screwball idea came in the form of a tiny little ebook. It was all of about 30 pages of unimpressive, scribbled-together gobbledygook, written by some British dude who'd allegedly figured out how to beat his anxiety, and more specifically, his panic attacks. It was aptly titled *Panic Away* and the author of this Looney-Tune literature was a man who went by the pseudonym Joe Barry.

The gist of this ebook boiled down to three main points that were supposed to help you stop your panic attacks in their tracks. Whenever you'd have an attack, you were to follow one after the other in successive order to end it. These three main steps were as follows:

1. Do Nothing When You First Get The Symptoms Of A Panic Attack

2. Welcome Your Panic In With Open Arms

3. Ask For More Of It

I know, I told you this book was fucking nutty. That's exactly why I completely dismissed it for the horseshit it was the second I first came across it.

First of all, why would you want to do NOTHING when you start getting a panic attack? Everyone who's ever had a panic attack knows you can't just sit still and do fucking *nothing*. This is ridiculous and it seems like the perfect start to a totally useless strategy for stopping attacks.

Secondly, why on God's good green fucking Earth would you want to welcome the panic attack in? And with open arms? *Is this Barry guy really that much of a fucking fruitcake? This is just getting absurd now.*

Finally, and this is where it really gets good, Barry, in all his exuberant wisdom, recommends you actually ask for—I shit you not—MORE of your panic! Literally. (I couldn't have made this pea-brained process up if I'd smoked all the laced-up marijuana in the world.) The final and most important step to his unbelievably stupid approach to beating panic attacks . . . was to call for more of them! How the fuck can that possibly make any sense!?

It didn't. At least that's exactly what I'd thought, those months back when I'd read it. I'd gone through the little book in just a few minutes, shocked at what this man was telling me to do the next time I got a panic attack.

I actually went back through and re-read it again (because it was so short, and because I was so perplexed), looking to see where my eyes had misconstrued the information I'd absorbed. But no, my initial assessment was correct: This dude was fucked.

For some reason, however, during this latest life-altering beatdown by the bully, I found myself thinking back to Mr. Barry's fucked-up technique. And in that moment of absolute despair, I decided to give it a shot.

PANIC AWAY IN ACTION

Fuck it, I thought to myself. *Let's try out that wacky Barry Method. I got nothin' to lose.*

And anxiety-laden though I was, I started rattling my brain for the info I'd read months earlier, recollecting the key points of this shot-in-the-dark attempt.

Welcome it in? I asked myself silently. *No, challenge . . . no, the first step is doing . . . nothing. Yeah, just observe the panic. Okay,* I thought, as I dubiously began the three-step process.

"Just observe your thoughts," I repeated out loud, reassuring myself that I had control of at least that much in that volatile moment. "I can observe this panic attack for a minute and see where it takes me."

"Welcome it back," was my next thought aloud. "Oh. Shit. This is where it gets real." I remembered in that moment the full extent of this next, exponentially harder step, and though it scared me even more than I'd already been in that panic-dominating instant, I proceeded.

"Welcome back, panic," I began. "Welcome back, feelings of going crazy. Welcome back, thoughts of being a loser. Welcome back, thoughts of being a porn-addict who can't get any girls to like him. Welcome back, butterflies in my stomach. It's good to feel you again. Welcome back, shaky legs I missed you. Welcome back, sweaty palms, heart-racing, mind-racing, and light-headedness, I fucking missed you all!" I continued with this new litany, growing bolder and more enthusiastic in my hospitality.

"I missed you, thoughts of ending up in a mental hospital. I missed you, feelings of being a fucking reject. Wow, I missed you so much, thoughts of losing my mind and going fucking crazy. Welcome, welcome, welcome back!"

After this, I moved right into the third and hardest step of them all, the asking for more part. Surprisingly, no, *shockingly*, I'd been building a brave momentum toward the end of my dialogue in step two. Really getting into it, I grew louder and gutsier with my welcoming proclamations to the panic. But when it came time for step three, I'd be lying if I said I didn't hesitate for a moment, knowing this was really where shit could hit the fan and backfire big time.

But nonetheless, I continued.

"Give me more," I mumbled out. "Give me more of this anxiety. Give me more of this terror. Give me more of this fucking panic," I said each sentence louder, with a little more conviction. "Give more of these thoughts of being a fucking loser. Give me more of these thoughts of ending up in a mental institution. Give me more of these sweaty palms, these shaky legs, these butterflies doing motherfucking backflips in my stomach! Give me more of this fucking goddamn panic!"

I was yelling now, and continued, blood beginning to boil. "Fucking give me more of everything you got! Give me more of these thoughts of going crazy, of being a loser, of having no friends, of not being liked by girls, of not getting a date, of having no fucking idea of what I'm doing with my life! GIVE ME MORE OF FUCKING ALL OF IT!" I was now shouting as loud as I possibly could, calling the fuck out of the bully who'd been picking on me for so long. I'd had enough of his torment and in that moment I decided, "Fuck him, I don't care if he beats me even harder, I'm not taking any more of his shit. I'm sick of it!"

And I kept yelling and calling him out with every ounce of energy in my bones.

This lasted for a few extraordinarily intense minutes: Swears, cusswords, made-up words, and pure vernacular garbage issued forth from my lungs and tongue in those stark moments of profanity-laced nonsensical diatribe. It made about as much sense as a misbehaved schoolboy trying to speak with a massive bar of soap in his mouth. But it didn't matter. It was powerful.

In those frantic moments of releasing these copious amounts of pent-up frustration, fear, and anger, something incredibly profound happened without me even realizing: The panic went away.

That's right, it disappeared.

I was so focused on getting all of my thoughts out, and so tired of failing in the fight against my panic-attack bully, I actually forgot that I was supposed to be scared.

It was almost as if something had magically switched ON in that moment, and I'd literally flipped the bully around and gotten on top of him. I didn't understand it right then, or truly realize the magnitude of what'd just occurred, but it hit me soon after:

This batshit-crazy, totally-fucking-out-there, and completely-fucking-nutty technique by Joe Barry actually worked. In fact, it was the only thing I'd come across that'd been able to stop my panic attack right away.

It not only worked, it worked fucking fast.

I WAS WRONG

I realized later, upon deeper reflection of that profound moment, exactly what had transpired.

And here's what I learned about the *Panic Away* method and why it works.

Actually, first let me say, I was totally fucking wrong about my initial assumptions regarding this ebook by Joe Barry. All that shit I said earlier, yeah, I take it back.

He's not mad. He's a genius.

But now, let's break down the *Panic Away* process and see just why.

WHY MOST TECHNIQUES FAIL

Typically when you get a panic attack, your first instinct, like mine, is to run, hide, suppress, or pretend the panic attack doesn't exist altogether. Essentially, the go-to strategy for most is to do everything possible to avoid facing the panic attack and all its accompanying symptoms. But that's the first mistake.

General anxiety can be effectively lowered or even removed when you use a strategy like any of the ones I just mentioned. A low-level rise in fear or a meager gust of anxiety can usually be resolved with a technique like shifting your thoughts onto a different topic or distracting yourself[1] with an arbitrary activity. This works decently enough for these occasions, because here you're still in control, and the anxiety is not overpowering your thoughts and emotions yet. An approach where you actively and quickly change the course of the anxiety is actually not a bad option and can often be pretty effective for some.

However, when we're talking about panic attacks, these techniques almost always fail.

That's because panic, just like the word implies, is a frantic state of mind, where you're not in control of your thoughts. It's actually the reverse. Your thoughts have taken over your mind and are controlling YOU. They're dictating your feelings, your emotions, and your bodily processes: your heartbeat, upset stomach, and sweaty palms, and everything else you so badly wish you could take back under control.

In this moment, we have to resort to something far more drastic and far more direct. And that's essentially what the *Panic Away* technique teaches you: how to fight the panic attack head on.

WHY THIS ONE WORKS

Instead of running or hiding, as our natural impulse usually dictates we do, we pivot our energy in a different direction. And we don't react. You may think the first step in this method, that of just sitting back and observing your thoughts, is a submissive one, but it's not.

On the contrary, it's a *powerful* first step.

It proactively calms us down (similar to meditation, wherein you're just observing things and focusing) and gears us up for the next couple of actions. Doing nothing actually means pausing for a moment from your intrinsic penchant to react and therefore increase your fear. This critical step number one is perfect for initiating the takeback of your overthrown mind.

The second step, welcoming the panic back, is where things really start to take shape. This little act of verbalizing the panic attack's symptoms and the personification of its idiosyncrasies allows you to begin to reveal the true nature of what's causing your trouble. It's like putting a face to a cloaked figure in the darkness, and you start to feel differently about what you're up against. Your battle, for the first time, actually appears winnable.

But by far the most profound step is the third and final one, of asking for more of the panic attack symptoms. This is what initially drew me to the conclusion that this method was maniacally flawed, and made me not want to ever try it. But again, this is the game-changer in this process, the key to why it works.

When you ask for more of the panic attack's symptoms, you challenge the bully. You're intrinsically saying, "Fuck you!" and calling him out for what he is. And that is nothing.

You see, most people get so tangled up in their emotions and thoughts that they slowly let the panic take over their reality. The bully becomes an overpowering and insurmountable symbol of their greatest weakness, one they fear more than anything. And the more they become afraid, the worse the fear gets.

Just like any bully, panic thrives on fear, and it thrives on those who cower down to it. By doing everything else *but* standing up to the bully, you feed into it, and make it worse with time.

There's only one true way to get rid of any bully. Every schoolyard kid who's ever been in a fight will tell you: you've got to punch him, right in the fucking face. And that's what this last step does. It's a mental left uppercut right to the bully's fucking chin!

By calling for more of everything the panic has to offer you, you take all the symptoms that previously terrified you and bring them to light. You expose the panic exactly for what it is: a mental fabrication that holds absolutely *zero* power over you. And when you do this, it disappears.

Panic, and any fear for that matter, cannot exist when we stand up to it. Just like the schoolyard bully it yields its power from our intimidation.

To end your fears, you must face them head on.

The Wiz

The Wizard of Oz is one of my all-time favorite movies. It's got everything you could possibly want in a film (minus naked women and guns): great actors, cool characters, an awesome storyline, action, mystery, suspense, munchkins, witches, and even a wizard. Not to mention, the effects are still cool and realistic enough even in this day and age of high-tech resolutions and CGI.

Not bad for a film made in 1939.

Among the many impressive scenes throughout the movie, the one that stands out the most to me is the part near the end, where Dorothy finally meets the great Wizard of Oz.

If you haven't seen it, I'm not sure what planet you live on, but the whole point of the movie is for Dorothy and her friends to go to the Emerald City, where the Wizard resides. They embark on their quest to meet him because he's said to hold immeasurable power and is the only one who can help them get what they each seek most in their lives.

Long story short, Dorothy and the gang arrive and get to meet the Wiz, only he's not who they'd envisioned. He's actually quite an asshole. He's mean, he's rude, and he tells them he doesn't want to help them as he towers over them menacingly from a gigantic projection of himself displayed supernaturally over an even more gigantic veil.

With his thunderous voice, his ability to conjure flames from the ground, and his constant outbursts of intimidating threats, the Wizard terrifies the hell out of Dorothy and her friends, especially her miniature 10-pound Cairn Terrier pup named Toto.

To put it quite simply, the Wiz is a fucking bully. He preys on those who fear him and obtains all his power from doing this. The more people feared him, the more power they handed over to him and the more he assumed the role of dominance over them. Sound familiar?

The best part in the entire flick, in my humble opinion, comes when the tiny little terrier named Toto, in a moment of weakness and fear, runs off to seek shelter from the Wiz' insults. But in an ironic twist of fate, the little dog tries to hide behind a grey curtain inconspicuously off to the side, and in doing so drags open the drape to reveal the true identity of this great Wiz.

What he reveals is both shocking and hilarious. This great and powerful Wizard of Oz is actually just a great big fraud. He's no wizard at all, just a charlatan with an elaborate setup of special effects and gadgets, to give off the illusion that he's larger than life and more powerful than anyone can fathom.

In reality, the Wiz is a little old man, who'd have a tough time punching himself out of a wet paper bag.

Dorothy and the gang soon realize all of this, and in their moment of instant clarity take back all power the Wizard previously held over them. They take over, demand justice, and end up getting what they want—all because, with the help of serendipity, they have realized this bully, who was causing them so much anxiety and fear, was really nothing to fear at all. He is exposed as a concoction of their minds' beliefs, a fabrication of their reality, and when this happens they take back control.

Anxiety and panic attacks are just like the Wizard. They are not to be feared and something that when you expose to the light, reveal themselves as truly NOTHING.

Or, even better, a wrinkly, feeble, and ball-sagging old man.

THE ILLUSION OF FEAR

In his first inauguration speech in 1933, during a time of great economic anxiety in America, the great president Franklin Delano Roosevelt, better remembered by history as FDR, declared this: "So, first of all, let me assert my firm belief that the only thing we have to fear is . . . fear itself: nameless, unreasoning, unjustified terror which paralyzes needed efforts to convert retreat into advance."

I couldn't have said it better myself.

The man was dead-on with his assertion. Fear is an illusion. When you can get past your fear of the bully, when you can take action against him, when you can punch him right in the fucking face, he will never bother you again.

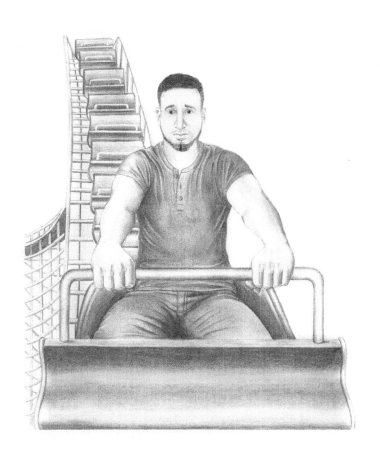

Chapter Fifteen
Facing My Biggest Fear

After implementing the bizarrely effective *Panic Away* method discussed in the last chapter, I never had a panic attack again. Sure, I've had many close calls, anxiety rushes that bordered on almost becoming a full-on panic, but never again have I had an actual *attack* in the true sense of the word. Armed with the skill of defeating them, I have never had to fear doing battle with panic again, and with this omnipresent confidence, I've never had to.

Make no mistake about it, though, the sword remains in its sheath, always ready and willing to be wielded if necessary.

MEETING THE NATURAL

Soon after this unbelievable self-discovery of panic-attack mastery, I began hanging out with a buddy of mine to whom I often refer in story-telling situations as *The Natural*. I came up with this moniker for him years back, as it was the only thing that could accurately depict his extraordinary social aptitude (especially when it came to women). My friend was a certified fucking ladies' man and could naturally meet, attract, and date almost any woman he laid eyes upon.

Yeah, he was pretty fucking badass, to say the least.

Anyway, The Natural (Bobby, as he was known to most layfolk), along with being an immaculate social communicator with women, also just so happened to be an astonishingly adept persuader—with all genders, and all creatures for that matter. He could talk a starving Rottweiler off a meat-wagon and then persuade it to become a diehard vegetarian, and probably even a loyal PETA member given enough time.

Oh, and if that wasn't cool enough, Bobby also happened to be a *bona fide* daredevil. He was a true adrenaline junkie who loved doing crazy shit, not because he had any addictions or anything, but because he was just a fucking extreme limit pusher. He'd constantly be testing to see how far he could take things in life. Some people are just fantastically crazy; The Natural is one of these people.

SIX FLAGS

One day I find myself with Bobby at the Six Flags theme park in Agawam, MA. We're walking around the park, just shooting the shit, joking around and eating food, enjoying life. I was probably 18 at this particular point in time (it was several months after my *Panic Away* experience), and like all 18-year-old men was in the peak of my sexual yearning. As a matter of fact, if a strong breeze blew by, my dick would quickly engorge to the sturdy equivalent of a granite rock. That's the level of testosterone and lust I'd built up over the years (makes sense, considering how unsuccessful I'd been with women up until that point). I know, it's pretty sad, but also quite impressive.

I mention this fact, not because it directly contributes to the moral of this tale, but because it describes my main purpose for going up to Six Flags in the first fucking place.

My sole motive for driving up two and a half hours to Western Massachusetts, to visit a park full of rides and roller coasters I had no interest whatsoever in going on, was to meet some girls. That's it. I hated crazy rides like the ones that flung you out of the atmosphere or freefall-dropped you from the clouds, and I especially, unequivocally, absolutely fucking hated roller coasters.

They had been the bane of my existence for the entirety of my early life, and the root cause of numerous vomiting episodes over the years. Carnivals, theme parks, festivals, fairs . . . they'd all induced regurgitated moments of pure agony more times than I'd like to admit, and they'd all derived back to one true culprit: the roller coaster.

Every single time I went on any roller coaster I'd immediately get a rush of fear. Followed promptly by those fantastic butterflies inside my stomach that always seemed to want to show up at the most inopportune times and throw a Thanksgiving-like parade. Subsequently, I'd get incredibly nauseous and start regretting the last meal I'd consumed, as the ride would commence.

The fears would expatiate with every passing second, and the nausea would smolder up with every unnatural twist and turn. By the time the ride would conclude, I'd have garnished myself with everything I'd consumed in the last three to four hours. And then I'd mortifyingly step off the death mobile and attempt to play it off like I didn't have grotesque-looking puke stains all over whatever soon-to-be-discarded shirt I was wearing.

However, this charade would quickly be exposed, as I couldn't keep up the fruitless act for long. Like clockwork, I'd only make it a few steps before tossing up last night's dinner too.

Yes, it was not only embarrassing, but fucking disgusting.

I would promise myself every single time to never go back on another roller coaster again. But inevitably, someone would challenge me to go back on and of course I'd go back on one. I guess I'm kind of like the serial drinker who gets a terrible hangover and swears off alcohol for the rest of his life, only to be pounding back tequila shots the very next Friday when his buddies invite him out for a night on the town. (Or maybe I'm more like Marty McFly in *Back To The Future*: when someone calls me a "chicken," I have to do everything possible to prove them wrong. Either way, it's definitely a major character flaw, and a painful one at times.)

Bobby, being the master communicator and manipulator—I mean . . . *persuader* that he was, seized on this weakness of mine. He played off the, "Let's just walk around and hit on girls" idea and made it seem like that was the plan all along. But *The Natural* had something else up his sleeve the entire time. And little did I know, his plan would not only work, it would inadvertently change my life.

THE PERSUADER

As Bobby and I arrive, we do just as we planned for maybe the first 30 minutes or so. We walk around, check out and talk to two really cute girls for a bit, and then get some food.

All is well at first.

After finishing up on some chicken tenders and fries, however, Bobby's plan slowly starts to take shape.

"Hey bro," The Natural says. "What do you think about going on just one roller coaster today?"

"Fuck that," I defiantly say, thinking to myself, *Here we go, already pestering me, I should've known.*

"Come on, man," he quips back. "They're really not that bad here. I know you were saying before how you got sick on those carnival and shitty fair roller coasters before, but these one are different. Six Flags has the safest roller coasters in the world. Little kids go on them all the time. My little brother (who was like seven at the time) rides on them too."

"Nah, I can't, dude. Trust me, I wish I could, but I know I'll just get sick," I reaffirm, trying to hold strong in my sternness, though starting to feel The Natural's pressure.

"Justin, I know you'll be fine, bro. Trust me. I go on these rides all the time. I've never gotten sick once, and like I said, my little brother's been on every one of these roller coasters a bunch of times with me. You're gonna' be fine, man. Just one, and I won't bother you again. I promise."

Adamant, though clearly wilting, I make one last attempt at holding off his insistence. "I don't know, I don't think it's a good idea," was all I could come back with. Then, like a masterful car salesman who sells a brand new Lexus to the ambivalent customer who only went in the dealership to "look around," Bobby goes in for the kill. "Come on dude, one ride. We'll be done with the whole thing in five minutes and I won't bother you again. If you do throw up, which you won't, I'll pay for your food on the way home." *Son of a bitch*, I think to myself. *If I throw up I won't even want any food after.* But after a few seconds of pondering his offer, I inevitably give in. "Okay, let's do it," I reluctantly reply.

The Persuader has done it again.

I MEET BIZARRO

We walk around for a few minutes, trying to find a suitable ride. I point out a couple of small, baby-sized roller coasters as I make a joke about riding them. "Let's get on those little midget ones over there," I laugh, as I point and chuckle.

"That'll be a blast," I add, trying to play the cocky-guy role now, and trick myself (and Bobby) into thinking I have things under control. Little does he know (or maybe he actually did) that I would love nothing more than to get on those baby fucking roller coasters in that moment. Actually, as I look back at them, I am almost contemplating turning around and coming clean on how fucking petrified I actually am. I'm a midget-roller-coaster rider at best; what Bobby is looking for is something far out of my league.

A minute or two later I realize just how far.

We come upon what can only be described as the biggest and most sinister-looking roller coaster I have ever seen in my life, Bizarro. Just as its name insinuates, this ride was an absolute freak of nature. It towers over all the other rides in the park, and looks like a skyscraper among teepees. It has so many ups and downs and twists and turns, and every few seconds you can see and hear the cart carrying its screaming occupants whizzing by.

I start motioning away from this monster, but Bobby, sensing my desertion, immediately begins his reassurance. "It'll be over in a few man. Trust me, you're going to like this. It's such a fucking blast."

"This is the fucking fastest ride in the whole park, dude. Let's do *any* other besides this one." I am pleading now.

"Come on bro, you said we could do just one. Like I said, I won't ask you again the rest of the day if you don't have fun. I promise!"

I think for a moment, but decide this is just too much for me right now. I really could get a heart attack or something if I go through with this. "How about we do that one we saw at the beginning of the day? The one that was like a little smaller than this (it was a lot smaller, but still formidable for me)? That seemed pretty fun."

"Nope, you said you would go on *one*, and this is the one. It's too late too, we're already in line." He motions over to the steel railing protruding from the ground behind us, and the people that have, without my knowledge, filled in the space to where we were just standing moments before.

With all my fear and premonitions the last few minutes of dying a thousand different deaths on this monstrosity, I've had no idea we've actually stepped into line, and even less idea that we've advanced in it. But Bobby does. That sly bastard. I have played right into his hands.

There really is no turning back at this point. I'm caught between a rock and a hard place. I can either hop over multiple guard railings and completely wuss the fuck out, in front of Bobby and the number of ever-growing people in line (especially a few cute girls next to us), or I can suck it up, pretend to not be a pussy, and then blow my cover in about 15 minutes when we're coming off the ride. (Normally, I would choose the former, but I think because of those girls next to us, I choose to stick it out.)

God bless that teenage sex drive.

BEING LED TO THE SLAUGHTER

For the next 10 minutes or so, I'm freaking out inside. I don't show it, as by now I've gotten used to dealing with copious amounts of anxiety and mitigating its effects on me, but internally, I'm terrified.

Superficially, I keep my cool and try to crack a few jokes, but in reality I feel like a man being led to the gas chamber. Each step I take closer to stepping into the coaster car is a moment closer to my demise.

Finally, after the longest 10 minutes of my life, we reach our turn. We step up to be seated, and Bobby naturally requests the front row of this leviathan. *Great*, I think to myself sarcastically. *As if this couldn't get any better.*

I sit next to him, dreadfully awaiting the end of my life. *I've had a good run. Sure, I could've done some more things, could've kissed some more girls, went to some more parties, tried some new adventures . . . but I did alright. It was good while it lasted. And I'll miss it, but it was good.*

"Whoo! Fuck yeah, baby!" The Natural is shouting and waving his hands up and down. "This is going to be fuckin' awesome! We're so fucked!" And he laughs and shouts some more. "Haha. I can't fucking wait, baby! Whoo-yeah!" The Natural continues his frantic yelling, screaming incessantly, and excitedly thrusting his arms into the air.

Finally, with just a moment or so before we are about to take off, I decide I've had enough. "Dude, will you shut the fuck up!?" I proclaim audaciously at him. "We're about to fucking die here, at least stop acting like a fucking fool. Stop yelling and pounding your hands and shit. You're making us look like fucking idiots. Save me some dignity before my death, at least give me that much!"

What Bobby says next is perhaps the most profound declaration I've ever heard up until that point and ever since. And he totally does not mean for it to be. "Dude, this is how you *have to* ride these things. You gotta' put your hands up, and fuckin' yell and scream and get hyped up for this. It's a fucking roller coaster, man. If you sit back and do nothing you're going to hate it. But when you get all pumped up and yell, it's so much fun! Try it."

Now, ordinarily I would have carried on a debate with Bobby about the illogical bullshit he was trying to spew on me: Why putting my hands up, losing control of the only thing I had control of in that moment, was a horrible idea. And why yelling and screaming, and hence wasting my energy and precious last few breaths of my life, was an even worse fucking idea. But for whatever reason I refrain from doing so.

Maybe it was the point in life I was in at that time: The fact I'd been going through a transitional period of self-discovery and exploration; the fact I'd just recently beat my panic attacks and anxiety problems and was looking to master all other weaknesses. Or maybe, it was the fact that the ride started moving and I'd had no time to continue on with conversation.

Instead, I decided to do what he was doing.

STARING DEATH IN THE FACE

At first I felt stupid as the ride crept up the first few hundred feet of its elevation. But I continued on with it. And Bobby was pleased I was copying his actions. "Yeah baby," he yelled. "Keep yellin', brotha! We're fucked, but this is awesome! Whoo-yeah!"

"Fuck it! We're so fucked, bro! This is fucking crazy," I was screaming louder and louder now as the peak inched closer.

"I know! I love it, baby!" The Natural went on. "Fuck all you motherfuckers! Fuck all you bitches!" he yelled from atop the highest point in the park, at no one in particular.

"Fucking pussies!" I added, piggybacking off his crazy antics. "Fuck your mothers and fuck your sisters you little assholes," I got that in once more, just before we made the descent down from the heavens.

And then, we came flying down at an ungodly rate of speed. *Holy shit!* I thought for a second. *This is really happening!*

"Fuck, yeah!" The Natural continued. And I looked over at him quickly, hands up, yelling and screaming like a madman, and laughing too, like an even madder man.

And then I too started laughing. "This is fucking awesome, bro!" I yelled between cackles. "Holy fuck, we're so fucked!"

"I know, I fuckin' love it, bro! Fuck all those pussies! The fuckin' boys are here, baby!" Bobby continued his nonsensical diatribe of pure brute excitement.

"I love it, baby! This is fucking awesome!" I threw my hands in the air, screaming as loud as I could.

Facing My Biggest Fear

And we continued this offensive, coarse, and vulgar behavior for the next two minutes, yelling, screaming, cursing, and laughing in intermittent periods of utter enjoyment.

Then finally, the ride came to its concluding halt.

And with it, my outlook on life would never be the same.

A NEW MAN

I stepped off the ride a new man.

Something incredibly powerful had just occurred and I knew it. Up until that point, riding roller coasters had been one of my biggest real-life fears. As I mentioned before, they were a torment to my existence. But now, using this unbelievably archaic technique borrowed off Bobby, I'd learned how to actually enjoy them.

We got off and my first reaction was, "Let's go back on again!"

Bobby was equal parts shocked and equal parts thrilled at my announcement. "Fuck yeah!" he said. "I knew you'd have fun, bro. Let's hurry up and cut those people off before the line fills up." He motioned for us to head back over to the start of the line.

And so we waited a few more minutes, and did it all over again. And then when we got off, we went to every other roller coaster in the place and rode them too. Actually, by the end of the day, we'd ridden every roller coaster in the park at least five or six times, making sure to ride the better ones a couple times extra over the others.

It was truly a remarkable day, one I will never forget.

I'd not only learned how to ride roller coasters, but how to face my fears down head on. It didn't dawn on me until a little while later, but what I was actually doing when putting my hands up, yelling, screaming, swearing, and acting like a complete jackass, was the same concept I'd used to beat my panic attacks.

It was the exact same technique, just applied in a different manner.

Exposure Therapy

Almost 100 years ago (1924), Mary Cover Jones, "The Mother of Behavioral Therapy," demonstrated that by progressively exposing a three-year-old boy with a terrible fear of rabbits, to the rabbits themselves, she was slowly able to get him to overcome his fear.[1] She did this by training him to challenge himself more and more, and condition his emotions to get used to the fact that the fear of being around rabbits was irrational. This seminal work laid the framework for further innovative behavioral therapy in the years to come.

In particular, Cover Jones' experiment on the leporiphobic boy set the precedent for treatments like exposure therapy, which can be very effective for overcoming fears and mental traumas like PTSD.[2] In exposure therapy patients are assisted with confronting their fears head on, albeit in a safe and controlled environment. By doing so, they're able to change the ways they view and experience their fears, and thus get over them.

Recently, a research team led by Dr. Johannes Gräff, was able to identify, with never-before-seen clarity, the brain's neuronal activity at work during a fear-inducing moment. By studying the neurons of mice, Gräff and company were able to see neurons coming together and forming what they call engrams, small clusters of connected neurons. They believe these engrams are the actual physical representation of our memories.

The scientists concluded that when people remember things, these engramatic neurons fire together, and the more they do so, their connections become more solidified. But they also noted that during this process of bringing together these neural molecules, also called reconsolidation, there exists a purgatorial window where change can occur. And this is where it gets interesting.

> Gräff's team found that by studying the mice's fear response, they could not only pinpoint the engrams being formed, but also, by using the technique of exposure therapy, they could actually condition the mice to overcome their fears, and clearly see the new engrams being created when they did so.[3]
>
> They also noted that when they tried to condition the mice to get over their fears without accurately using the exposure therapy technique, they had virtually no success. But when they used this emotional approach, it was remarkably effective.
>
> In short, by facing your fears, you can literally rewire your brain into overcoming anything. These trailblazing rodents have shown the way.

A NEW POWER

You see, when I'd historically cowered down in my seat while on any roller coaster before that day, I was giving into the fears and allowing them to have power over me. I was quiet, reserved, and timid, and trying to avoid the fear of riding on the coaster, even though you literally can't escape it.

Essentially, I was handing over all my power and giving the roller coaster the keys to my emotions. Basically saying, "Hey Bully, kick my ass real quick, and oh yeah, make me throw up all over myself midway through. That's my favorite part."

And like clockwork, by trying to avoid the fear, I only got more of it.

But by using Bobby's little tactic, I took back control by facing it head on and going with it, as opposed to being scared and attempting to block it. For the first time in my life, I figured out the secret to defeating any fear that pops up in your life. And that's this: To get over your fears, you have to embrace them fully. When you do this, they no longer become your enemy but your ally.

All fears will go away when you face them head on. They have no choice but to because your mind is the only instrument that dictates your emotions. If you tell your mind to be afraid, you will be. If you tell it to embrace something and call it out, it will too. But actions are necessary here. It's important to take action into facing your fears, so your mind can truly process your new belief of embracing them.

Without action, you're just making a hopeful affirmation, and this rarely helps. But a powerful action combined with a powerful assertion completes the equation and leads to magic every single time.

The roller coaster of life will always have its ups and downs, twist and turns, and fears and anxieties lurking just around the corner. You have two options: You can either curl up, feel like shit, and hope for the ride to end as quickly as possible, like I did for many years. Or you can embrace the chaos, face the fears, and enjoy the excitement of it all. To me the choice is obvious, and it's become a way of life for me every day.

Thanks Bobby, I love you, ya' fucking prick.

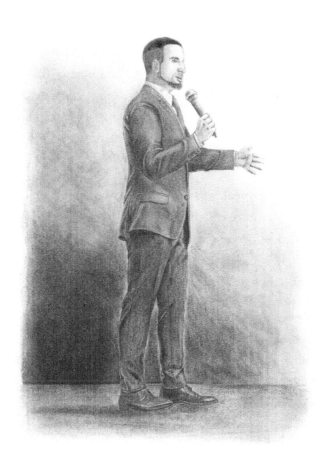

Chapter Sixteen
Taming the Beast

I can hear the voice of the guy on stage, but I'm not listening to a word he's saying. He's really just a blur, noise in the background. I'm pacing confidently around the outside walkway of the audience, my movements an expression of the excitement inside. I'm nervous, but I don't let on or give in; instead I go with, as I learned long ago.

"And now, we have my friend who came all the way down from Boston, Massachusetts to deliver this incredible speech on how to quickly gain confidence in your life. The Elite Man himself . . . Gentlemen, and ladies, please give a warm round of applause welcome to Justinnnn Stenstrommmm!" The host of this 300+ men's conference enthusiastically boomed his introduction to the cheering crowd of business men (and a few women). The audience clapped with excitement and my butterflies did a few backflips as I approached.

I'd been invited to speak at one of the largest men's conferences in the world. A conference called StyleCon, which featured many of the top men's business professionals in the world. It wasn't my first time speaking, but it was one of the bigger audiences I'd spoken to up until that point. So naturally, the nerves were fired up.

As I walked on stage and took the mic from the conference organizer, however, I stepped back into the moment and focused my attention on performing what I'd traveled over 1,000 miles to do. This was no time to get caught up dwelling on the fears surrounding anything but delivering a knockout speech.

I'd been practicing my speech for the past few days, and I'd presented it before to many other crowds. I knew it like the back of my hand, and I knew it was good. Just as I turned to face the audience, I filled my mind with one more thought, *My speech is really fucking good and these people are going to love it.*

And with this, I was ready.

After that quick little reset, I was able to tame the beast and end up delivering an epic fucking speech. By the time I was finished the whole room was lit up with energy and they thanked me in the form of thrilling applause.

Witnessing a sea full of cheering people, loving what you've just given them, is one of the coolest feelings in the world. I can only imagine what rock stars feel like after a concert. Although not on the same level, speaking to an audience has many parallels, and the feeling you get is truly special. It's also unique in the sense that, had you not created the speech through brainstorming, preparation, and crafting your ideas together, this moment would've never happened.

Just like when you write a book or a blog post, or make a viral video or own a successful business. All of these examples are the brainchild of your exceptional ability to craft and shape your imaginative mind into constructing something tangible, something real. And when others recognize this and give you appreciative feedback on something you've given your time, energy, and focus to, the feeling is, quite simply, *amazing*.

But anyway, the badassery of this particular speech would not have been possible without the countless years of prep work done beforehand. You see, this event took place just a couple years ago, in early 2017, many, many years after the conquering of my panic attacks and anxiety. The confidence I'd built up over the years (don't worry, grasshopper, we'll be covering all of this later in the book) allowed me to get on stage and perform at my best in front of a shit-ton of people. But the key strategy I used—the last one I want to mention when it comes to mastering your anxiety—is how to shift your perspective on it.

SHIFTING YOUR PERSPECTIVE

The truth of the matter is, you will always have some kind of anxiety for the rest of your life. This isn't an admission of failure or a surrendering of your power over it, but actually the opposite. Anxiety, in the right dosage, can actually be a good thing. There's a time and a place for everything. And there's a time and place for anxiety. A bear jumping out in front of you whilst jogging at the park? Yeah, good place to get a surge of anxiety, or else you can consider yourself bear fucking bites.

Furthermore, going up on stage, believe it or not, is also a good place to get a rush of anxiety. That's right, just think about it for a sec. Would you rather have slight nerves flowing through your veins before you go on stage, or would you rather have the same amount of blood boiling through your body as you do when you're having tea and crumpets with grandma? I think we both know you'd prefer the nerves option. Grandma's great and everything, but typically our energy isn't exceedingly high when we're lounging back sipping tea and listening to her reminisce about the glory days.

No, without those moderately sprinkled nerves of stimulation coursing around inside us, we wouldn't be able to get excited for the speech. We'd be flat, we'd be boring, and we'd be fucking talking about nursing homes and canes. (Well, maybe not, but you get the point.) Anxiety, in a situation like stepping on stage in front of a massive crowd of people, is actually a great fucking tool. You need it to light a fire under your ass and get the crowd excited. And it does this job fantastically.

What you want is not to eliminate anxiety, but to get it under control, and to use it to your advantage. Just like when riding roller coasters or demolishing panic attacks, work with the anxiety and move toward it, not away from it.

It's really just a shift in perspective here. By recognizing that the anxiety holds a solid purpose[1] this alone can start to engrain in you the need to work alongside it. It may take some time to master this of course. But when you do, you can do just about anything you want.

Nine times out of ten the only thing holding you back from success is your fear of failing to achieve it. Getting past this fear and actually using it to your advantage is often what separates the wildly successful from the astonishingly mediocre.

APPLYING THIS NEW PERSPECTIVE

This concept of shifting perspective and using your fears to your advantage can be applied to just about anything: going on a date with a beautiful woman; leading a business meeting; or maybe taking an important test of some sort.

For a date, the anxiety forces you to put your best foot forward. It forces you to pick out a great outfit, iron your clothes, shower up, wear your best cologne, hit the gym the week leading up to it (and hopefully continuing to go thereafter), wash your car, show up on time, and bring your most charming and attractive personality. (Assuming you're really into the girl, that is.)

If you are, you'll definitely do these types of things. If you aren't into her, you could not care less, and wouldn't put in the effort to be at your best (in which case, you should stop wasting your time and find someone who does light a fire under your ass!). But the fact that you invest all this time into showcasing yourself means there's some bit of anxiety there to make it happen. This anxiety is your driving force, and is most certainly on your side here.

The same thing goes for a business meeting. If you're not worried about being at your best, and have *zero* anxiety surrounding a very important conference with your company's top-dog execs, you're not going to do well there. You probably won't care how you look, you'll most likely show up late, and you certainly won't be the least bit fucking charming. You might even get your sorry ass fired, because you'll demonstrate how little you care.

However, if you do all things right, and take the time to be at your best, you're going to shine. The bosses will love you, and you'll be closer to that raise and promotion you covet. Anxiety of course being the true catalyst for your splendor. Once again, you can thank that anxiety for compelling you to greatness.

Say it with me now: "Thank you, anxiety, you're a real friend!"

And just to complete the trifecta, for the example of taking a test, it should be obvious by now, but having anxiety for something like a big test, although it stresses the hell out of us sometimes, is an ally and a key component to our success. The anxiety of failing or not getting a great score keeps us up late at night, studying our balls off. It makes us put in the extra time and energy needed to really learn that which needs to be learned. And it gives us that added drive to stay dedicated to comprehending even more.

Without anxiety we'd get lazy, procrastinate, and spend a significant portion of our precious time dicking around on Snapchat or watching reruns of *Family Guy*. But because of our fears of failing in our goals, we're driven by this anxiety to work hard and stay committed. And by doing so, we're able to succeed. (Again, you can thank that pesky son-of-a-bitch called anxiety; just don't let him take over like before.)

There's a balance here as you can see. Too much anxiety and our minds become overthrown. Too little, we become lazy and flat. Don't think of anxiety as the enemy, think of it as an ally (or a tool) you use to your advantage from time to time.[2]

With this changing outlook on anxiety you can really begin to implement it favorably in your life: more excitement, more energy, more dedication, more commitment, more determination, more passion ... anxiety, when used correctly, can offer you all of this and more. Just remember, you hold the power over it. You're the boss.

Tame the beast and the world is your oyster.

PART III
Depression

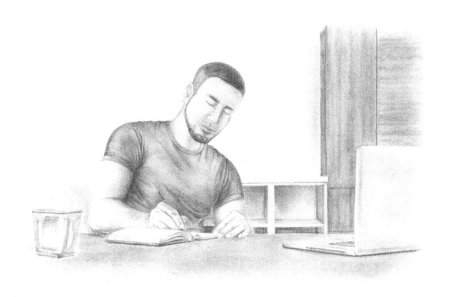

Chapter Seventeen
Cultivating Gratitude

As I sat on the couch, replaying the many ways I could end my life, I grew more and more depressed. I had nothing going for me: no friends, no girlfriends, no direction, and no fucking purpose. Every day was like the one before it, meaningless and boring. *I could jump off the Bourne Bridge, that might not be so terrible.* I thought. *It's only like 20 minutes from here. All I'd have to do is drive down there and walk off the side. Seems pretty easy . . .*

Sons of Anarchy was playing in the background. My dad and I watched it regularly and, it being a new show at the time, I thought it was pretty cool. But on this day I wasn't paying attention at all. It was probably a good episode, but I couldn't recall a second of it. My thoughts were entirely consumed in my self-desired extinction. *Maybe I can just take all of those pills in the medicine cabinet*, I pondered.

There's gotta' be dozens of different bottles and I think those anxiety ones are still in there. If I take the whole thing at once, that would probably work too . . . I don't know, so many options . . . Fuck! I nearly blurted aloud. *What the fuck am I doing? I can't keep thinking about this stuff, this is nuts! I have to knock this shit off or I'm really going to end up dead. I can't wait around anymore and do nothing. No, I've gotta' figure this out now!*

I stood up and stormed out of the room, determined to find an answer.

MY PROGRESSION

I'd like to say I'd been working diligently on my anxiety and depressive issues at the time of this suicidal moment in question. But the truth is I actually hadn't been. I'd tried a few things for my anxiety, but hadn't really gotten better at managing it, and the panic attacks were still popping up regularly and whoopping my ass.

Needless to say, I'd done little to quell the depression, either. But that day on the couch, I knew it was something I could take lightly no longer. If I did, I probably wouldn't live long enough to see my next birthday.

As I mentioned before, my initial focus after storming off the couch was to figure out how to stop my panic attacks and drastically reduce my anxiety. Having an inclination that these offenders were feeding my desire to not want to live, they seemed like the perfect culprits to go after.

Don't get me wrong, it's not like I accurately formulated this extravagant plan and came up with a Pattonesque strategy for success. I didn't say to myself, *I'll focus on anxiety and panic for 90 days, and then shift my attention to the depression issue, whereupon my concentration will be primarily directed on alleviating the feelings of despair for 90 additional days. And I will use this tactic, this tactic, and this tactic, to effectively enact change in my life.*

No, it was more like: *Let me really focus on reducing the panic and anxiety at first, but also, let me slowly chip away at the depression, both directly, and indirectly* (as a result of lowering my anxiety, and from the carryover of many of the anxiety-fighting strategies).

In fact, even if I'd wanted to construct a flawless game-plan to divvy up the attack, the bond between the anxiety and depression siblings is far too strong to ignore one while battling the other.

So it certainly wasn't 90 days until I took up arms against depression. If I had to guess, though, it was probably a few weeks into my tussle with anxiety before I really began diving into some specific tactics for conquering my depression. And once more, although anxiety was the star in the beginning of my re-awakened quest, as I got better with it over time, depression took front and center stage and warranted more of my attention. Anxiety and panic's fight was won sooner; depression would last a while longer. But in the end, they'd both fall to the elite mind I was cultivating.

PRESENCE

It was around this time that I discovered the whole *Power of Now* concept I mentioned before, pioneered by the enlightened hobgoblin/saint, Eckhart Tolle. Living in the present moment is incredibly helpful for both anxiety and depression. Like many strategies in this book, it benefits an array of conditions. And it just so happened to be one of the first things I found while seeking an escape from my depression.

It worked incredibly. I started focusing myself in the moment, as opposed to dwelling on all the things I hated about myself or things that hadn't gone my way over the last few years. It was sort of a way to erase and reframe the bad shit that had happened, without actually having to expunge any of it.

I just focused on the negative things less and less. And it kept me grounded. It kept the pessimistic thoughts from shaping into harmful feelings, i.e. suicidal depression. Living in the now is a truly powerful concept, and though it may take some time to fully grasp, it can be a complete life-changer when you do.

Along with focusing on what's in front of you (hence not focusing on the negativity of your past, which only brings depression), you can even add to this, and focus on positive things. By doing so, you implement the practice of gratitude, which is an essential tool for conjuring feelings of happiness and content.

THE GRASS IS ALWAYS GREENER

Everyone has the belief that the grass is always greener on the other side of the fence, that other people have things easier and that their life is so much better than ours—especially in this social media age we currently live in. If things were bad a few decades ago, they've gotten infinitely worse with the advent of social media (what I call "vanity media").

We're all guilty of constantly checking our vain social metrics: *How many likes did my Facebook post get? How many hearts did my Instagram selfie get? How many people viewed my Snapchat video?*

These questions and many others run through our minds daily, conditioning us to want to display more and more of how fucking incredible our lives are and how fucking cool we are for having them. We see all of our friends, or people we look up to getting hearts and likes and views, and we think we need to get them too. It's a constant battle for social supremacy and recognition on our profiles. We want to fit in with our friends. We want to seem hip. We want to appear attractive to the opposite sex and show them how awesome it would be to date us.

But when does it stop?

Post a picture and check it every five minutes for the next two hours, getting a slight boost of dopamine with every artificial "like" you receive. Then feel disappointed when six hours later you didn't get as many likes as you wanted, and that girl you thought was really cute didn't give you that like you so desperately craved from her.

Fuck, it never ends.

Not to mention those "friends" of yours and those celebrities you follow all seem to live the most epic and badass lives imaginable: Fancy cars; nice watches; boatloads of money; beautiful women; great clothes; funny statuses; gorgeous scenery; tall, jacked, muscled, handsome, perfect . . . yup, better-than-you, in-every-possible-way. With every post you see comes another reiterating fact that their life shits on yours. You feel like the guy who's left out in the cold while everyone else is inside partying. It's always winter in your world.

You simply can't win.

Or can you?

HOW TO WIN

As much as it may be hard to cease focusing on other people and how great it seems their lives are, you must. It's important to understand how life really is. And how it really is for *everyone*.

So many people hide behind the mask of social media pretending they have everything going for them. It's so easy to post pictures or videos and sugarcoat (or Photoshop) your ideal reality. But the truth is, most people are unhappy. And typically, those who seem to have everything going for them on their social media platforms? They're often the saddest of all.

In fact, the more perfect, done-up, and complete the posts of those you idealize, the greater the chances of their discontent. Narcissists, for example, tend to persistently post attention-seeking pics of themselves.[1] Whether it's to show off their sculpted arms, thin waists, big butts, six-pack abs, or pretty faces, their continuous yearning for approval is actually a reflection of their unhappiness. One recent study demonstrated a strong correlation between those who frequently post selfies and those who have body dysmorphic disorder, a mental condition where individuals obsessively focus on a perceived flaw in their own appearance.[2]

Sounds crazy that people who are insecure with how they look would want to display more of themselves to the world. But it actually makes sense. These people need constant reassurance in the form of likes, comments, and views, to tell them they're okay and to placate their anxieties about their own bodies. It's a useful coping mechanism, and one that can be employed at any moment.

But it's not just body dysmorphics and narcissists, and it's not just you who's unhappy with how you look or how your life really is. It's just about everyone. With the regular distorted feedback we're receiving on how inferior we are compared to others, it's becoming increasingly challenging to not feel down about ourselves.

To buck this trend and break out of this vicious cycle, it's important to recognize the insecurities that so many others face, and the unrealistic posts and pictures that don't accurately depict their reality. Cropped images, filters, retouching, a hundred shots of the same picture, many crafted takes and re-takes, it all adds up to the façade of flawlessness. But don't let it fool you, it's still just a fucking façade.

Everybody walks around with a mask on, molded to the way they want the world to perceive them. Whether that's on social media or whether that's in person. It doesn't matter. The grass is not always greener, people just like to pretend it is, and in turn trick others into buying their bullshit. Don't buy what they're selling; understand it, and live your own life. It's the only way of breaking this cycle.

BEING GRATEFUL FOR WHAT YOU HAVE

Along with stopping the cycle of wanting to compare yourself to others all the time, it's important to get in the routine of practicing gratitude. It's essentially the opposite of vanity and narcissism, and practicing it is like taking your clothes off before hopping into the shower. When you apply gratitude, you strip what's truly important down to the bare bones, and leave all the other bullshit behind. Instead of consciously dwelling on ego-driven forces, you intentionally reflect on meaningful facets.

The easiest way to start practicing gratitude is to simply think about all the good you have in your life throughout the day. Our thoughts are the catalyst for our emotions, and by having positive thoughts continually, as the day goes on, you drive home the desire for positive output.

It's important too because for most people upwards of 70%[3] of their thoughts are negative during the day (for depressed individuals this can easily exceed 90%). We're constantly bombarded with negative stimuli, so it's no wonder we feel like shit all the time. Our go-to unfortunately, is to be negative.

Knowing this, taking small breaks throughout your day to be positive for a few minutes can make a big difference. Even if you're changing just a few percentage points on that negativity scale, this can be huge.

Moreover, here's a few good strategies to help you implement more gratitude in your life and boost the positivity points instead.

TELL YOURSELF YOU'RE GRATEFUL

To be grateful, tell yourself you're grateful. I know it may sound a little lame and a little too simple, but it works. Start with something like, "I am grateful for _____." (And say this aloud.)

Then repeat it, but choose something else you are grateful for as well. And continue to go down the line, calling one thing after the other, until you run out of things to think of. This may take a minute or a few minutes, but by the end of the exercise you'll literally feel better about yourself. Your mind will be dwelling on the positive aspects of your life as opposed to the standard fuckery it marinates in about 90% of the time.

Some things I can remember being grateful for, even in my darkest times of depression, have included things like my mother, my father, my grandmother, my siblings, my little nephew who was just born, my dog, my physical health, my intellect, my determination, the house I grew up in, the fact we had heat, the fact we had electricity, my car, the food I had every night to eat, the laptop I used to search for cures to my problems, and a bunch of other essentials I hold near and dear though have often overlooked if I didn't make a point to do so.

As you can see, it can be anything and everything. It doesn't have to follow any order or adhere to any rules; just call out loud the things you're thankful for having. And trust me, if you have your hands on this book, there's plenty to be thankful for. (Not just because this book is so incredibly phenomenal and life-changing, although who in their right mind could argue against that? But also because, if you're reading this, the chances are you probably live in a developed country, and it's certainly past the year 2018, so even if you're not, you still have it better than the billions of people born before you historically. Even the poorest fuckers in the world live better than most kings did just a few hundred years back.)

There's always thanks to be had.

Any time I've started to feel a little down about my life, I immediately begin thinking about everything I'm blessed with. And rather than continuing to feel like shit, I start to feel better, knowing that I truly am blessed in life.

Mark Twain famously once said, "When you find yourself on the side of the majority it's time to pause and reflect." Thanks Marky, I agree. And I'll add to your assertion now by affirming something equally wise, "When you find yourself on the side of the negative, it's time to pause and reflect gratitude."

JOURNAL YOUR GRATITUDE

Instead of audibly pronouncing your blessings in life, you can write them down. This may be easier for some, and also, more helpful to others. Also, it can be done as an addition to the verbal exercise, not solely as a replacement.

I love journaling. Whether it's writing out my grand plans, reflecting on the day's events, brainstorming random shit, or counting my blessings, like I recommend here. It's powerful and effective for getting you to consider things in a different manner. It's almost like utilizing a second brain because you're better able to map out your thoughts and piece information together perceptibly. Oftentimes alone, you're unable to do this.

My journals are a fucking mess. They're almost thief-proof because my handwriting is award-winningly awful and because I'm all over the place with my thoughts. A scribbled plan here, a brilliant theory there, a cross-out of a shitty concept nearby, and tons of random ideas inundated throughout. It's a smorgasbord of the illogical and the genius and that's what makes it beautiful.

And effective.

Journaling is something I recommend whether you're depressed or not, but especially if you're depressed. Use it as a way to focus on all the good you have in your life. You can literally use the same set up as you did for the exercise above, acknowledging your gratitude aloud. But feel free to add in some additional things, make it messy, and deep-dive into areas that arouse more interest.

So for instance you could start with writing, "I am grateful for _____." And of course go right down the line and list one thing after the other in succession. This is helpful, and naturally, I highly recommend you do this. But you could also switch it up and maybe list just one or two things, and then really dive into what it is about these things that you really love.

You could be grateful for your dog, and talk about how the dog makes you feel, how much you love his companionship, how beautiful he is, how much fun it is taking the dog for walks and playing with him, how much you love lying down on your couch with him . . . Really, anything that comes up surrounding your joy in having the pup. Or, if you hate dogs (you're probably a cat weirdo), you can choose some other domesticated animal of your fancy, or something else entirely different you're thankful for, unrelated. This is just one of the many examples that abound.

The Man and the Squirrel

On a completely off-topic and outlandishly fascinating side note, I recently met a young man, in person, who harbored a squirrel as a pet. Yes, a

> squirrel, as in the little tree-dwelling rodents that so famously munch on acorns the way fat kids devour Twinkies. This particular tame squirrel was in the man's hand for the duration of my encounter with him, which was well over an hour.
>
> I could comment on the psychological bond the man must possess with such a rare, undomesticated creature like this squirrel, and go on about how close they must be despite the animal's instinctively feral nature, noting its apparent docile temperament that extended throughout our entire interaction. And I could continue still about the love that expands past environment and knows no bounds, and ultimately the beauty of how friendship can be shared between two such contrasting species, and what this could mean for the hope of all humankind, and all life for that matter. But I won't. Instead I'll keep my assessment of the squirrel and the young man brief.
>
> Here it is: Squirrel boy was a fucking wacko. Infinitely weirder than any cat weirdo I've ever come across. His personality was beyond strange, he smelled as if he hadn't taken a bath in years, and he housed fewer teeth in his mouth than the old lady from the supplement shack years back, setting the dubious new record for least amount of molars in one mouth I've ever seen.
>
> And the squirrel? The wild varmint was repulsive and sickeningly malnourished. If there existed a heroin epidemic in the squirrel community comparable to that in the human world at the moment, this distinguishable critter would be the poster child for laying off drugs.
>
> But I digress. Very much so indeed. Let's get back on topic.

The point is to think of something you're grateful for and bring that to the forefront of your mind. It's a great technique for getting you to focus on what you have and what you're blessed with, as opposed to having those pesky negative thoughts take over and dictate your day.

I recommend journaling once a day, maybe right before bed, as a way to initiate this good habit. Start by journaling all that you're grateful for, then dive deeper into each, and subsequently allow yourself to focus on these things more and more throughout your days. You'll soon discover the ratio of positive to negative thoughts balancing out and your mood improving.

LEAVE OTHERS BETTER THAN YOU FOUND THEM

A simple practice to implement gratitude into your life is to assume the mindset of always trying to leave people and situations better than you found them. This doesn't mean you have to walk around like Ned Flanders from *The Simpsons* and constantly get walked all over by everyone you come across because you turn yourself into an ass-kissing do-gooder. No, don't act that way at all, it's cringeworthy. But rather, have a positive outlook on life and try (your best) to make those you come across in life a little happier.

You, just like me, know how shitty life can be. If you're reading this book, chances are you've faced some really bad anxiety or depression problems and can relate to the struggle of being miserable all the time. It sucks, and we both know it. With that in mind, do society, and more importantly *yourself* a favor, and be a positive energy in this world. With so much drama, and hate, and division constantly flooding our communities, be one of the few who cheers others up.

Lead with this attitude first, but you don't have to marry it. If someone is blatantly rude or rejecting of your kindness, it's okay to move on from them without wasting your time. You don't have to be Superman and attempt to save every soul you come across; leave that for Clark Kent. If someone's an asshole, let them be and carry on unaffected.

Nevertheless, implementing this attitude is as simple as walking into different environments with the belief that your presence is a gift. Your goal is to elevate the mood of people around you or to improve a negative situation into a positive one.

So throughout the day this may mean saying "Hi" to your mail lady and chatting her up about her day. It may mean bringing up an upbeat topic to chat about with your co-workers. It could also mean complimenting an old woman sitting next to you on the bus. Or it could mean sincerely thanking and maybe even offering to write an exceptional review for the barista who did well handling your order at *Starbucks*—even if she's not cute and you don't want her number. Lastly, it could mean helping family members or friends with problems they're having trouble figuring out. The possibilities are quite literally endless.

The point of this exercise is to adopt the new belief that you have something to offer other people and it's your job, no, your *duty*, to leave these people better off than you found them. By having this mindset of giving and improving, your gratitude, and your life for that matter, will improve radically.

COMPLIMENT OTHERS

There's something truly special about putting a smile on another person's face. It's rather magical in a sense. They're happy, hence the displaying of their pearly whites. And you're happy, because you made them smile, and are granted the same gift in return.

Smiling is contagious, as they say.[4] As well as laughter, and just about every other emotion humans have. When we see others doing something we naturally want to mimic that emotion in an attempt to build rapport. "We've known for some time that when we are talking to someone, we often mirror their behavior, copying the words they use and mimicking their gestures," says Sophie Scott, a neuroscientist at the University College London.[5]

So why not make them smile? Why not add to their day and in return your own? Make them smile and you'll actually really be making yourself smile. It's selfishly helping others. Which is probably one of the few areas in life where it's good to be self-absorbed.

Personally, I love complimenting people all day long. I suppose I'm very selfish in this regard. It makes me feel fucking fantastic when I offer up a genuine, well-placed compliment to someone and I can tell immediately I've just made their day.

I'm impartial to whom I'll compliment too. Now, it's probably more often than not a woman I'll make smile, but trust me, I throw a lot of dudes compliments as well. In a typical day, I may tell a woman I know and come across that her new hairstyle looks really great. Then I may tell another lady that her eyes are really pretty. Then I might bump into a male friend and tell him his shirt looks fucking great on him. And if I see another guy, I might tell him he's looking jacked and the new workout program he's on is crushing it. And if I bump into an older lady walking her dog down the street I'll almost always tell her what a beautiful pup she has and ask her if it's okay to pat it. And, if granny's been hitting the gym doing her squats and she's in fantastic shape I may even tell her what a nice a . . . just kidding, that I will not do.

The objective here is that you sincerely notice things in people you come across and that you express back to them the good you see. Whether it's a physical attribute, a personality trait, something they own, or anything else that catches your eye, tell them and let them know you admire whatever it is they possess. This concurrently makes them happy and brings joy into your own life as well. It's a glorious win for all.

SEEING THE GOOD IN OTHERS

Sometimes it can be hard leaving others better than you found them and it can be really tough trying to find a way to genuinely compliment someone. And, like I mentioned before, sometimes you

Cultivating Gratitude

gotta' say, "Fuck it, I tried." And move on. However, before you give in and swear off this hypothetical person for life, try to see the little good they have left.

I get it, some people are complete assholes and seem like they were raised by a pack of blood-thirsty wolves. They'll act inappropriately, obnoxiously, rudely, and in every other offensive manner you can think of. But here me out, *it may not be their fault*.

Actually, it's almost certainly not their fault. People, adults, don't choose to be assholes. We'd much rather fit into society (most of us anyway) than be condemned by it. Just like in the study mentioned before about smiling being contagious and people mirroring each other to fit in, it's a way for people to connect and it's a survival mechanism passed down from our ancient ancestors who had to get along and help each other out in their small tribes and communities in order to survive.[6]

We're actually wired to connect with others.

So when you see some dickhead actin' the fool—pity the fool, as Mr. T would counsel. Give him a break, at least at first. He was either raised in a broken home and developed maladaptive traits for early childhood survival (the most likely of all scenarios), has health or mental conditions that have gone untreated, or is simply ignorantly unaware of the customary etiquette of your particular geographic location (rare, but possible).

Either way, give the guy a chance.

Try to see through his detestable behavior with a glass-half-full lens. Find whatever redeeming quality he may possess and ruminate on that. You may be surprised at, upon realizing that most people have issues and aren't choosing to be blatant fartknockers in society, you're actually becoming more forgiving of things that might ordinarily drive you up the wall. And with this open mind and open heart, you're able to see the good in what they have to offer.

Maybe it's a homeless man on the street who usually boils your blood every time he comes up to your car at a particular intersection. Or maybe it's a loud and irritating subway passenger who loves rapping out loud for the rest of the train's occupants to enjoy (or more accurately, hate). Or perhaps it's the bitch-faced cashier who never says anything except, "That'll be ten bucks," in an I-hate-my-life-and-you voice every time she rings you up.

Just *try* to see some good here.

I'm not saying you have to give the smelly bum a five dollar bill every time he comes around. I'm certainly not saying you have to enjoy the musical ineptitude of Grandmaster Suckass. And I'm certainly not advocating you become best friends with the Kathy-Bates-looking cashier.

But give them a break. Try looking at them in a slightly different light. Again, not just for their benefit, but really for your own.

Maybe you offer the poor man the other half of your sub that went untouched, and that you were probably going to throw out anyway. Maybe you view The Grandmaster as someone who actually provides entertainment every day, albeit circuitously, and you can appreciate the fact that he's *so bad*, he's actually good (he makes you laugh, goddammit, and that's just as good). And maybe next time, instead of playing into Mrs. Bates' shitty attitude and giving her that mean mug you so frequently go to, you smile at her, and ask her how her day's going. (You don't need to sleep with her, or any of the others for that matter, but try putting a spin on the negative emotions they've previously instilled in you.)

You more than likely can make their day better, while also making your own that much better too. And that's the key here. Selfish gratitude, the gift that keeps on giving.

HELPING OTHERS

Perhaps the epitome of selfish gratitude is helping others out, which is why I want to elaborate on this particular gratitude exercise. Whether that's volunteering your time at a charity, helping with children at a school or old folks in a nursing home, or working with veterans, animals, homeless people, shelters, hospitals, churches, disaster relief, or any other persons in need. It doesn't matter what you choose, but choosing something where you can help others is one of the best ways to help yourself.

Numerous studies show that those who volunteer to help out others are much happier and have better mental and physical health[7] than those who do not. It's that contagious good-will quality again. When we know we're making a positive impact in other people, we get a sense of fulfillment and feel those positive emotions returned back to us. There's something to be said about the power of offering our services and time to help those who truly need it.

If you are able to, I recommend volunteering for something in your community. Help others out and you'll help yourself out. Trust me, it's one of the best feelings in the world when you can make a direct impact on someone else's life.

TAKING EACH MOMENT AS A LEARNING EXPERIENCE

No matter how bad a situation may suck, or perceivably suck, there's always a silver lining to be found. Every dark cloud holds a possibility for growth. It's a fact. When you realize this, you can begin to look more favorably at negative experiences.

A person who annoys you every day. A job firing. A break-up. A loss of a loved one. They all have their silver-linings. They all come with a lesson to be learned and an opportunity for growth.

Now hear me out here, I'm not saying that every one of these things doesn't come with some level of pain. Trust me, it does. Especially the loss of a loved one. But what I am saying is, no matter how shitty the situation may be, there's always an opportunity to mature from it.

The purpose of our entire existence, in my humble opinion, is to learn and grow as human beings. Whether you believe in God, Allah, Buddha, aliens, science fiction writers, or nothing at all, our purpose in this world is to experience life at its fullest and become the best individuals we can be, leaving this world a little better than we found it and becoming a better person in the process.

We're all going to die one day. It's just the way it works. You'll be dead. I'll be dead. Your wife will be dead. Your father, your mother, your brothers and sisters, your children, your pets, everyone and everything you love will be gone. As George Harrison famously sang, "All things must pass."

It's not a somber sentiment but actually a joyous one. Life is perfect in that we all have an expiration date. If we didn't, nothing would have meaning. It's like playing chess against a baby. It's no fun when you don't have to even try or there's no challenge. You don't get excited and you know the outcome before you even begin. Life's the same way. It becomes boring when everything is guaranteed.

When it comes to situations or times in your life that suck or cause you true pain, look at them as a part of the overall journey. For someone that you lost, in particular, appreciate all the memories you had with them and be thankful for all the time you got to spend with that person. Again, we all have to go at some point, and just because someone leaves a little earlier than you thought, it doesn't change the wonderful moments you got to share with them. And, if you believe in an afterlife (I happen to believe there's something beyond what we see now), rejoice in the fact you get to see that person again, you just have to wait a little while.

For smaller, more common instances, like say getting stuck in traffic, or getting annoyed by the same person daily, or your power going out in your home, or you spilling milk all over the floor, yes, it's okay to get upset or even pissed-the-fuck-off for a moment, but after giving yourself a minute or two of feeling this pain, look for the good in it.

The traffic can allow you time to listen to your favorite songs a little longer. The annoying person in your life can afford you the virtue of mastering your patience. The power going out in your house can allow you a chance to read that book you've been holding off on reading and that's been collecting dust for six months. Spilling milk all over the floor can present you with the chance to have a new breakfast that doesn't involve lactose and that may be a much healthier option.

No matter what it is, there can be some immediate good to take out of any situation. And there's always some long-term good and some lesson to be learned from all of life's experiences. We grow from everything we experience. What doesn't kill you really does make you stronger. It's not just some stupid Kelly Clarkson mantra.

GRATITUDE IN A NUTSHELL

With all of the gratitude exercises the goal is to recognize how much you have going for yourself and how much you have to offer the world. It sounds cliché but you have so much to fucking offer and you were put on this Earth for a reason. We all were. I truly believe that with every fiber of my being. It's not just some hoorah, woo-woo crap that you might hear some online charlatans spouting with their motivational posts and videos. It's true. You are unique and you are special. Give yourself some fucking credit. You deserve it.

It took me a long, long time to give myself credit too, but when I did, my whole life changed. Start being grateful and start helping others out more and you'll begin to see just what I mean here. Gratitude is a powerful tool. Use it often and use it wisely.

It's a great first step in beating your depression. This next step though, might be my favorite.

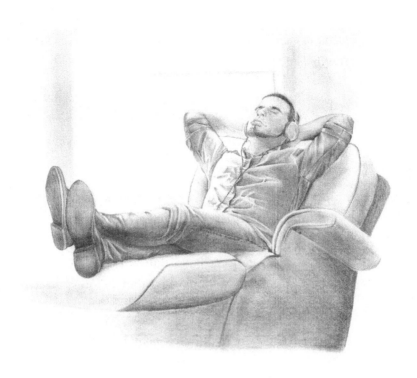

Chapter Eighteen
Hypnotizing Your Depression

"You're getting sleepy . . ."

"Follow my watch back and forth, back and forth."

"Get sleepier and sleepier with each swing left and each swing right."

The crazy, old hippie-looking man whispers these directions to you in a soothingly quiet, yet creepy manner as he swings his ancient pendulum back and forth, left and right.

He uses his allegorical magic to whisk you into hypnosis and take over your mind, doing with you whatever he pleases. Maybe he'll decide to have you kill on command or maybe he'll order you to rob a bank under his control and give the entire loot to him and him only.

Whatever he chooses, you'll have no say, because you're hypnotized, and hypnosis is the one sure way to take over someone's life and make them do whatever you want. It's like having a voodoo doll, only with more power and potential.

This is what most people think of when they think of hypnosis. They conjure up the image of an eccentric, wizard-like dotard who has mystical powers and uses them to take over people's minds. They think of the man swinging a pendulum or pocket watch and whispering weird shit into the subject's mind before pouncing on their cognitive prowess and seizing it as their own.

Well, let me be the first to say hypnosis is *nothing* at all like this.

First of all, you can't take over someone's mind like some *Manchurian-Candidate*-related novel. It just doesn't work like that. Subjects in hypnosis, as it's primarily used and in the setting that I'll be referring to, must choose to enter hypnosis by their own accord and must allow themselves to be hypnotized.

Contrary to popular belief, people don't lose control of their minds whilst in a hypnotic state. They can, at any point, decide to end the hypnosis session or otherwise do something else consciously. They're not under the control or manipulation of someone else; this is a complete falsehood and an all too common misconception surrounding hypnosis.

No, people undergoing hypnosis have complete control over everything, so don't be fooled like I was at first by the Hollywood notion of some peculiar old dude making you do weird shit against your will.

Secondly, you don't need a pendulum, an old man, or anyone else for that matter, to reap the benefits of hypnosis. And yes, the benefits are amazing, but we'll broach that matter in a few.

Just know that the typical association that most people have of hypnosis is way off and is not an accurate depiction of it by any stretch of the imagination.

Before I dive into what hypnosis really looks like, let me first reveal various real-life examples of the phenomenon to convey its routine existence in our daily lives. Yes, that's correct, hypnosis is already being used in your life right now, you just never realized it. You and everyone else enter into hypnotic states multiple times throughout the day.

ENTERING INTO HYPNOSIS

Let me set the scene: You're driving down the highway on your way to a doctor's appointment a few towns over. It's a regular day, partly cloudy, mid-sixties, nothing special, nothing out of the ordinary.

Anyway, you're driving down the freeway thinking about how awesome sex was last night (or anything for that matter, but we'll say sex just for fuck's sake) with your wife. You're in the middle lane cruising along at about 65 or 70, not really thinking about much else aside from how beautiful your wife's ass looked in the candlelight glow.

You're fantasizing about that black lingerie outfit she was wearing and how it instantly turned you on, and how she seductively danced when she first walked in the room. You're getting unbelievably aroused, and yes, your schlong is turning more and more into a rock-hard phallus with every passing moment. *Wow, I can't believe she's still so fucking sexy, even after all these years,* you think to yourself. *I'm such a lucky guy. That new thing she did last night with her tongue, holy shit, that felt so good! I can't wait to do that again later.*

You envisage your wife's pure beauty for a few more moments and think of how much you love her and how happy she makes you. "Goddamn I'm a lucky fuck," you pronounce once more, before focusing your attention on the upcoming exit to your doctor's office.

Looking back on the road, it hits you like a bag of bricks, however. Stunned, you come to the realization that you've already passed the doctor's exit!

"What the fuck? How can that be possible?" You say out loud, in utter perplexity. "How the hell did I go past it . . . and past two other exits?"

For a moment, you question your sanity, but then you realize this type of thing has happened before. Not only to you, but to your friends and people you know. You hold off on the Alzheimer's Google search for now, and take the next exit to head back to your physician.

What's happened here, and what happens in situations like this all the time, is that our brains enter into hypnosis. We may not have realized or been able to put a name to a phenomenon like this in the past, but that's what's going on.

We're so distracted by something we're consciously thinking of that our subconscious minds go on autopilot and take over the situation. Sometimes the autopilot will lead you to pass your intended exit (and keep going for two more), and other times you'll get lucky and arrive at your destination without really even remembering the drive to it. In either case, your subconscious mind (the most powerful part of your mind) was the one directing things, and hypnosis (your ability to distract yourself) was the facilitator of this process.

Hypnotizing Your Depression

Other examples of everyday hypnosis include: watching a compelling, edge-of-your seat movie; reading a novel that enthralls you with its storyline, making you feel like you're one of the characters; playing a video game that captures your attention to the point where if someone calls your name you can't hear them; being so focused on your work that you aren't distracted by a phone call, text, or naked woman walking by; or, lastly, perhaps daydreaming about your rich and famous future and forgetting where you are for several minutes.

All of these moments are instances of self-induced hypnosis. They all alter your perception of reality and tap into the autopilot part of your mind known as the subconscious mind.

If you've previously partaken any of the aforementioned activities, you can be hypnotized, and you can therefore prosper from its laundry-list of benefits.

HOW IT WORKS

Hypnosis, as mentioned before, is a technique for tapping into your subconscious mind. You do it naturally throughout the day, but the easiest way to enter into hypnosis is through what's called an induction.

The Subconscious Mind

You have two parts to your mind as we currently understand it: the conscious mind, which is what's used by you to consciously think of things in every waking minute of your day; and the subconscious mind, which works in a behind-the-curtain sort of way (kind of like the Wizard of Oz without the bullshittery and fraud). Your subconscious mind controls your unconscious mental and physiological processes (heartbeat, blood pressure, breathing, digestion, the body's chemical distribution, and your feelings and emotions, to name but a few of its countless functions).

It essentially presides over everything you can't consciously direct.

For instance, you couldn't deliberately tell your body to pump 55ml of blood from your aorta artery and deliver it to the rest of your cells. It wouldn't listen to you. (Not to mention, it wouldn't be practical.) You can only consciously focus on one thing at a time. If you had to worry about distributing 2,000 gallons of blood throughout your entire body in a day, you wouldn't get anything done.

The subconscious mind is all-knowing and all-powerful.[1] It knows exactly what it has to do and is able to do so many things at the same time. It truly has an unlimited and infinitely exceptional ability to keep us alive and healthy.

A couple of the aspects you may have noticed that the subconscious mind takes care of are both our emotions and our feelings. These again are not something you can consciously manage (though with exercises like those in the gratitude chapter you can take conscious actions that positively affect the subconscious mind, and therefore your feelings and emotions).

You can't tell yourself, "I want to snap out of my depression," and then, poof, your depression disappears. You can't say, "I want to feel happy and alive and over my misery," and then, like the wave of a magic wand, you're in a great fucking mood and everything's awesome.

Unfortunately, it doesn't work that way. These are conscious thoughts and cannot possibly affect your feelings and emotions (at least not immediately) which reside in the subconscious part of your mind.

The only effective way to willfully tap into the subconscious mind, as of this writing, is to use a tool like hypnosis. That's why hypnosis is so effective. It grants us access to a resource which is all-mighty.

THE INDUCTION PHASE

An induction can be brought on by a professional hypnotist in person, in the comfort of your own home by listening to a professional hypnosis recording, or, to a lesser but fairly effective degree, by reading aloud a hypnotic induction script, and hypnotizing yourself.

Having a hypnotist take you into hypnosis is probably the best way, but it's also by far the most costly and least realistic as far as everyday use. Hypnotizing yourself via audibly reading a hypnosis script (this includes the entire hypnosis session's words; similar to a movie script it's got the beginning—which is the induction—the middle, and the end) can also work well for many, but it may take some time to get used to. And quite honestly I believe it's not as effective, at least in my experience, as my favorite method for using hypnosis, listening to an MP3 recording.

Using an MP3 is very simple, and comparable in many cases to seeing a professional in person. It's also very practical to utilize every day, as all you have to do is find a quiet, comfortable place to relax for around 20 minutes or so. You then simply plug in your headphones, sit back, and hit PLAY. From here the hypnotist will begin doing his job and taking you through the hypnosis session, each section at a time, beginning with the induction.

The induction is the phase of the hypnosis session that gets you comfortable and incredibly relaxed. It's the part where you focus your body, and then your mind, on becoming very calm. (It's best to do hypnosis either in the dark or in a dimly lit room, to induce a more relaxed state of mind.) A good hypnotist will spend between five to 10 minutes allowing you to feel enjoyably at peace and tranquil. It's very similar to a guided mediation, or the feeling you'd get if you were doing a slow-paced and soothing yoga session.

This unloading and de-stressing stage is a critical first step in prepping your mind for entry into the subconscious arena.

You can think of your subconscious mind as your castle. Inside the castle you hold all your books, all your weapons, all your supplies, all your secrets, and everything else that's critical for survival. Naturally, the castle is heavily guarded by armed soldiers surrounding the perimeter, has a deep water-filled moat separating the castle from the rest of the world, and past that, several watchtowers and additional guards on the land separated by the gully, ensuring the castle's protection.

These security measures are important and necessary. They keep you safe. But sometimes you need to come inside the castle and make a few changes. Maybe you want to fire a few unruly staff members, add some tough and trustworthy watchmen, or redesign several rooms to your liking. It's important to have the ability to walk into your castle and enact change whenever you wish to.

Enter the induction.

The induction is your way of getting past the security. By relaxing your mind to the point of utmost tranquility and peacefulness, you metaphorically lower your castle's fortification. The drawbridge is brought down, the front gates are opened up, the guards have gone to sleep, and the front door of your magnificent castle is wide-open and waiting for your entrance.

Once you're inside the castle, you can implement your change. And this is where the next part comes in.

THE THERAPY PORTION

The therapy part of the hypnosis session is where you give the orders (to your subconscious mind) and provide optimistic directions for change in the area of your life you want to improve. This could be whatever you want, but relating to its application on depression, it would mean giving your subconscious mind positive affirmations and directions on being happy. Statements similar to the following would work well:

"You are grateful for all you have in your life."

"You are unique and wonderful and you have incredible gifts to offer the world."

"The present moment is the most important moment we have. Your past is already written and over. Leave it in the past."

"Focus on all you have now and be happy with what you are blessed with and where you are heading."

Phrases like these and many others would be spoken to you by the hypnotist during this part of the session. It's important to note that this would seamlessly be read from the script the hypnotist has created, and would naturally flow. The random affirmations listed above are just examples of the types of things that would probably be said at some arbitrary point during the hypnotic trance. Also, if doing the self-hypnosis by reading your own script, you'd read it aloud in first person. So you'd say things like "I am grateful" and "I am blessed," as opposed to "You are . . ."

These positive declarations are used to reprogram your unconscious mind into functioning in a way that's conducive to what you want. It's kind of like programming a computer with code. You give it a shit-ton of instructions and it just does whatever you tell it to. That's really how your subconscious mind works.

It's not good or bad, it's indifferent; it just uses what it's given.

You, through your stimuli all day long, feed your subconscious mind programming codes on a very minuscule level. Your environment, your thoughts, your conditioning, what you do, what you see, what you experience, the way people react to you, it all adds up in the back of your mind, and over time it programs how you feel on a day-to-day basis.

Whether you realize it or not, you're constantly programming your unconscious mind. If you're inputting good, healthy codes, your output is going to be a happy one. But if your inputs are negative, your output is naturally going to be depressing.

So many people become depressed over time for this very reason. They unwittingly program themselves in a very insidious manner to actually be depressed.

So if a kid is getting bullied and picked on all the time, and being called "fat" and "stupid" and "ugly," chances are his subconscious mind is going to be indirectly programming itself from this negative feedback to have a negative output. If all his inputs are negative, all the codes his mind is receiving are negative, and in return, this poor kid is probably going to be severely depressed, have low self-esteem, no confidence, and probably even some anxiety and panic-attack issues.

A good first step to helping this kid out would be to stop the bullying (and beat the fuck out of those little assholes picking on him). However, if that weren't an option, it would be best to remove him from that harmful environment and put him in a more nurturing one, where his subconscious mind could get the right inputs and the boy could have a much better external output and livelihood.

But if for some reason this opportunity wasn't possible, or if the bullying has done a real number on this child's unconscious mind (essentially taking over and running amuck on all his internal emotions and feelings) a great way to hijack his subconscious mind and take it back would be to implement hypnosis daily.

The hypnosis would allow new codes to be reprogrammed into the child's mind and would be a way for him to have positive outputs (i.e. positive feelings and emotions), even when his environment wasn't ideal. It's a great way to override the system if it's been programmed the wrong way, or if it has contracted a virus. You can beat the virus if you know what you're doing; in this case, hypnosis is your antiviral solution.

So the therapy portion of hypnosis is where all the good shit happens. It's the feeding of your mind the positive codes it needs to enact change in your conscious reality.

And it works.

Just make sure you get a good quality hypnosis MP3, or work with a highly-trained hypnotist. Some guys, like in all industries, are morons and should be avoided like the plague.

When used correctly, hypnosis is perhaps the most powerful depression-fighting tool of all.

THE AWAKENING

Oh, and lastly, the final part of hypnosis is the awakening component.

This is exactly what it sounds like it is.

After the relaxing induction phase (about five to 10 minutes), and after the reprogramming, therapy portion (around five to 15 minutes in most cases), comes the awakening phase, which is about a minute or so long, and just brings you back up to consciousness.

It's the approach used for you to come back to being fully conscious and alert after implementing changes in your subconscious mind. It's leaving the castle and waking up the guards on your way out.

On this note, the state of actually being in hypnosis is very similar to meditation. It's a feeling between being fully conscious like you are right now, reading this book, and being fully asleep, like you were last night. It's a cool, relaxing place to be in and obviously makes you feel pretty calm, being that you're in a meditative-like headspace.

If you fall asleep hypnosis doesn't seem to work, and if you're fully alert, it doesn't seem to work either. But don't worry if you don't find that in-between sweet spot right away. It may take a few sessions before you get the hang of being in a hypnotic state. Also, some people feel very little if anything while under hypnosis, whereas others seem to have a profound sense of tapping into that Zen-like state of mind.

Personally, I'm usually pretty alert for the first five minutes or so, but then I slowly let my consciousness drift into the background, and then don't really remember the therapy parts of the session afterwards. I'll recall bits and pieces of the hypnotist's voice throughout, but overall, I don't recollect the things he's said as I would if I were listening to him fully awake. It's kind of an esoteric experience, but one I very much enjoy.

Time seems to get a bit distorted throughout, and you almost feel like you've fallen asleep by the end of it, but you haven't, and you know you haven't, because when the awakening part arrives and the hypnotist directs you to wake up at a specific moment, you wake up.

One point I want to drive home is that you're in full control at all times. So there's no need to worry or fear anything negative happening as a result of the hypnosis session. There's never been any side effects[2] attributed to hypnosis and to tapping into your subconscious mind, and there never will be. It's one of the safest practices you can try out.

MY EXPERIENCE WITH IT

From the minute I first put my earbuds on I knew I was in love.

I felt like a kid getting his first kiss. The hope and promise of improvement that permeated throughout my being alone was enough to make me feel good. Never mind the actual benefits of using the hypnosis MP3 that were soon to follow.

I'd been searching desperately for a true weapon against my depression, and after trying numerous other experiments to no avail, I was certain that hypnosis was FINALLY the answer.

I researched it assiduously and eventually stumbled on a book called *Instant Self-Hypnosis: How to Hypnotize Yourself with Your Eyes Open*, by a man named Forbes Robbins Blaire. This, as I alluded to earlier, is a method for hypnotizing yourself, simply by reading a hypnosis script aloud. This book had everything from Stress Relief to Immune System Boosting to Memory Improvement to Confidence Improving scripts and everything else in between. It also explained the fundamentals of hypnosis and how it all worked.

It was a really good place to start and I practiced daily using some of the scripts for stress relief, which had a lot of anxiety crossover; I dabbled with the confidence scripts too, as I surely needed more of that.

The book was a great place to begin, but it lacked what I'd really sought at the time, a script to combat depression. So I continued to search a number of places online until I finally came across a site called MindFit Hypnosis that happened to have both CD and MP3 formats on releasing depression (it was aptly titled *Releasing Depression*). The site was (and still is at the moment) run by a man named Dr. Andrew Dobson, who's actually a hypnotherapist (a highly-trained hypnotist, oftentimes, as in Dobson's case, one who holds a doctorate in a relating field like psychology). I looked around his site for a while and although it wasn't the most visually appealing configuration I'd ever seen, I decided to give him a shot.

So I ordered the *Releasing Depression* MP3 and received the email to download it minutes later. After popping that baby on, I was reborn.

Okay, maybe not literally, but seriously the impact it had on me was remarkable and it came relatively quickly. I'm not saying my depression completely went away after my first session, because it did not, but I did feel better after my first session (probably a combination of the hope and optimism I had for it to work, the meditative-like state it put me in for 20 minutes, and the hypnosis itself reprogramming my mind with positive suggestions). And I continued to feel better and better with every session thereafter.[3]

I would play the hypnosis track every morning when I woke up, religiously. It was the first thing I did to start my mornings. I'd go in my basement in a small, quiet room, dim the lights by facing a small table lamp down and away from my direction, sit on an old beat-up couch, and put the headphones in my ears and relax. After 20 minutes I'd feel refreshed and revitalized with happiness.

A NOBLE TOOL

Now, it's important to note that these suggestions were great for making me feel good and for cuing up the code for positivity in my day, but using them alone and doing nothing else, is almost certainly not enough to beat depression. At least not for me, and I'd surmise for just about everyone else.

It's a wonderful tool, and as I like to say often, probably my single favorite of all the tools for fighting off depression, but defeating an adversary like this typically requires a more comprehensive approach. There's so much going on in depression, both psychologically and physiologically, and attacking it in multiple ways is the most prudent blueprint for victory.

Hypnosis does a noble job in laying down the ideal inputs to start off your day, but you've got to make sure the rest of the inputs and stimuli going into your mind thereafter are also positive, or at least not horribly negative, for the hypnosis effects to take shape.

It's like planting the best seeds in the world but then forgetting to water them. Or worse yet, planting them next to weeds or in a swamp. They're bound to die. You can keep replanting them all you want and giving yourself hope that maybe they'll grow, but optimizing the conditions and choosing a nourishing environment is truly the best approach.

WILL IT WORK?

Hypnosis works on almost everyone, but not quite. It's estimated that around 80% of the population have a medium or moderate susceptibility to hypnosis; meaning it's fairly easy for them to be hypnotized and with a little practice they can use hypnosis effectively.[4] It's probably where I fall, and obviously where most people fall too.

It's also estimated that about 10% of the population[5] is highly susceptible to hypnosis; meaning they can easily be hypnotized and reap the benefits very quickly. But then there's approximately 10% more who are very poorly susceptible to hypnosis; it's tough for them to enter into hypnosis (not that they can never obtain its benefits, it's just much harder for them to use it, and it may not be in their cards to do so).

Most people start to feel good after a few sessions (if you're lucky you'll observe effect rather quickly like me), but to really notice the positive suggestions from hypnosis take shape it more typically takes a few weeks to a month. 21 days is often the timeframe for habits to form, so it's a good benchmark to go for, at a minimum.

MY RECOMMENDATION

I'd recommend using hypnosis every day, preferably around the same time. Right before bed or as soon as you wake up are both great. 21 days in a row should be the initial goal, but there's no limit to when you should stop. Go for four weeks, six weeks, eight weeks even, and see how you feel. The more you do it, the better it's going to work as far as consecutive days are concerned. And like with any new undertaking or novel habit, it takes some time to really see the results, so be patient.

Even now, many years since overcoming my major issues with depression, anxiety, confidence, and a host of other challenges along the way, I still, every so often, power up my iPod, kick back on my recliner, and listen to a mesmerizing hypnosis track on some varying topic of choice. I do it because it works and I feel good after, and because I like taking back my castle sometimes and whipping the minions into shape.

Moreover, hypnosis works incredibly for a number of conditions besides depression. The crossover for anxiety[6] and confidence amelioration is well documented, and it can help tremendously for sleep improvement,[7] energy levels, procrastination, focus, phobias, and so many other aspects of life you wish to enhance. Its potential for optimal daily performance throughout all spheres of life is nearly limitless.

One thing it will not do, however, is make you taller. I tried this. It failed. I wasted $70 and I'm still five foot fucking seven and will remain so until my death, 100 years from now, whilst sharing my last precious moments in the same bed with a 22nd century Playmate of the Year.

Yes, I just predicted my own glorious demise. And yes it will be 100 years from now, following marvelous intercourse with a future big-titted babe. If my anti-aging genius buddy Dr. Michael Fossel can crack the code[8] like he says (and I believe he can), this is all but a certainty.

But on a final hypnotic note, there are many great hypnotists and hypnotherapists out there. Along with Dr. Andrew Dobson, whom I often recommend, there's others I've used over the years who are great as well. Paul McKenna comes to mind as being another esteemed hypnotist and a favorite of mine. And Dr. Dave Hill, considered by many to be one of the greatest living hypnotists in the world, and whom I've had the pleasure of chatting with and befriending over the years. These men are just a few of the exceptional ones that I can vouch for at the moment, but there are so many others out there to choose from. The list of quality practitioners goes on and on. Just pick someone who's legit and someone you enjoy listening to.

Whoever you choose is going to be let into your castle, so you should probably trust and have some level of fondness for your guest. But even if you don't, you can always boot there ass out and find someone else. After all, you're in charge here, it's your fucking castle. If you decide someone isn't a good fit or if they seem like that creepy old guy I described earlier, toss them headfirst into the moat.

You're the king here. Remember that.

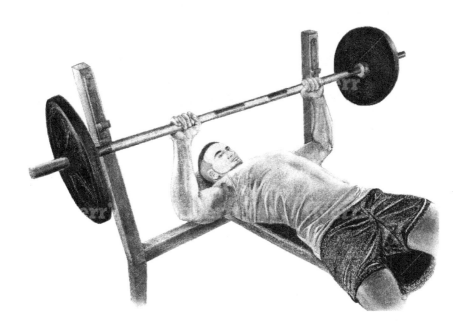

Chapter Nineteen
Working out Your Blues

From the second I walked into the prestigious institution I knew I'd found my new home.

I gazed about in awe of all that befell my eyes and was consumed by sheer beauty in that magnificent moment. As I glanced around at all of the facility's divine structures I couldn't help but feel like that fat fuck boy, Augustus Gloop, when he first stepped inside Willy Wonka's chocolate factory. I was brimming with excitement, but I promised myself I wouldn't do anything rash like dive into a chocolate pond or get sucked up through a chocolate pipe like portly Augustus.

As my highly-esteemed tour guide (named Billy) escorted me down the breathtaking corridors which led to the true source of all my enthusiasm, I grew more and more giddy with each fleeting second. Every step I took closer to my destination revealed the further elegance of this already enchanting architectural masterpiece I so fortunately had the pleasure of exploring.

Secret passageways, undoubtedly leading to more wonder, encircled me on all sides as I continued my trek. What wonder they held behind their doors I could only imagine, but they filled my yearning with even more fervor, and added to my growing infatuation with the place. I committed to circling back as soon as I could and unraveling their mysteries the instant I got a chance.

At about a few dozen yards out from reaching my Mecca, I noticed a beautiful bright light radiating from the core of my intentioned journey's end. I've never had a near-death experience, but I can only imagine it being somewhat equivalent to the phenomenon I witnessed in this moment, only less majestic.

Instinctively, I picked up my pace and nearly started running toward the light, and Billy, my tour guide, kept right up. Bursting with exhilaration I passed those last few dozen feet in seconds and arrived upon what I'd come here to behold all along.

It was absolutely beautiful.

As I regarded the idyllic scene before me I couldn't help but feel an overwhelming sentiment of euphoria. I felt like a severely dehydrated man in the desert who, after days of searching for even the slightest drop of water, stumbles upon a pristine oasis of crystal-clear river water. I swear for the next few seconds I heard that heavenly angelic "aweeeeeeeee" sound that so often accompanies these sacred moments.

By now you may be wondering where I was. What type of place could illicit such a profound response and have me feeling so deeply emotional?

Was it some mysterious yet majestic museum, filled with all kinds of curiosity and intrigue?

Could it have been an ancient site of fantastic prestige like a famous cathedral or monastery?

Or was it something even more renowned, like say a prominent historical landmark of worldly acclaim and marvel?

Well, in reality, it was none of these.

In fact, to most people, the basis for all my spectacular excitement might seem rather unsophisticated, perhaps even downright callow. The truth, as it turns out, was that the real origin for all my emotional exhilaration in that celestial moment was derived from . . . a gym.

MY HOLY PLACE

This wasn't just any gym though. This was a work of art.

The layout of this body-sculpting arena was unprecedented. Every type of machine and exercising apparatus you could possibly imagine encompassed the vast space of this consecrated ground. It housed equipment that looked as if it belonged 100 years in the future. And all of the contraptions looked as though they'd been thoroughly washed before and after every single use.

"Clean," would be the biggest miscarriage of sanitation in history. This place was immaculate. Everything, and I do mean *everything*, was the most polished, sparkling, and shiny object you'd ever lay eyes upon. Even the floors were gleaming.

The members of this illustrious fitness center were quite extraordinary as well. Peering about I saw some of the fittest and most attractive individuals I've ever come across in my entire life. Drop-dead gorgeous women with hour-glass bodies adorned most of the elliptical and stair-master machines. Hulking, magazine-cover brutes decorated the free weight benches and squat racks. Yes, there were dozens of people crafting their already nearly perfect physiques at this particular hour of day, and not one of them looked like they'd ever been on the wrong side of a romantic rejection.

Naturally, I fit right in.

Okay, maybe not.

And actually, I have to come clean. Perhaps I went a little too overboard with the flawless description I so generously depicted of this facility. In complete honesty it was kind of, um, *unspectacular.*

Alright, no more games, I'll be really honest. It was a fucking dump.

The machines were vast in quantity yes, but most of them were like 50 years old and looked as though they'd needed an upgrade for the last 49 of those years. They were tough and durable, but they also held rust stains and chipped off pieces of metal and plastic from obvious wear. And yes, admittedly, everything wasn't all that clean or unblemished. There were countless spots on the floor, dust on all the machines, cracks and fractures on much of the equipment, and visible holes on many of the benches. Lastly, those model-like gymgoers I'd previously described? Ah . . . yeah, they actually really didn't exist.

But in genuine transparency, what I truly saw when I looked around that day was just as appealing to me as the aforementioned Barbie-doll clones would be to most. But they were far from what you and I would consider ideal. Instead, what I viewed was more comical than attractive, but nonetheless fascinating.

Scanning around, I spotted a middle-aged, balding fat dude with an obviously chocolate-stained wife-beater tank top reading the newspaper while collapsed atop a squeaky exercise bike. Judging by the lack of sweat which escaped any part of his brow, or anywhere else on his grotesquely misshapen figure for that matter, he'd probably only been on the machine for a few minutes. I knew his perspiration wouldn't hold off much longer though, as he was pedaling away with the same intensity someone who'd actually stolen a real bike might display. As he flapped his pork-filled legs up with each cycle, his paper bounced up and down off his lap with the same ardor a Kevin-McCallister-shoved toolbox might have if thrust from the top of the *"Rocky* Steps" outside the Philadelphia Museum of Art. The fact that this bloke could discern anything from that paper was really the most impressive aspect of it all.

If the bicycle-boy-of-wonder's intensity was any indication of the overall effort this gym lodged, don't be fooled. Over on the treadmill, about 30 feet away, stood an older than middle-aged, but not quite decrepit older lady, who trudged along the treadmill's conveyor belt with the same tenacity a feeble 98-pound man might have if he walked alongside her on an exact same treadmill with a Steinway grand piano strapped onto his back. Her grey, crinkly old hair sat undisturbed in a bun and wasn't in any jeopardy of falling out anytime soon. Sweat too escaped this woman, but unlike her contemporary, it was absolutely for a lack of trying. Just as impressive as the bicycler's ability to read the newspaper was this woman's ability to mimic the pace of a dying snail.

Other than these two captivating creatures, the rest of the gym was actually quite forgettable. Scattered throughout the rest of the cardio area, the weight machine portion, and the free weight section, numerous fairly ordinary and otherwise plain individuals sat, stood, or laid, pumping weights or pumping their legs in a modest effort to look a little better or otherwise improve their health.

Again for me, a teenaged boy, who wanted nothing more than a place to lift weights and do cardio throughout the week, I could give a shit less if this place was packed with sexy, young and seductive women or if it was loaded up with frail, wrinkly, old grandmas. As much as this place may not have held the same worldly acclaim as a finely crafted architectural institution like say the Taj Mahal, to me it was just as astounding, and all I'd ever wanted.

BEFORE I STARTED REGULARLY GOING TO THE GYM

Before my foray into this humble abode I'd spent most of my time in the boxing gym getting my face punched in. Yes, I did enjoy the boxing gym to a certain degree, minus the face-punched-in part; but even at its pinnacle, I longed for a place where I could build up my skinny frame and become more attractive.

After I hung up the gloves I dug out a little workout room in the trodden-down old shed in my backyard. For about a year or so I'd irregularly go out to that shack and pump iron in an effort to put on some size. I'd installed a pull-up bar in there, a rundown but free flat bench press set with rusted red plates that my neighbors were throwing out one day, and a smorgasbord of other random dumbbells and free weights I'd collected from various charity-related sources. Though my muscular gains were pretty decent (all things considered), after a while, I plateaued out and wanted more.

I knew my little personally-constructed gym just wasn't enough to satisfy my motivation to get in tip-top physical shape and really pack on solid muscle. And after searching for the solution, I stumbled upon my holy grail.

MY USE OF THE GYM

During this period, the gym was used as a means to grow larger muscles and look more appealing to the girls I wanted to date. But it also helped me improve my self-esteem, and was unwittingly one of the best anti-anxiety and anti-depression tools I stumbled across.

I'd always been active in my life, but never felt like I was doing things I really wanted to do as often as I wanted to do them. When I was really little I loved playing baseball, but as I grew older, I stopped enjoying the game, though I still kept playing it years after I found any fun in it. Soon after this I picked up basketball, and really loved the sport, but had to stop after just a couple of years because I just wasn't that good at it. Then I turned to boxing. Again, I liked boxing to an extent, but really, like most people, I didn't enjoy getting beat up from it (although I made myself believe I did), but took it up for several years because of the misguided belief that I had to be tougher.

Lifting weights and working out was really the first time I got to freely do something I actually enjoyed. I didn't have to quit because I wasn't good enough, and I didn't have to get beat up to continue to enjoy it. I made my own rules. I made my own schedule. And I chose to do whatever I wanted and not do whatever I didn't want. It was fucking awesome.

On so many levels.

Of course the physical improvements were what stood out the most to me at that time, but the myriad of other advancements were just as profound, though admittedly more subtle. The stress that lifting weights alleviated for me was incredible. The depressive feelings that it got rid of for hours after a good workout were a much-appreciated gift. The positive physical gratification it induced for my self-image was a daily joy. Exercising did all of these things and more. I didn't recognize the breadth of its power at the time, though I'd notice little bits and pieces of its various benefits, but looking back at it now, it played a major role in helping me overcome my depression. Now, many years later, I can see just why it harbored such an integral role.

THE SCIENCE OF EXERCISE AND DEPRESSION

Study after study demonstrates the benefits of exercising every day. Even as a standalone, it's a natural and very effective treatment for depression.[1] One hallmark study done in 1999 on 156 men and women comparing the effects of exercise with antidepressant medication concluded after 16 weeks of observation that exercise alone was just as effective as taking antidepressant medication in the study's participants.[2]

Dr. Michael Craig Miller, an assistant professor of psychiatry at Harvard Medical School, said this about exercise, "For some people it works as well as antidepressants. In people who are depressed, neuroscientists have noticed that the hippocampus in the brain—the region that helps regulate mood—is smaller. Exercise supports nerve cell growth in the hippocampus, improving nerve cell connections, which helps relieve depression.[3]"

It also appears to regulate and increase feel-good hormones like endorphins and neurotransmitters such as serotonin, dopamine, and norepinephrine.[4] Exercise is the perfect prescription for depression as it works on a number of areas in the brain directly improving the chemistry and functionality of it, while at the same time helping to improve your feelings regarding your self-image, which in many ways can be just as powerful as any of its physiological effects.

Working out has also proven to be very effective in both short and long-term alleviation of depressive symptoms, with studies showing unlike many prescription drugs, you don't have to increase the "dose" of your exercise, and it won't lose its effectiveness over the long haul.[5] Not to mention, the only side effects you'll ever get from regularly exercising are positive ones. (Unless of course fighting off the wild yearning for your newfound lusciousness by the opposite sex is something you spurn. I guess in this bizarre case you'd be shit out of luck.)

Lastly, one study conducted in 2006 demonstrated the many benefits of exercise from a mental health standpoint. It included everything from improved sleep, to increased interest in sex, to better physical endurance, to stress relief, to improvement in mood, to increased energy and stamina.[6]

I could not make up the innumerable windfalls of good fortune exercise offers if I possessed the science fiction imaginative prowess of H.G. Wells himself. It's unfathomably terrific.

BACK AT THE GYM

So to me, walking into that gym that first day was as good as anything I could've walked into. I mean it. There was no place in the world I would've rather been. This beat-up, old-school, filthy, and pretty goddamn ugly-looking gym was the most beautiful sight conceivable. I knew that day that I'd be making that gym my second home. I couldn't wait to start pumping iron and sweating my ass off right alongside bicycle boy.

Hell, I was so happy during that time I even sort of befriended the oversized bicycle boy shortly after joining.

I didn't hang out with him or anything, or invite him over for tea and crumpets, but I'd say "Hi" and casually give him the courteous nod and half-smile every time I'd come across him. No matter how much he'd sweat all over the cardio machines or how many chocolate-stained tank tops he'd offensively parade his repulsive chest and misshapen arms in, I was always happy to see him. Fuck, I was always happy when I was in the gym, no matter who I saw.

WHAT I DID

I started going to the gym every day. I didn't know much about working out but I slowly picked up a lot along the way (I did know that when I exercised I felt great thereafter). So with a little research and a lot of implementation I slowly honed in on a pretty solid workout routine. One that had the twofold effect of helping me pack on some serious muscle, and consequently feel fucking great whilst doing it.

It's important to note that I tried just about every workout routine imaginable. From the one-set High Intensity Training of weight-lifting trailblazers like Mentzer and Yates, to the numerous set volumetric teachings from the likes of titans like Schwarzenegger and Coleman, to the fast-paced CrossFit-style workouts mimicking the theories of Glassman, and so many of the other variants which lay in between the philosophies of these icons. Some of it resonated with me and I noticed good results, others didn't and I soon discarded it for something else. Even now, after all these years, I still switch things up occasionally and mess around with different weight-training programs. It keeps things exciting.

The truth is, they can all work in some fashion, so do what feels right. Not what your genetically gifted and naturally-jacked buddy tells you to do. Nor what the juiced-up magazine models who're consuming copious amounts of steroids advise either.

You have a unique body and will respond distinctively to what most aligns with it genetically. Don't be sold by someone's looks or credentials; but on the same token, don't be afraid to experiment and try a number of different teachings. Anything can work when done right, and some better than others.

The most important thing to remember is to work out, no matter whose plan you follow. (Except for Paul Reubens. If he ever comes out with an exercise program don't buy it.)

MY RECOMMENDATIONS

Exercise regularly. That's my number one most important tip. Whether you're pumping iron or running a few miles, break a sweat often. Typically, five to six days a week is best for general fitness and optimal brain and mental health.

Before you cringe, it's really not that tough.

Walking for 30–60 minutes alone can be considered a day's exercise. Is that too much to commit to for adopting such a powerful, natural anti-depressant lifestyle? I think not.

Top brain docs like Dr. Daniel Amen typically recommend walking 30–45 minutes a day, three to five times a week, for the many health benefits it can offer, including that of improving your mood and having anti-anxiety and anti-depressive effects.[7] This, or another comparable steady-state cardio exercise (bicycling, running, swimming, stair-climbing, ellipticalling, etc.), should definitely be added to your weekly workout routine.

Naturally, strength training should also be incorporated into your routine. Lifting weights isn't just good for improving your chances with babes on the beach, it's also good for alleviating your depression and anxiety.

One recent study published in 2011, and conducted on 58 adults, showed a significant improvement in depression over a four-month period in participants of the study who adhered to a resistance training protocol compared to the control group who did not perform any weight training exercises.[8]

Lift weights three to five times a week, just like your cardio. If you are a complete novice in the bodybuilding space, start simple. Don't fret about trying to be sophisticated or thinking about all the other guys at the gym who seem to be doing a ton of random shit. I am one hundred percent serious when I say that approximately 95% of the men at any given gym have absolutely no idea what they're doing.

Some of them may have bigger muscles than you, but that's more of a happenstance than a reflection of their brilliance, and simply them spending a lot of time doing something repeatedly, not by any means because they're enlightened and know some secret you do not. Most of the time these guys actually do more harm than good by thinking they know more than they actually do.

So stick to the basics.

If you want an easy routine to follow that can work great for many, simply do a Push Day, a Pull Day, a Leg Day, and a Core Day. That means you dedicate 30–60 minutes, one day out of the week, to working on your "Push" muscles, another day working on your "Pull" muscles, another on your "Leg" muscles, and finally, another day on your "Core" muscles. From there you can either fill in the gaps on your days off with some cardio, or add the cardio at the end of your lifting sessions, either way works.

A FEW KEYS TO REMEMBER

Form is critical. You want to remove all of your natural momentum and focus instead on only using the muscle groups the lifts are intended to stress.

Working out Your Blues

Also, in regard to time, try to spend between 30–60 minutes during your lifting days and then get out of there (or add in a few minutes of cardio at the end, but not too much). You really shouldn't be in the gym lifting for much more than an hour because after this general threshold, you start to see less and less return on your investment. In fact, if you continually spend well over an hour, even multiple hours lifting, like some, there's a good chance you're overtraining and thus spinning your wheels. By doing this you're not actually allowing your muscles to recover and grow.

Additionally, for the most part, three sets of each exercise is pretty good for most. Three to five reps per set builds strength, eight to 12 gets you hypertrophy, and 15–20 gets you more of the toned look. The science is still coming out on this, and I often think it's a little over-hyped, but generally speaking, it's something to shoot for.

Furthermore, put enough of a heavy weight on where you're failing (you can't do any more reps in good form) at around these rep ranges, but not too much of a load that you have to start using your momentum to cheat. But yes, you do need an actual decent amount of weight on to stress your muscles sufficiently and to cause the muscle fibers to tear, so they can then grow when you're resting.

If you curled a beer bottle 1000 times you probably wouldn't tear a single muscle fiber, as the mass of the container is just far too light. However, if you curled say a 30-pound dumbbell 12 times with that same arm, you'd be tearing a ton of fibers, as that stress is sufficient enough to cause this type of muscular response. The point here is to lift heavy enough so that you're "failing" between your desired rep ranges whilst still maintaining good form, and that you stop when you can't lift any more reps or when you lose your good form.

Rest time in between sets, again, generally speaking, should be a minute or two. And the total number of sets for your Push, Pull, or Leg Days can be anywhere between say 15–20, give or take a few.

Finally, when it comes to exercise order, it doesn't really matter, but usually it's best to do the more complex exercises first. This means the ones that take the most energy out of you. So think your barbell flat bench press, or dumbbell flat bench press, your barbell or dumbbell shoulder press, your pull-ups, your bent-over rows, your squats, your leg press, and your deadlifts. The isolated exercises like say your tricep pull-downs, bicep curls, and calf raises would be done toward the end of the workout, as they're already being used for the complex movements, and they're much easier to do and take less out of you.

WHY YOU REALLY SHOULD EXERCISE

As human beings we're wired to move around, to exercise, and to sweat. It's part of what makes us human and part of what balances all of the processes in our brains. Among many threats, one of the biggest risk factors for depression is our sedentary epidemic we as a society are currently undergoing. With the popularity of TV, smartphones, and computers continuing to climb, it really must be a conscious decision to get your ass up and exercise. One 2015 scientific meta-analysis of over 110,000 patients who've undertaken sedentary behaviors in their lifestyle showed a significant increase in the risk for depression because of their inactive behavior.[9]

It's simple—sitting around is a surefire way to get depressed no matter how many seemingly fascinating cat videos you binge-watch.

Exercise is so effective for depression that it's almost too good to be true. As New Zealand physicist Sir Paul Callaghan put it several years back, "Throughout history many societies, ancient and modern, have used exercise as a means of preventing disease, and promoting health and well-being. There is evidence that exercise is beneficial for mental health; it reduces anxiety, depression, and negative mood, and improves self-esteem and cognitive functioning. Exercise is also associated with improvements in the quality of life of those living with schizophrenia. However, exercise is seldom recognized by mainstream mental health services as an effective intervention in the care and treatment of mental health problems. There is evidence to suggest that exercise may be a neglected intervention in mental health care.[10]"

Well said, Sir. Well said indeed.

The fact that mainstream medicine has neglected this powerful and natural antidote is a travesty. But this sham can end with you. Get up off your couch, take action, and start exercising. Your mind will love you for it.

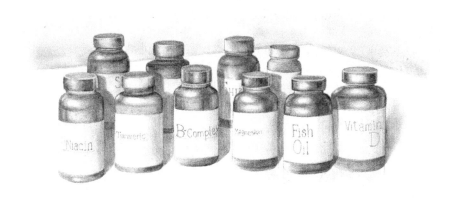

Chapter Twenty
Supplements for Depression

This chapter contains neither witty introduction nor anecdote of humorous lore. It dives straight into the marvelous capacity of natural supplements as a means to alleviate and overcome depression. Piggybacking off the last section's brilliance in describing agrestal approaches to defeating anxiety, it gives you a multitude of magnanimously terrific suggestions for trumping your blues.

As before, I'll go right down the line and rattle off many natural compounds, explicating their ability to assist in mental health optimization, and in particular, their ass-kicking capacity when facing off against depression.

Also, in the same reflection as before, I've listed the forthcoming supplemental recommendations from the safest to the least safe, though again, even the least safe ones are infinitely safer than just about any prescription drug on the market, and even these least safe nutrients are ridiculously fucking safe when taken correctly. But once more, I'm no doctor, so if you're looking to blame someone if you fuck up royally and do something stupid, look somewhere else.

Consult your own doc for this and all other medical advice.

Okay, legalities aside, let's jump right in.

THE RIDICULOUSLY SAFE

Magnesium

Magnesium is the one nutrient above all others I have taken that has helped most with my anxiety and depression, and since researching it more and more I've only grown fonder of it.

The studies on magnesium's usefulness for depression have been well documented for some time. It might be the safest and easiest way to get rid of your melancholy, and by some accounts even one of the fastest. In one particular study subjects displayed rapid recovery from major depression in less than seven days while taking between 125–300mg of magnesium.[1]

My Recommendation: I recommend taking 200–250mg one to three times per day as needed. With that last serving hopefully coming right before bed to put the cherry on top for a good night's sleep. And yes, the citrate and glycinate forms are typically best.

Turmeric

Turmeric (Curcuma longa) can help fight infections, some cancers, dementia, inflammation, digestive problems, and most pertinent of all, the double-headed beast that is anxiety and depression.

In one recent double-blind, placebo-controlled study, 56 individuals with major depressive disorder were treated with curcumin (from turmeric) 500mg twice daily or a placebo for eight weeks. Between the four to eight-week mark a significant improvement in depression was found in only the curcumin-treated patients, suggesting that after the first month, the curcumin started to really take shape and help relieve symptoms.[2]

My Recommendation: I'd suggest taking 500–1,500mg a day of turmeric. Start at the 500mg or 750mg dose (some products have 500mg per cap, others offer 750mg) and go to 1,500mg if desired. Turmeric is incredibly safe, and extremely difficult to overdose on. I've periodically taken up to 4,500mg a day of this herb for various inflammatory bouts, like acute aches and pains and headaches. It's purportedly safe in some cases all the way up to 6,000mg (or even 12,000mg a day in a few rare instances), though I wouldn't recommend going this high.

There's two schools of thought when it comes to choosing your turmeric supplement. The first is that the turmeric you consume should be kept as close to its original form as possible (*Curcuma longa*). Meaning you should not isolate any particular compounds or generally mess with the way nature created this wonder-herb, as it can take away the synergistic effects that this plant offers when keeping all of its key components together.

The second school of thought is to take turmeric as a standardized extract that contains 95% curcuminoids (the part of turmeric on which most of the studies have been done[3]). Look for 500mg–750mg of standardized turmeric extract that's made up almost entirely of curcuminoids. So if it's 500mg per capsule and it's 95% standardized for curcuminoids, you'll be getting 475mg of curcuminoids per cap.

In either case, you want to get a supplement that has BioPerine or black pepper extract (standardized to contain 95% piperine) at 5mg for every 500mg–750mg of regular turmeric or the 95% curcuminoid turmeric, as this increases the bioavailability of the herb in your body.

Both types of turmeric work great in their own right and the choice is ultimately yours.

Fish Oil

Fish oil contains the omega-3 fatty acids eicosapentaenoic acid (EPA) and docosahexaenoic acid (DHA), which are the precursors to eicosanoids—signaling molecules that are known to reduce inflammation in the body.

Further research should be undertaken but it grows ever more apparent by the day that proper omega-3 intake coincides with a healthy and happy brain. One 2016 study published in the *Nutritional Neuroscience* journal showed a 40% decrease in major depression disorder symptoms and a significant improvement in amino acid and nutrition content in the prefrontal cortex[4] in participants who took a high-dose fish oil supplement over the course of 10 weeks.

My Recommendation: I recommend taking one to three grams a day of triple strength fish oil. Look for the total omega-3 fatty acid count on the back of the label. And then look at the DHA and the EPA content of those fatty acids. The EPA and the DHA should add up and get to as close to one gram as possible and should comprise at least 70% or more of the total fatty acid makeup.

Finally, if possible, try to get the fish sourced from Alaska as this seems to hold some of the cleanest fish available.

Niacin

Niacin has a wonderful ability to increase the production of feel-good neurotransmitters like serotonin, dopamine, and norepinephrine without compromising the balance of them.

Recent studies have also indicated that niacin helps initiate the production of BDNF[5] (brain-derived neurotrophic factor) in the hippocampus which leads to neurogenesis, the creation of healthy new brain cells. Low levels of BDNF have been strongly correlated with major depressive disorder in both human and animal studies.

Perhaps most impressive of all, niacin appears to be a natural and safe alternative to treating schizophrenia.[6] More studies need to be performed on this, but according to experts like Dr. Andrew Saul, and pioneering health innovators like Dr. Abram Hoffer, schizophrenic individuals possess an excess of a chemical called adrenochrome (which is adrenalin in oxidized form) and niacin, in all its astounding brilliance, actually reduces the body's production of this harmful chemical.[7] This adrenochrome compound is purported to have hallucinogenic-like effects in the brains of schizophrenic people, thus removing it seems to stabilize the condition.[8]

My Recommendation: For general health I'd recommend taking 250–500mg of niacin one to four times a day. For more serious depression (or anxiety for that matter) you may want to consider taking 500mg five or six times a day. For schizophrenia, I'd start at 500mg five or six times a day, and go from there, depending on how you feel (you can either taper down, or go up a bit if necessary). Dr. Hoffer gave patients more than 10,000mg of niacin at times (though typically just transiently) if they really needed it. This was often only for new patients who were extremely sick, but it just shows how non-toxic niacin truly is.

B-Complex

Deficiencies in any one of the B-complex vitamins can lead to depression, but especially deficits in niacin, B6, B12, or Folate,[9] which seem to be more common these days.

The collaboration of all the B-vitamins in maintaining homeostasis in the brain cannot be overstated. Neurotransmitters like serotonin, GABA, and dopamine are dependent on all the B-vitamins, so do not neglect the consumption of any one.

In one recent double-blind, placebo-controlled study of 60 adult patients diagnosed with major depression and various other forms of depressive disorders, the patients who consumed a B-complex supplement showed significant and more continuous improvements in depression and anxiety symptoms after 30 and 60-day follow-ups over the placebo group who did not.[10]

My Recommendation: Take a good (activated) B-complex supplement every day. Usually a B-50 complex once or twice a day will do just fine.

THE VERY SAFE

Lithium Orotate

Lithium can work wonders on anxiety, but it may be even better for major depression, bipolar depression, and even schizophrenia.

Though lithium carbonate has been studied extensively for conditions like bipolar depression,[11] and has demonstrated substantial reductions in depressive symptoms (albeit at the cost of many undesired side effects), lithium orotate on the other hand, has not been as extensively researched in a clinical setting.

But knowing that lithium, when combined with orotic acid (as in orotate), readily crosses the blood-brain barrier to deliver its profound brain-nourishing effect, it's quite clear that the unwanted side effects of massive doses of lithium carbonate are not necessary.

My Recommendation: I recommend taking 5mg of lithium orotate, if you decide to use this supplement for depressive symptoms, one to three times a day, or as needed. Also, after looking at the literature on this, I'd feel very comfortable with taking up to 25mg a day of lithium orotate. But you can go a little higher still if needed. Just be careful, as with any supplement, and use your best judgment.

Probiotics

Probiotics can have a beneficial effect on depression as they perform an infinite amount of functions throughout the body. Studies have suggested that strains like Bifidobacterium longum can lower depression scores over the course of about 10 weeks.[12] Meanwhile, Lactobacillus rhamnosus strains of bacteria have been shown to decrease depression-related behavior.[13] Furthermore, the probiotic Bifidobacterium infantis has demonstrated the ability to reverse behavioral deficits.[14]

But exactly how it all works and exactly which strains to supplement with and in what dosages, currently eludes the medical establishment. One recent 2017 meta-analysis review conducted by researchers[15] examining a number of other probiotic-for-depression studies, noted that, "The majority of the studies found positive results on all measures of depressive symptoms; however, the strain of probiotic, the dosing, and duration of treatment varied widely."

My Recommendation: Play around and try a few different supplements with varying bacterial strains. Choosing ones that include some of the strains from the studies specifically on depression and mental health is clearly a good idea. Look for probiotic supplements with depression ameliorating qualities like Bifidobacterium longum, Lactobacillus rhamnosus, and Bifidobacterium infantis, and also some of the more popular and universally beneficial strains like Lactobacillus acidophilus and Streptococcus thermophilus. Overall, try to get a decent variety of strains, maybe a handful or so, to hit on some diverse aspects.

I recommend taking in a minimum of 25-50 billion CFUs (colony forming units—the number of good bacteria) per day. But you can easily go up to 100 or even 250 billion CFUs if you'd like. Just make sure you buy from a reputable company.

Chamomile

Chamomile (specifically the *Matricaria recutita* variety, or German chamomile) is a potent anti-inflammatory and helps to lower oxidative stress throughout the body, which in elevated levels can lead to depressive-like effects in the brain. It also appears to be a potent GABA-increasing herb, using specific phytochemicals like chrysin and apigenin to bind to GABA receptors in a similar way as benzodiazepine drugs like Xanax and Valium do (minus the side effects), and thus facilitates the upregulation of GABA.

New research further indicates its depressive and anxiolytic improvements can also be attributed to its wonderful ability to increase the effect of other key neurotransmitters like serotonin and GABA.[16]

There aren't many studies on chamomile at the present time. But one recent double-blind, placebo-controlled study of 57 depressed and anxious participants showed a significant improvement in mood for all the chamomile-taking patients versus the placebo group.[17]

My Recommendation: Chamomile seems to be incredibly safe and very effective. I've never used it, but I would recommend trying it if you've exhausted some of the other options mentioned before. Look for a 220mg chamomile extract, standardized to 1.2% apigenin (what researchers have used in the studies) and take it once or twice a day as needed. Perhaps take one at night, right before bed, as it may induce drowsiness and then see how you feel the next day.

Chamomile can also be consumed as a tea or inhaled via aromatherapy as an essential oil.

THE SAFE

Sam-e

Sam-e (S-Adenosyl methionine) is a critical compound used ubiquitously in the body and fuels over 100 metabolic reactions, but has its highest concentrations in the adrenal glands, liver, and brain. People who are depressed tend to have lower circulating levels of Sam-e and supplementing with this compound has been found to be quite beneficial. In some studies it even out-performed antidepressants,[18] without the side effects, and it appears to work much faster than antidepressants do.

One of its main mechanisms for combating depression, naturally, is its ability to boost the feel-good neurotransmitters of serotonin and dopamine, as well as other important neurotransmitters like acetylcholine.

A cautionary note on taking Sam-e must be made, however, about its rare, yet documented nevertheless, effect on some people with a history of mania. It's been noted that for these unfortunate individuals, it can make their mania worse in some instances. So caution must be taken, as well as a doctor's consultation.

My Recommendation: If you do not have a history of mania and would like to try this supplement out, it's generally regarded as well-tolerated and very safe. The dosage for Sam-e varies between 400mg–1600mg a day. Some people take 400mg once or twice a day, going up to 800mg in total. Others take 800mg once or twice a day, going up to 1600mg in total. As always, I'd start at the lowest dose and see how you feel. Try 400mg once or twice a day for two weeks. If you feel good with that stay there. If you don't, try upping the dose to 400mg three to four times a day thereafter. Take this baby on an empty stomach, and do not exceed more than 1600mg in one day.

5-HTP

5-HTP (5-Hydroxytryptophan) is a chemical the body creates from the intake of the amino acid tryptophan. After tryptophan becomes 5-HTP, 5-HTP is readily converted into serotonin, the natural feel-good neurotransmitter of the brain. Of all the supplements to consume, 5-HTP is probably the best serotonin creator of them all.

You definitely want to supplement with tyrosine, however, if you're going to supplement with 5-HTP. This is because 5-HTP is so effective at raising serotonin levels that it actually can lower your other equally important neurotransmitters like dopamine (serotonin and dopamine share the same receptors in the brain, so if your receptors are being used to produce a bunch of serotonin, the dopamine isn't being sufficiently created and you're going to have lowered dopamine levels, as well as other neurotransmitters like epinephrine and norepinephrine which are actually produced from the dopamine itself[19]). Generally speaking, you want to supplement tyrosine to 5-HTP at about a 10:1 ratio, meaning you'd take approximately 500mg of tyrosine for every 50mg of 5-HTP.

Studies for depression are mixed for a number of reasons (one of them being this lack of dopamine compensation that many don't know about), however, there are some studies that have properly balanced the neurotransmitters in the brain and other studies as well that have demonstrated its efficacy.[20]

My Recommendation: If you decide to give this a try because it is a very effective serotonin booster, start at 50mg one to three times a day as needed. I'd start with one 50mg pill at bedtime (as it can undoubtedly promote a better night's sleep) and see how you feel from there. Maybe you'd do better taking it a few times throughout the day, but start at the minimum dosage. And remember, take tyrosine with the 5-HTP at all times (ten times the amount, i.e. 500mg of tyrosine for 50mg of 5-HTP or 1000mg of tyrosine for 100mg of 5-HTP, etc.).

5-HTP is pretty safe in limits up to about 400mg a day in divided doses (you can move up to taking 100mg doses instead of 50mg if needed). I wouldn't go any higher than that though. Also, one more final caution: Do not take 5-HTP with SSRI drugs unless otherwise directed by your doctor. This combination can be extremely dangerous.

St. John's Wort

St. John's wort (*Hypericum perforatum*) contains the chemical hypericin (as well as hyperforin and a number of flavonoids that add to its medicinal effects), which many scientists believe is what gives the herb most of its value. St. John's wort seems to improve the availability of neurotransmitters like serotonin, dopamine, and epinephrine.[21]

A few years back Cochrane researchers reviewed 29 different trials of St. John's wort for the treatment of depression. These 29 studies had participants totaling up to 5,489 patients with symptoms of major depression. At the end of their review, their lead researcher Klaus Linde, of the Centre for Complementary Medicine in Munich, Germany, concluded, "Overall, we found that the St. John's wort extracts tested in the trials were superior to placebos and as effective as standard antidepressants, with fewer side effects.[22]"

The one major caveat with St. John's wort is that it can interact with many medications. It's not like others harmless nutrients and supplements, where you can safely take it without really thinking much about it. St. John's wort does not go well with many different medications, especially, other antidepressant drugs. Do not, I repeat,

DO NOT, mix this with antidepressant meds as the side effects can be incredibly dangerous, even fatal.

But warnings aside, the side effects, although higher than say most of the other supplements listed in this section, are still generally low. This is a pretty safe herb to take when you take it the right way and when you don't mix it with anything known to react negatively with it.

My Recommendation: I wouldn't start with this herb personally, but if you've tried a few of the others and haven't found relief, this may be a great supplement to try. Its benefits on mild to moderate depression have been well documented, and again, when consumed properly it's generally pretty safe.

If you want to take this, take 300mg of St. John's wort extract one to three times a day (make sure it's standardized to contain 0.3% hypericin). As always, start off at the minimum dose and work your way up if needed. The most common dosage per day for depression is 900mg, but people can go all the way up to 1800mg in divided doses if necessary. But don't go any higher and make sure you monitor your feelings while on this. This herb is powerful.

FINAL THOUGHTS ON SUPPLEMENTS

Taking a vitamin, mineral, herb, or natural compound can help alleviate your depression, and may be a massive component to your recovery. They alone may not defeat depression, but they can be a solid weapon to add to your arsenal for the battle.

It's foolish not to consider taking supplements, especially when there's so much research establishing their efficacy, and equally significantly, so much research proving their safety. Especially in regards to the first few supplements mentioned in the beginning.

Supplements for Depression

Not only can natural supplements like the ones covered in this chapter help your mental health, they can also improve your general, everyday wellness.

Fuck it, I say. Join me on the bandwagon of supplemental splendor. Just be safe and only bear the nutrients of time-tested diligence. And oh yeah, don't turn into a froggy-handed, smelly witch doctor. The world does not need more of them.

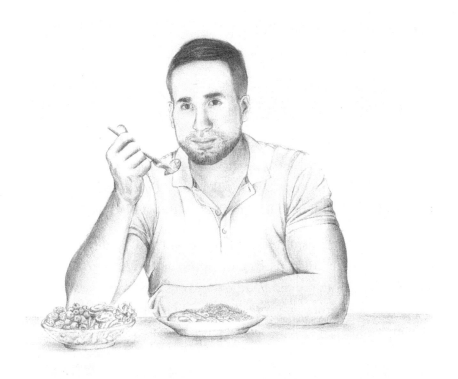

Chapter Twenty-One
The Antidepressant Diet

"And would you like to make that a large?" The mid-40-year-old, heavy-set black woman behind the counter asked, with a friendly smile.

"Absolutely," I emphatically replied, as I returned her smile with a grin of my own.

"Perfect, that'll be *[who the fuck remembers?]*, sir," the jolly, fast-food worker chimed back.

"Here you go," I said, handing her the precise amount of necessary currency for this fast-food feast.

Then, several minutes later, as I peered down upon my order as it arrived, an even bigger smile crossed my face.

On the tray before me lay three double cheeseburgers, one enormous container of French fries, one giant 20-piece assortment of chicken nuggets, and one massive goblet of Sprite, courtesy of the opportunistic upsell from the kind but cutthroat black woman.

Oh, and if that wasn't enough, the blood red, high-fructose corn syrup I liberally dispensed into approximately 20 mini ketchup containers with the unfettered goal of consuming just seconds later, topped off this grotesque spread I so enthusiastically couldn't wait to devour.

And devour I did. Not one microscopic grease drop of that exorbitantly slimy meal was spared. I went to town on all of it in just minutes, and then licked my fingers afterward for good measure. I could not let a single iota of caloric sustenance go to waste, not at this time in my life, anyway.

I was on a misguided mission to get big. Being a short, skinny kid at the time, and weighing maybe 135 pounds soaking wet, I knew I needed to add mass to my frame. In all my exuberant yet naïve wisdom, I'd decided I needed to eat like a complete slob. I figured I had to eat as much as possible and as often as possible, and then train like there was no tomorrow . . . to put on size. I don't know if I'd read this stupidity somewhere or just taken the advice of some juiced-up meathead asshole at the gym, but whatever the source, I'd listened to it.

I'd eat five to six times a day of everything I could get my hands on. I became a human garbage disposal. Being young, active, and working out often certainly helped me stay relatively fit, but the insides of my body were vastly aggrieved with my lifestyle decision.

Muffins, donuts, corn bread, protein shakes, weight gainers, processed peanut butter, fried chicken, colossal amounts of red meat, sodas, juices, chocolate bars, and just about every sugary confectionary you could think of, I'd ingest. My goal was to get as many calories into my frail body as I could, trying relentlessly to stuff my face with as much protein as possible, but being indiscriminate when it came to carbs and fats, as I knew they too offered up the precious calories I sought and I presumed could only assist a skinny, frail boy in his quest to become a more burly young man.

Yup, in those days, my caloric intake rivaled that of a medium-sized African elephant. And though I certainly packed on some pounds and added some mass, it wasn't healthy. Not by any means.

This one particular McDonald's-feasting day actually carries with it more story to be told, as later that day a subsequent series of events followed that indirectly altered my dieting in the ensuing months, and for the rest of my life thereafter.

So let me continue.

LATER THAT DAY

That night, as I was eating my sixth meal of the day, I had in front of me a gargantuan homemade plateful of fried chicken in the form of numerous drumsticks, several breasts and thighs, a separate side dish plateful of white rice with some corn and peas, a large glass of orange juice, and a mountain-sized blob of ketchup, brimming from the top of an oversized utility bowl most ordinary human beings might use for cereal and the like.

And I'd be derelict if I didn't include my dessert, which lay just a few feet away from all the deliciousness before me. My after-meal snack included a large chocolate chip muffin from the local grocery store and a family-sized bag of Funyuns, which was essential to balance out the inevitable salt-craving that would immediately supplant the sweet-tooth indulgence.

After plowing through all the treats, and stopping myself only after killing more than half the bag of Funyuns, I decided I'd consumed a sufficient amount of nutrients for the day. I proceeded to relax on the couch for a bit and unwind, and maybe an hour or so later, went to bed.

Sleep came rather quickly, but it didn't last. About two hours after dozing off in my room, I awoke strangely, and immediately felt weird. I noticed a throbbing pain emanating from my stomach and as I rolled from my right side onto my left, a feeling of nausea went coursing through my abdomen and up to my head. Instantly, I knew something was terribly wrong. Call it a Spidey-Sense if you will, but something was telling me (probably my gut) that something really bad was about to happen.

However, being the delusional optimist that I am, I rolled over a few more times over the next several minutes and tried to ignore this premonition. I even tried shutting my eyes and going back to sleep, but I couldn't. The pain was getting worse and the nauseating feelings were becoming more pronounced. After another moment of reluctant questioning I gave in and decided to go to the bathroom, at the very least, to examine myself and appease any potential acts of sickness that might befall me at any moment.

But my best laid plans were not meant to be.

As I lumbered out of my twin-sized bed I stood up, hoping to miraculously shake off the ill feelings that had roused my otherwise peaceful slumber. For the tiniest millisecond, I swear to this day, I felt great. But as I took two steps to the door, that all changed.

After landing my right sock-covered foot down on my blue carpet, and having traversed a mere three feet or so toward the door and closer to the bathroom destination, it hit me like a ton of bricks. Without warning, and with no ability to control any of it, my stomach viciously expelled what felt like the entirety of my six-meals-worth of half-digested food particles from earlier in the day. I brutally vomited all over my floor, all over my shirt, and all over my previously fresh white socks, which had now become brown contaminated stockings.

After a moment of brief calm, I thought for a second I might be in the clear. But after composing myself from this appalling experience and picking myself back up (having fallen down in the same manner as one might collapse after being shot in the back of the head, execution style), I realized it was only the beginning.

I took a small, stutter-step forward but even this elementary motion was too sophisticated for my fragile state to handle, and I collapsed back down whilst unloading another mass of projectile vomit, this time unintentionally aimed at my half-opened bottom bureau drawer, which quantifiably filled up, drawing in that repulsive moment a sickeningly strange comparison to how I'd measurably filled my large-sized cup at McDonald's earlier that day with Sprite.

I'd love to say this was the end of my puking escapade, but unfortunately it was not.

Over the next six or seven hours, I continued to orally excrete the remnants of my previously devoured treats, crawling my way to the bathroom at one point in an effort to remain somewhat dignified in my futile attempt to partially mitigate the horrific mess that had already been bespattered throughout my room. But this was simply a moral win and nothing else.

My bedroom was covered in puke. My bed, my blankets, my carpet, my bureau, my shoes next to the door, my hat which had sadly fallen into a great puddle of puke, numerous books shelved close enough to the periodic discharges to get a fair amount of ricochet-like splatterings . . . even my beloved iPod, which had unwittingly been left on the floor next to my bureau, was not fortunate enough to evade the onslaught. All were drenched with the macerated debauchery from the day prior. The iPod in particular was so ensconced beneath a mammoth mound of vomit, there was no way its batteries would ever complete another circuit and power back on to transmit the joys of music, to me or anyone else again. Nope, that little eight-gigabyte baby was toast. Not even it could survive this apocalyptic catastrophe . . . And even if it could, there was no fucking way I'd ever want to use it.

Yup, I must've thrown up about 20 or 30 times during that time span, and then a good half a dozen or so more times thereafter, from the aftershocks of it all.

And adding to that momentous celebration, about an hour into the puke-fest, I got the obligatory explosive diarrhea that typically accompanies such a merry event, because God knows, if you're going to go for it, you might as well go all in. This shit-fest lasted just as long as the puking, perhaps a little longer, and I honestly couldn't tell you which was worse. They were both hell.

It got so bad at one point, I had to just lie in bed naked, with a giant black trash bag covering the lower half of my body, and another one spread open and resting beside my face. It was not uncommon during these deathly hours to both shit and puke at the same time, so this ingenious setup was both necessary and welcome.

The expulsions of both my throat and ass tapered down to a reasonable limit probably eight or so hours after they'd begun, and then maybe at like the 14 or 15-hour mark they stopped altogether. It took me a good 24 hours though before I really felt like a human being again, and then at least 72 hours before I felt somewhat normal.

After cleaning up the atomic-bombish calamity that had formerly been my room, I wondered why I'd gotten so sick in the first place. To this day I don't know exactly what it was. It could have been really, really bad food poisoning from the great assortment of shitty food I'd consumed in that 24-hour period. It could've just been a stomach flu going around that I'd been lucky enough to catch. It could've been something else entirely unknown. I'm not quite sure.

But I do know that in all my life, that was the sickest I've ever been. And what I also know, and realized a couple of days after this horrible experience, was that whatever it was, my gargantuanly excessive ingestion of unhealthy foods had certainly compounded its effects. All that junk I was forcing my body to break down and use for "nourishment" had been damaging my health in more ways than I could imagine. But I knew enough to realize I had to stop.

I slowly, over the next few months, stopped eating like the world was coming to an end, and started choosing healthier foods to replace in my diet. It wasn't an overnight shift, but slowly and surely I adopted a much healthier routine that not only kept me from frantically vomiting like that again, but also gave me more energy, better workouts at the gym, and most importantly, better and more sustained feelings of contentment and well-being throughout the day.

The diet I adopted over time supported me both mentally and physically, and absolutely had a beneficial effect on my anxiety and depression levels.

HERE'S WHAT I DID

Cut Out Fast Foods

The first thing I did was stop eating the obvious dogshit I'd been so frequently stuffing down my throat via the fast food restaurant chains. No more McDoubles and grease-laden garbage for me. (Surprisingly, this was actually rather easy to remove from my life.)

Cut Out Almost All Junk Food

I also stopped eating about 95% of the junk food I'd previously been so happy to indulge in. Cookies, muffins, candy, chocolate bars, cake, brownies, ice cream, and every other type of sugary or sweetened snack were all completely removed from my diet. The only thing I really still allowed myself to have (hence where most of that remaining 5% came from), though in moderation, were chips from time to time. They were just too delicious to give up for good.

Drink Only Water

Furthermore, I began drinking absolutely nothing but water. Throughout the day and with every meal, water was my beverage of choice—no soda, no Gatorade, no orange juice, just plain old fucking water. And I have to tell you, I loved it. To this day, the only time I ever drink anything but water is if it's some form of alcohol (I certainly enjoy a couple of beers or a few mixed drinks every now and then, just like the next guy).

Actually, on a side note, alcohol in moderation can not only be healthy for getting you to open up socially and connect with others, but recent scientific research is demonstrating an actual physiological benefit as well. One study found that alcohol can be an excellent anti-inflammatory and can assist the brain's glymphatic system in removing waste by pushing more cerebral spinal fluid (CSF) through the brain. Toxins, waste, and damaging proteins like beta-amyloid and tau (both found in Alzheimer's) are cleaned out during this process.[1] (Of course if *moderation* is not in your vocabulary you might be better off eliminating it altogether as it's probably going to get you into more trouble than good.)

Eat Better Carbs

Additionally, I cleaned up my carbohydrate intake and eliminated (or drastically minimized) a lot of the foods I'd come to realize weren't healthy. I stopped eating cereal, bagels, and pizza, and radically lowered my intake of pasta and bread. Instead, I replaced these meals with healthier carbs like veggies and fruits.

Fibrous complex carbohydrates became a staple in my diet. Vegetables like broccoli, cauliflower, spinach, kale, cucumber, lettuce, tomato, and zucchini were regularly consumed. Starchy complex carbs (oatmeal, brown rice, and potatoes) were also consumed, but not as frequently as the former, fibrous type. And natural simple carbs in myriad fruits were also eaten, and rather generously. Apples, bananas, oranges, grapes, blueberries, strawberries, and more were gulped down frequently throughout the week.

Eat Better Protein

I continued to thrive on protein, as I always had, but cleaned up its source. I eliminated the urge to mow down anything just because the protein content was listed as high on the Nutrition Facts panel, and instead started eating protein from sources far superior in terms of nutritional content. Lean proteins like chicken or turkey breast, various types of fish like salmon, sardines, cod, and tuna (which I later removed because of its high mercury content), along with beans, lentils, quinoa, steak, Greek yogurt, ground beef, and some seafood (shrimp, clams, lobster, etc.).

Protein-rich foods like these were my favorite. They became the linchpin to most of my meals and what I looked forward to tasting the most. I probably still was eating too much protein, but overall, I'd certainly improved its quality and thus my overall health.

Eat Better Fats

And lastly, in regards to macronutrients, I started eating much healthier fats. The trans fats found in all the horrible foods of my past gluttonous days disappeared. All the cookies and brownies and snacks loaded with trans fats (the unnaturally produced chemical resultant of the hydrogenation of oils) were completely detached from my diet. Also, saturated fats, previously consumed from sources like double cheeseburgers and ice cream desserts, were mostly replaced by better sources like grass-fed meats and coconut oil.

And yes, saturated fats, when sourced from the right foods, can absolutely be healthy for you. Numerous modern studies reveal that the dogma purported for the majority of the 20th century on all saturated fats is just simply not true.[2]

Along with cutting out trans and optimizing my saturated fats, I started eating a ton of healthy polyunsaturated and monounsaturated fats. For my polyunsaturated foods I ate things like fish (omega-3's), walnuts, sunflower seeds, and flax seeds; for my monounsaturated foods it became almonds, avocados, peanuts, hazelnuts, and olive oil.

Smaller Meal Sizes

Perhaps most importantly, I began to eat more proportional meal sizes, appropriate to that of a human being. Although I still desired a large, muscularly-defined frame, I no longer craved it, nor would I risk my health in trying to achieve it. I kept my meals in greater balance, and overall dramatically lowered the burden on my digestive system.

I still maintained a relatively high protein intake, but as I mentioned, their profile came from better sources, and so did my carbs and fats. And instead of having a roller-coaster-like consumption of disproportionate amounts of these macronutrients, I refined their intake and leveled them out.

So instead of dropping in say 1500–2000 calories in one voracious sitting, arbitrarily throughout the day, I was spacing it out to something like 400–600 calories per meal, over four to six meals every three or four hours. This way I still got my protein fix for my muscle-building goals, but my blood sugar wasn't skyrocketing (and then plummeting), my digestive system wasn't being torched, and my inflammation wasn't soaring through the roof. Overall, it was a pretty happy medium.

WHAT THIS DID FOR MY HEALTH

By adjusting my diet in this manner I noticed a change almost immediately. I stopped having gas from all the unhealthy crap I was no longer forcing myself to wolf down every day. My energy increased noticeably, and seemed to steady itself more throughout the day. I wasn't perpetually walking around bloated. I wasn't getting random headaches from consuming poor quality foods loaded with additives, artificial sweeteners, and neurotoxins (like MSG). I leaned out in a good way, while still keeping my muscle size and tone. And most importantly, my mental state improved dramatically. My depression was noticeably lowered and my feelings of general anxiousness all but disappeared for good.

What I'd effectively done was replace harmful foods (for the most part anyway; I didn't get unbearably strict to the point where I wouldn't be able to maintain this new diet) with beneficial ones that promoted a nourished brain, and consequently a healthier mind.

HOW I EAT NOW

Taking into account the science I've learned over the years and the wisdom I've acquired, I now eat even healthier than I did when I first began making changes to my diet way back when. Even though I saw great results by taking out the basic evils, like shitty fast food and soda, I've since learned a lot more about tightening things up even further.

Anxiety and depression have been gone for many years, but my overall sense of contentment and enjoyment of life have continued to grow with time. I attribute this in large part to the improvements in my diet and my enduring self-mastery of health.

Don't get me wrong; I cheat from time to time. I'm neither a saint nor a health-freak by any means. I definitely still wallow in the occasional restaurant cheeseburger or pizza, but overall, I maintain a pretty healthy diet.

At the time of this writing I still mainly practice a Zone-like diet (eating balanced, smaller-portioned meals, every two and a half to four hours). I'd say about 50% of my meals come from carbs, 30% from protein, and 20% from fats.

Most of my carbs come from healthy veggies like broccoli, cucumbers, cabbage, carrots, spinach, cauliflower, cilantro, lettuce, or tomatoes (and sometimes even the disgusting but ridiculously healthy consumption of kale). Along with the veggies, I opt for brown rice, white rice, potatoes, or quinoa, though in reasonable amounts, and yes, I currently still revel in the deliciousness of whole wheat bread (my kryptonite) though this too may change very soon as I'm going to test my own abstinence from wheat[3] and dairy[4] soon,

The Antidepressant Diet

considering all the research against their consumption. Lastly, I still love my fruit. Blueberries, strawberries, apples, grapes, raisins, peaches, oranges, and bananas, are all consumed regularly and copiously.

My proteins come from a variety of sources, but generally from chicken, steak, beans, lentils, fish, shellfish, mixed nuts like almonds, cashews, and peanuts, as well as Greek yogurt (but again this may be gone when dairy goes) and a number of other household foods that offer solid nutritional value.

My fat intake is a mixture of all the good saturated, polyunsaturated, and monounsaturated fats I talked about earlier. I get most of the good saturated fats from my beloved meats and coconut oil. My polyunsaturated fats come from my ingestion of fish like salmon, sardines, and mackerel, along with sunflower seeds, walnuts, and other mixed nuts and seeds. And my monounsaturated fats primarily come from cooking with olive oil, and eating almonds, avocados, peanuts, hazelnuts, pecans, pumpkin seeds, and all the others that give me that healthy dose of good fat my body craves.

Right now, as I revealed earlier, I try to focus on eating fairly healthy the overwhelming majority of the time (like 95% of the time) but do allow myself to have some fun too. There's a balance to this diet thing, like anything else in life. And I find that people who always have to be so strict with everything are typically some of the most miserable and unhappy people around. I choose not to be one of them.

Take care of yourself by eating healthy, but indulge and have some goddamn fun sometimes too. Sure avocados, one of the healthiest foods you can eat, can taste great most of the time. But so can a brownie-infused ice cream fucking sundae. Enjoy one every now and then.

CONCLUSION

Diet plays a massive role in the way we feel. You hear it all the time, but it's true: "You are what you eat." As the great philosopher Hippocrates so eloquently noted, "Let thy food be thy medicine and thy medicine be thy food."

From energy fueling your life, to the neurotransmitters being created in your brain, to the vitamins and minerals involved in so many cellular processes, to the balancing of our gut microbiome, and so much more. Food is at the center of it all.

The cleaner you eat, the better you will feel. It's really that simple. Food can either harm you or help you. It's up to you to decide which.

For me, the choice is quite clear. Yeah, I'll occasionally wolf down a greasy cheeseburger and fries, but most of my days I'm content eating cauliflower and steak.

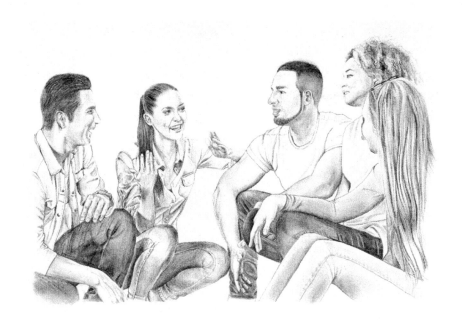

Chapter Twenty-Two
The Power of Community

I looked up at the clock every couple of minutes as I halfheartedly separated the meats, the bread, the produce, and all the other perishable shit from the non-perishable fuckery strewn out before me. *This shift is draaaaaaaagging,* I thought to myself. *I can't wait to get the fuck out of here.*

"Thanks," I managed to mumble back to a customer as she walked by and categorically caught me off guard by saying, "Thanks so much," and adding in, "Have a great day," smiling all the while and revealing a genuine kindness and sincerity not found in most. *Wow, do I suck,* I thought. *That lady was actually really nice and I couldn't even smile or think of anything polite to say back.*

I carried on, separating more endless piles of groceries for people I didn't give a shit about, counting the ticks on the clock, hoping that somehow they'd speed up. But of course they didn't. And after some further time passed I turned my frustration onto the checker, the one ringing in and sliding all of this grueling work down to me.

She's so ugly, and boring. Why doesn't she talk? If she's going to be that fucking ugly and out of shape, she should at least get good at talking to people. She hasn't said anything all day and she's boring me to fucking death! She only talks to the stupid customers when they come in line. Oh man I can't wait to get the fuck out of here . . .

This was the norm, a pretty standard day in my life for the first few months of my occupational tenure at Shaw's Supermarkets, a big supermarket chain in the Northeast region of America. I hated it there, and would incessantly torture myself throughout the entire shift with internal dialogues of hatred directed towards customers, co-workers . . . and myself.

Yup, I was a complete asshole for the first several months of my grocery-store career. But this vitriol came to an end, however, when one day, in the midst of my personal transformational period of beating anxiety and starting to have my way with depression, I decided to try something different.

A NOVEL IDEA

During my epic quest for cerebral salvation I'd unexceptionally come across a bit of humdrum on the power of connecting with others and regularly socializing to ward away depression. Naturally, assuming it was as stupid as it sounded, I waved it off as nonsense and carried on searching for *real* help. (Indeed it was quite similar in many ways to the *Panic Away* reaction I'd had.)

But I guess I must have stored that thought in some infinitesimal brain cell in the back of my mind, because one day it dawned on me, out of the blue. With my newfound outlook on life and my wins starting to build upon one another, I was now seeing things in a more positive and progressive light. I remember just deciding, one day at work, in the middle of some additional ire clandestinely directed at another co-worker, that I was going to start trying to be nicer, and actually (as much as I knew it would suck) more social. *What the hell, I've got nothing to lose.*

I knew I wasn't a bad person, but it seemed like acting the way I was acting at work was turning me into one. I hated going there and resented my time being wasted. I felt like I was slaving away for just a few bucks and could be doing much more productive things with my time. But I needed the job, and in the back of my mind I knew this new technique might actually help my depression, or at least my happiness in some regard.

So from that point forward I tried a new approach.

ENTER MR. SOCIAL

You have to understand something about me. I'm a diehard introvert through-and-through. I'm one of those oddballs who loves spending a good amount of his day alone, because it charges me up. I love reading books, researching things, playing guitar, learning a new skill, writing, listening to music—all very solo acts. Trust me, it's not that I'm anti-social (not now, anyway); I love going out and partying, giving speeches, hanging out with friends, and making people laugh, and even being the center of attention in the right room. In fact, these are the moments I truly live for as they awaken the best parts of my soul.

However, that said, I'm naturally someone who charges up best when alone. It's just in my DNA. Spending time by myself allows me to get energized and balances the neurotransmitters and other physiological components in my body, allowing me to be at my best each day.

I love shooting the shit with friends and cracking jokes, just don't expect me to do that all day. I'll be fucking wiped and transformed into a character straight out of *The Walking Dead* by the end of it.

I say all this because as a natural, sovereign introvert, I've had the unfortunate predisposition to be absolutely fucking horrible in social situations. And I lived up to this penchant admirably for the first 17 years or so of my life. I sucked, really, really bad.

But like I said, I decided to at least try to change, and not be so socially awkward, if not downright bizarre, anymore.

I started off small, just talking to the girls who cashiered for me while I bagged. It was small talk, albeit nail-scratchingly painful small talk: asking them how their day was going, how school had been, their plans for the weekend, that kind of shit. It took some getting used to, but eventually the small talk became less and less awkward, and then more and more enjoyable. The more I practiced it, the more I got better at it.

Soon I was expanding my horizons and talking to the customers standing in line. Again, just small talk stuff about their day, the upcoming weather forecast, and plans for the weekend (that was clearly my go-to). Simple, basic, fairly fucking easy chatter. Nothing too complex, but it didn't have to be.

After a few months of progressively enhancing my social prowess, I started to notice how much I actually began to look forward to my days at work, as well as how much it was helping with my

The Power of Community

depression. I was feeling less alone and more fulfilled throughout the week, almost like I'd gotten a sense that I'd belonged. And this feeling only increased the more I socialized with others.

A little while later I began talking to *everyone* and got really good at doing so. I'd talk to the produce ladies, the deli workers, the fish guy, the meat guy, the teenagers my age who stocked the shelves, the service desk girls, the florist, all the cashiers up front, even my supervisors and the store manager (who took a particular liking to me and later became a great friend).

I'd stroll about and make the rounds during my shift, chatting up everybody I came across, and genuinely having great conversations with them. (Of course this meant doing less actual bagging work, which I was all too pleased to allow.) And nobody seemed to mind.

Even the supervisors and manager, after a while, stopped saying anything with regard to a blatant drop-off in bagging productivity, simply because they enjoyed my company and enjoyed shooting the shit with me. Yes, it was far easier for them to have some other guy, like the guy I used to be, pick up my slack while they chatted away with me and had a few good laughs.

I say all this for two reasons: One, it's absolutely one hundred percent true. And two, because it clearly exemplifies the complete 180 I'd taken in a matter of just a few months of working there. I'd gone from being a soul-sucking, miserable, quiet douchebag to a make-you-laugh and have-a-great-day-at-work kind of guy.

I say this in all modesty: People fucking loved me at that place.

And I loved working there.

But more importantly, it'd helped me in a profound way with my depression. It was one of the biggest missing pieces to the depression puzzle, one that up until that point I'd overlooked. But when I found it and really worked on it, it came together brilliantly.

THE POWER OF CONNECTION

Numerous scientific papers have demonstrated the intimate relationship between loneliness and depression,[1] and several more studies have identified the similar genes at play explaining why the two are so closely tied.[2]

One study conducted in 2001 on a diverse subset of individuals, including college students, the elderly, and psychiatric patients, confirmed the strong correlation between loneliness and suicidal ideation and actual attempts at suicide.[3] Additionally, as the degree of loneliness increased in these individuals, the prevalence for suicidal tendencies did so too.

Simply put: Being lonely makes us unhappy.

We humans crave social connection, *real* social connection that is, and when we don't have it, we're missing out on a crucial part of what makes us complete. You can do everything else right, work on yourself, and fix all your internal problems, but at the end of the day, if you're lonely, you're always going to have some depression in your life. You're always going to be incomplete.

Work on yourself as much as possible, but don't forget to take time out of your day to connect with others. It can be just as important as the self-work you do alone. Sometimes, it's even more important.

CHATTING PEOPLE UP

It might sound lame, but chatting people up is one of the healthiest things you can do. It's the best way to beat social isolation and stave off the leering effects of a lurking depressive state.

Talk to people everywhere and anywhere you go, and make sure you actually go out every day and place yourself into social situations (especially if you don't have the good fortune to work with an abundance of people). Converse with people on the train, the bus, walking down the street, at the grocery store, gym, bar, class, park, mall, nightclub, hotel, airport, post office—anywhere you go.

Become more of a social guy and embrace the intrinsic need to connect with others. Practice this skill and practice it often. In the 21st century and beyond it's not going to take much to get good at it. Believe me, this is a dying skill, so with a little effort you're going to stick out and really be someone people look to and want to socialize with.

Also, another great way to start connecting with people, aside from just chatting them up as you randomly come across them, would be to join some kind of group, class, club, team, gym, Meetup, organization like Toastmasters, or any other get-together where people bond collectively and share a common interest.

This is the perfect way to socialize with others even further and cultivate stronger relationships whilst getting you out of your house and out of your head. I couldn't recommend these types of activities any more highly. They are fucking awesome for getting you to enjoy your life by spending it with others, and consequently beat the hell out of your loneliness and depression.

One fairly recent research paper published in the *Journal of Experimental Social Psychology*, examining the effects of social isolation in various studies,[4] concluded: "People may search for meaning in many places. The current results suggest, however, that people find meaning from each other. Across four studies, we found that when belongingness needs are threatened—either by an instance of social rejection or ongoing feelings of loneliness—people perceive less meaning in their lives compared to when belongingness needs are met."

The power of connecting with others is real. It can help you obliterate your depression and make you feel more complete as a human being.

Beat back your depression today by becoming your own Mr. Social.

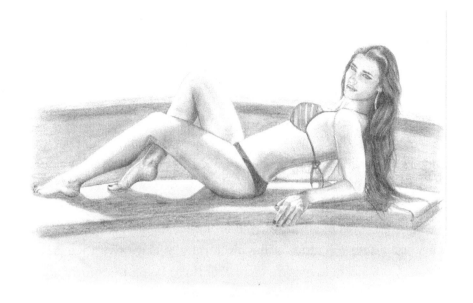

Chapter Twenty-Three
Having a Purpose

She was absolutely stunning.

Long black hair, dark brown eyes, a smile that accentuated her exotic facial symmetry, and a body that would turn even the most beautiful Hollywood starlet Incredible-Hulkishly green with envy.

I noticed her the instant she walked in, but instinctively I leaned on the darkish tint of my aviator sunglasses to conceal my visual fixation.

I was blown away.

She was easily the most beautiful woman I'd ever seen in my entire life up until that point. With every step she took she attracted the unbridled attention of more and more men, like a colossal super-magnet sucking up paper clips. As she seductively sauntered her way over to the pool's clear blue water, the sun glistened down on her olive skin, radiating her natural beauty even further and reaffirming my belief of her unworldly magnificence.

Like a kid praying to God for a miracle, every single man in that poolside gathering was wishing for the exact same thing in that moment. Smacks from wives be damned, every husband with a pulse wanted this Italian goddess to unrobe and step in. And so did every other boy above the age of seven and every grandfather below the age of 90. We were all in it together, like a stadium full of Red Sox fans hoping for a bottom of the ninth rally at Fenway. "Take, it, off. Take, it, off. Take, it, off." A silent chant was being murmured by us all.

And then she delivered.

As if her level of splendid beauty was not jaw-dropping enough, the proverbial cherry on top tipped (and possibly broke) the scale of attractiveness in her favor even further, in the form of her now nearly naked and exposed body.

She had the perfect hourglass waist-to-hip ratio, tightly toned legs, and a soft elegance to her perfect skin, and oh yeah, a nice pair of double-D breasts and a Jennifer-Lopez-like bum.

I was visibly floored. *What a fucking babe!* I thought to myself, as my buddy had just taken a nap moments before, and unfortunately missed out on this unbelievably generous gift from our Lord and Savior.

"She is so fuckin' gorgeous. I have to go talk to her," I whispered aloud to no one.

Having a Purpose

But then I considered it for a moment and decided to wait a couple of minutes, as I didn't want to scare her away.

And good thinking.

I sat back for about 10 minutes, playing it cool and becoming best friends with my sunglasses. I hid my infatuation like a champ, and acted as if my phone were more important than this walking *Playboy* model just a couple dozen feet away. In those 10 minutes, three different guys, who were all clearly delusional, went up and tried hitting on her. Each one of them got a kind but firm equivalent of the "talk-to-the-hand" rejection. And I giggled to myself each time.

After maybe five more minutes, 10 at the most, I decided it was time to make my move.

By now the hysteria had kind of died down and every wife and girlfriend in the vicinity had reeled her man back in and given him an earful to boot. The attention of the pool's occupants was no longer solely focused on her, at least not as blatantly as before, though I'm sure many guys were playing the same sunglasses game I was. Either way, I got up and confidently sauntered over to the pool too, although I doubt I had the same appeal that she did.

Instead of beelining it toward my target, however, I went in using the stairs about 20 feet away from her. I'd watched and learned from the failures of those three brave but foolish men, and wasn't going to make the same mistake. No, this required infinitely more finesse.

You see, what I'd picked up on, while most of the other men were too busy staring at her boobs, was that she'd quietly acknowledged a group of people on the other end of the pool when she'd first stepped in. It was very slight, and easy to miss, but she'd given the tiniest nod and revealed the faintest hint of a smile to a group of seven or eight pool occupants.

And judging by the dark black hair, the olive skin, and the relative similarities in facial structure they all possessed, they were almost certainly her family. I counted and surmised the possible relations of each person, going right down the line using their appearance: *That's gotta' be her father . . . that's her mother . . . probably her uncle and aunt . . . maybe a couple brothers . . . and that former babe, that's gotta' be another aunt, or maybe an older female cousin or a much older sister . . .*

No boyfriend or husband was spotted, so I knew I was good, and I immediately came up with a calculated strategy that Bobby Fischer himself would've been proud of.

MY GENIUS PLAN

A minute or two after I went into the water, I put my newly acquired social skills to work.

By now it'd been about a year or so of working at Shaw's and practicing my conversational proficiency, and I could strike up a high-quality chat with literally *anyone*. I was really that good at it. So naturally, instead of going right for this Mediterranean bombshell, I went for her family.

I began shooting the shit with them after tossing back a ball they'd been passing around wildly like some sort of Ancient Roman hot potato. I asked what they were playing and a couple of them responded back and said it was . . . well, I forget actually what they called it. But after describing it to me and after I'd examined it more closely for another minute, the game was essentially Taps, where you throw (or tap) the ball to someone else while in mid-air, and that person has to jump up and catch and throw the ball back to someone else, also in mid-air, or else be eliminated from the game.

Long story short, I get in on the game.

Having a Purpose

I start playing with this Italian family and laughing and cracking jokes, and we have a good time. We're playing for like 15 minutes or so, and I periodically, and ever so subtly, peripherally glance over at the missing family member with the knockout body and beautiful face.

She's watching us.

After a few more rounds of this game, the action kind of dies down, and though I was genuinely enjoying myself, I'm kind of happy it does.

A few of them exit the pool and we exchange some pleasantries, while a couple of the others kind of hang around and ask if I want to keep playing. I very thoughtfully decline and sort of swim away as if I'd been passing by the whole time, nonchalantly toing and froing my way around this massive pool.

And then I casually paddle my way toward the bombshell, who's now in the water herself, and ask her what I already know the answer to. "Is that your family I was just playing Taps with?" I say, with a slight smirk on my face.

"Yeah," Miss Universe responds back. "How'd you know?"

"I just figured you guys kind of all looked alike, and I noticed you were watching us play (plus I'd quietly asked the younger brother, during one of the game's breaks when the ball went sailing in her relative direction)."

"Yeah we're on vacation here," she replied. "We always get together and go on one family vacation every year, even now that we're all getting older."

"Oh that's cool. I like that," I replied, in a cool and collected tone of voice. "Yeah, I'm here on vacation too. I'm here with my buddy (I pointed to him, passed out on the beach chair nearby), but he had a rough night last night so he's in full recovery mode. I don't know when he'll be alive again." She laughed. "You're funny. Where are you guys from?"

And from there we hit it off, and the rest, as they say, is history.

Needless to say, I ended up hooking up with Miss Universe the next day and had one of the best days of my life.

One day many, many years from now, when I die and meet God at the gates of heaven, I'll undoubtedly replay the major moments of my life, both excellent and awful. And when this magical 24-hour segment of my life inevitably comes up in the highlight reel, I have absolutely no doubt at this point in time God will pause the apparitional film and say, "Wow! Well done my son. Well fucking done, indeed."

FINDING MY PURPOSE

You may be wondering why I've just described this little anecdote about hooking up with a beautiful girl while on vacation with a drunken buddy.

So let me explain.

It was around this time that I'd begun to really find myself and become happy again. I'd gotten past my problems with anxiety, ended all my panic attacks, and really gotten a hold of my depression. I was motivated again and optimistic about my future for the first time in years.

Through a combination of the different strategies we've covered earlier, I'd managed to completely change my life around. And one of

Having a Purpose

the final and most critical components to this success was the discovery of my purpose.

After getting good with socializing and connecting with people, naturally, I realized I wanted to get better with women. I loved chatting up women in the grocery store and flirting with the girls working on the registers, but I still didn't know how to start dating them.

So with a feeling of finally being back to my normal self, and with this newfound appreciation for self-improvement, I embarked on my newest quest: How to get good with women.

And this became my new purpose in life.

You have to understand, for someone who had gone 18 years of his life being a virgin, and who couldn't buy a date in high school, being able to date women at this point in time was a big deal for me. No, actually, it was a HUGE fucking deal, and something I desperately wanted to figure out.

So with anxiety and depression confidently under my belt, I took on the next challenge with a belief that I could and would be successful.

And just like my research in finding the solutions to my mental health problems, I hit the literature like a madman. I researched, studied, read, and watched everything I could find. Some of it good, some of it bad, and some of it downright ugly. But like before, I weeded out a lot of things that didn't resonate with me, and then tested the ones that did. And through a lot of trial and tribulation and times of me just looking like a complete moron, I was slowly able to put things together and learn how to attract the opposite sex.

And this was my passion.

As before, I became obsessed with mastering this area of my life and dedicated all of my free time into my improvement here. I'd spend almost every day, researching different dating strategies and techniques and listening to what the best dating coaches in the world had to offer in terms of meeting, attracting, and getting women to go out with you. I'd even regularly go out and approach women in public, working on my social aptitude, and picking up phone numbers in the process.

I sucked horribly at first and embarrassed myself many times over. I'm talking countless rejections, denials, humiliations, failures, and painfully awkward moments that would make Helen Keller herself cringe in disgust. But I stuck with it, and over the course of a few months, between talking to women when I went out, flirting with them at work, hanging around new friends who were good with girls, and learning key psychological and practical dating techniques from the dating coaches I studied online, I was able to slowly get better.

And then, after several more months of this, I started to get *really* good.

It was during this time that I'd met that Italian goddess while on vacation with my intoxicated friend. So at this point, it had become customary for me to go up and talk to her, even if she was the sexiest woman I'd ever laid eyes on. I had a purpose, and although I was petrified inside and would never in a million years have been able to walk up and pull that off before, I'd become motivated to follow through because of my inner mission. I was possessed in a sense to push myself and live out that purpose, even if it scared the hell out of me.

It's like one of *The Blues Brothers* used to say, "We're on a mission from God."

Having a Purpose

That's how I felt with my purpose, except it was less about God and more about my soul. My soul was calling for something to drive me, and at that point in time it was women.

UNDERSTANDING PURPOSE

For the next few years, getting good with women became the focal point of my purpose.

During that time I became exceptionally adept at wooing them. I don't want to sound egotistical, though it's hard to sound like you're not trying to boast in discussions of matters such as this, but I pretty much mastered the ability to court women.

Not to say I could attract and date any woman I came across in life, because I fucking couldn't, but thanks to this phase of relational life training, I now possess the ability to attract the highest quality of women on this planet. I'm talking women like the one I described earlier, who literally make every man in any room salivate and question his commitment to wedlock.

Do I still get rejected by beautiful women? Absolutely (and sometimes, by not-so-beautiful women too). But do I also now have the skill necessary to date them? You bet your ass I do.

Coming from a guy who got rejected copious times over in high school and never had a prom date, it's certainly been a gigantic leap. And it's not like I magically grew a foot taller or packed on 50 pounds of muscle either; I'm exactly the same short and skinny dude I was before, just a little older, and yes, much wiser.

But again, I'm not here to toot my own pontifical horn. I hate arrogant guys who go on and on about how much they've accomplished and how great they are. They sound like complete dickheads.

I merely want to emphasize just how fucking shitty my dating life was before, and how with some effort and determination, I was able to dramatically improve it thereafter. (By the way, anyone can do this too. I'm not special or unique here. Becoming more appealing to the opposite sex and cultivating the ability to attract the highest level of women, or men for that matter, is an altogether simple and replicable process.)

This was my purpose during that time. It motivated me and drove me into getting excited about life. And most importantly, it kept my depression from coming back.

Having a purpose is key to energizing your day. It invigorates your mind and spirit, and gets you to wake up and jump the fuck out of bed every morning because you can't wait to get closer to fulfilling your goals. It's truly what life's all about.

A number of studies have demonstrated the clear link between having a sense of purpose and having a higher quality of life.[1] Moreover, several additional studies have confirmed the ability of individuals who have a strong sense of purpose to be able to emotionally handle setbacks, traumas, and other negative stimuli that inevitably pop up in life.[2] In short, purposeful people are far more resilient.

At its finest, life's a series of goal-chasing, soul-filling, and success-achieving moments of growth and bliss, fused into one long journey of self-discovery. And your purpose fuels it all.

MANY PURPOSES

You can, and most likely will, have multiple purposes throughout your life. As you evolve and time passes on your journey, you'll learn and become passionate about many diverse things. You'll reach the pinnacle of one goal and decide to focus on another, or you'll evolve as a person and realize your purpose has progressed into something else entirely. Or you'll meet someone or have children, or any one of life's infinite unpredictabilities will steer you in another direction completely, and you'll be forced to pivot and come up with a new purpose once again.

Purposes come and go; sometimes they last years, sometimes they last months. Their duration isn't important. But the fact you have them is. We all need to feel like our lives matter. Having a purpose gives us that meaning.

My purpose has reshaped itself several times over the years. Beginning with my first articulated one beating my anxiety and depression, it subsequently evolved into getting better with women and becoming a more confident man. Then it was becoming a world-class life coach, then it shifted into running Elite Man Magazine and the Elite Man Podcast, then it went to successfully operating Elite Life Nutrition. Today, it's writing this book. Tomorrow it will likely transform into something else.

I should note, however, that I still spend a great deal of time on many of the abovementioned purposes. But I now consider them to be more like passions, as opposed to a specific purpose (which I define to be your main fucking reason for living at the present moment).

For instance, I still love running the magazine and the podcast, but those are now just some of my passions (formerly each had been my main purpose at varying points in time). My sole purpose at this current moment, and what gets me fired the fuck up each morning, is writing this epic tome. Why? Because I know it's going to help millions of people for years to come.

I don't dedicate hours and hours out of every day because I enjoy writing. Although it's kind of fun, there's a ton of other shit I can think of that I'd much rather be doing. No, I devote my time to this vessel because I'm excited about what it will bring. It's been my goal to share my story and my techniques for beating anxiety and depression, and for gaining true confidence in one's own life, for quite some time. And when I formulated the concept for this book, I suddenly felt invigorated, more than I'd already been, to go through with it and make this happen.

So I'm jumping out of bed every morning, and I can't wait to see this on bookshelves everywhere. I also can't wait to hold the finished copy in my hand. I'm beyond excited for this. And that's my current purpose.

Am I worried that when I finish this book I'll suddenly have no purpose again and may perhaps collapse back into a pit of despair and misery? Absolutely not.

I have other projects already in mind: Things that I can't wait to tackle at some point down the road. Novel goals and ideas that I will adopt and make into my new purposes all over again. Right now I'm loving this current purpose in my life, but I know there are so many others I can't wait to take on as well.

So yes my purpose is ever-evolving and your purpose will be too. Don't get hung up on trying to figure out a perfect reason for living, because that's not what this is about. It's about finding something, *anything* really, that gets you excited again. A goal that you feel utterly compelled to complete. Choose one and then get to completing it. Don't waste any more time; having a reason to jump out of bed every morning is one of the easiest ways to get over your depression—and keep it from coming back.

HOW TO FIND YOUR PURPOSE

So how do you find your purpose and get unbelievably passionate about your life again?

Having a Purpose

Well, to keep things simple, I've narrowed this process into three easy-to-follow, but incredibly effective steps. Here they are.

1. SELF-REFLECT ON YOUR PASSIONS

It's easy to get lost in the shuffle of life. To grow older and forget about the things you love doing. Job, kids, bills, health, stress, money, friends, politics . . . so many worries flood our minds on a day-to-day basis, dominating our thoughts and shaping our focus.

We get caught up in the grind and overlook our desires, and needs, to do what we enjoy. We ignore our heart's innate hankering to find and do more of what we love. And this leads to so much unrest and unhappiness.

Without knowing what you love, what you enjoy, and what you're passionate about, life becomes one big monotonous blah. You get stuck on autopilot, just sort of going through the motions and pretending to feel alive.

Fuck that.

If that's how you want to live life, go watch TV. You shouldn't be reading, and you definitely shouldn't be reading this book.

No, that's the shitty, old-school way of living. To act like you're happy and act like things are good, when inside you're crumbling.

To snap yourself out of this, you really need to focus on what makes you happy. You must concentrate on what gets you excited, I mean *truly* excited about life. Not fleeting shots of dopaminergic chemicals when two transgender women duke it out on a *Jerry Springer* rerun, but *really* excited, as when you are perfecting a new skill or taking up a novel hobby you've always wanted to try.

Take a long hard look at your passions. Really take a deep-dive into what you love doing in life and what gets you excited. And don't tell me nothing does, because if that's the case you just aren't rattling your brain hard enough (or you need to get out of your head and start experiencing a hell of a lot more in life).

Ask yourself questions, like: "What are my favorite hobbies? When do I feel most alive? What challenge or activity have I always wanted to try? How can I make an impact in the world? How can I help others and be fulfilled? How can I help myself? What areas of my life do I want to truly master? What do I want to achieve in the next two years, five years, 20 years? What do I want my legacy to be one day when it's all said and done?"

Questions like these and similar ones get you thinking about what really matters to you. They get you to open up and expand your thoughts into focusing on meaningful and often overlooked subjects. Most importantly, they get you to find some really critical answers to what your purpose is going to be.

I recommend jotting down these questions on a notebook and going to town on your answers. Feel free to go off on various tangents and pioneeringly traverse into areas of specific interest when you do this. There are no rules here, it's simply a method for you to explore your true desires.

By the time you're done, you'll have a good idea of a few of the areas you'll want to focus on. You'll have better clarity on what your passions are, and what your purpose may be. And you'll probably have a number of things jumping out at you, gently tugging you in one direction or another. This is a good thing.

It's better to have an abundance of passions, than no passions at all.

But I suggest focusing on the one thing that's giving you the strongest pull, right now, at least for the moment. Whatever sticks out to you as being the one thing you absolutely feel a burning desire to go forward with, that's the passion you want to focus on and convert into your purpose.

2. COMMIT TO YOUR PURPOSE

Whether you've pondered out passions you've already tried before and know you love, or whether you've conjured up ideas of new things you think you'll love and that get you excited when you think about trying them, the first brainstorming exercise is effective in getting the ball rolling.

The next step to figuring out your purpose, however, is committing to it.

Commit to creating a realistic but challenging goal: achieving, living up to, maybe even perfecting your purpose for a certain amount of time. Make this your only mission. If it's something you've tried before, great. Your commitment to its success should be very straightforward and concrete. If, however, you haven't tried your passion yet, but have an idea it might become something you absolutely fall in love with, at the very least, commit to following through on trying it out for a certain amount of time.

Say you have a passion for bodybuilding, and you've always wanted to do it competitively. Commit to signing up for six months of dieting and training, and taking it one hundred percent seriously. Make this your purpose for the next half year (you can decide to keep going of course beyond that span if you want), and then stick with it.

By setting a timeline and dedicating yourself to its completion, you're infinitely more likely to see it through, and consequently reap greater gain. So, it's an essential component to the commitment process.

But as far as the timespan itself, it's totally arbitrary. Your purpose-driven goals can be in increments of three months or six, a year or two, even 10 years . . . however long you want them to be. Just understand that when you set a goal, you should set it with absolute conviction that you will finish it and commit to the timeframe you have chosen. Don't break promises with yourself.

Conversely, if you're trying out a new passion, commit to the goal of just seeing it through for a certain amount of time, before committing to fully making it your purpose. You can consider this a trial period of sorts. If you've always wanted to try out say, a dance class, and you think you'll really love dancing, but aren't completely sure, commit to at least taking a new dance class for a month, twice a week, and seeing how it goes.

You might fall in love with it right away and know it's right for you; in which case you can immediately convert this into a longer-term, purpose-led goal of achieving some level of rhythmic excellence within it. Or, you might realize it's not quite what you expected, in this case you can shift to the next passion that popped out from your brainstorming session and try that instead. And so on, until you find your next true purpose.

Once more, passions and purposes are transient. Don't get hung up on the commitment or the decision to choose any particular one. Just pick something and commit to either testing it out, or better yet, making it happen.

Which brings us to the next and most important step.

3. TAKE ACTION

It's one thing to reflect on your passions and commit to achieving them. It's another thing entirely to take action and actually achieve them.

Having a Purpose

Without action, your ideas, your goals, your beliefs, your fucking life itself . . . it's all just philosophical abstract. It means nothing. Action is the only thing that makes your life have meaning.

Once you define your purpose and commit to fulfilling it, you need to take action every single day toward making that purpose a reality. And I do mean every, single, day.

Don't take this lightly. When you figure out what your purpose is, your true meaning in life, move the needle closer and closer to realizing that purpose every day. This will keep you motivated and excited about life, and give you something to look forward to each day.

Research, study, watch videos, buy programs, courses, books, get mentors, listen to podcasts (I hear that Elite Man Podcast one is pretty epic), go to conferences, go to Meetups, take classes, follow and listen to those who've already done what you want to, practice, put in the time, effort, and energy necessary, and do everything possible to make your goal a success.

By doing all of this your purpose has no choice but to succeed, and all the while, just the actions of going forth with your effort to achieve your purpose will obliterate any residual depression you might harbor.

PURPOSE AND HAPPINESS

As humans we thrive on having a mission to take care of. It gives us a reason for living.

It's why so many people who retire after spending their whole lives doing a particular job drop dead a week after hanging it up; they have no more purpose in life. It's why a widowed spouse sporadically dies of natural causes, a few days after her husband of

50 years dies from a losing bout with cancer. It's why people who sit at home and do nothing but eat bonbons and channel surf are some of the most depressed people on the planet, despite typically living in some of the most developed and supposedly happy countries on Earth.

Purpose is directly tied to happiness. Without purpose, we're mindless sheep, brainwashing our days away and robotically bahing to the cues of a society that couldn't care less about our well-being.

Don't be a sheep.

And definitely don't be a bonbon eater, lounging back and getting fat while your mind goes to waste. Once you have found your purpose, go out and do everything you can to fucking achieve it. Your happiness literally depends on it.

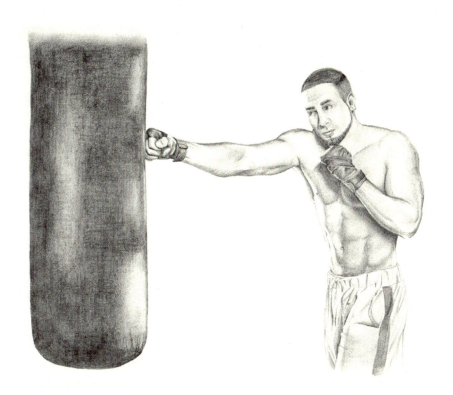

Chapter Twenty-Four
Loving Yourself

Boom!

"That's fuckin' nothing," I said aloud, as I pushed harder.

Wham!

"Quit being a pussy!" I yelled in defiance, this time louder. And pushed even harder.

Thuwump!

The 80-pound heavy bag came soaring back down, thanks to the velocity of my thrust and the basic principles of physics, smashing directly into my face just as I'd wanted, this time rattling my brain.

"That aint' shit," I yelled out loud, but inside I knew it was.

That was all for today. I knew that last one might've been a little too much.

I'd been in the midst of my boxing training, and to toughen up my chin I'd been hitting myself in the face with this massive punching bag I had out in my garage. I was 16 at the time and my one goal in life was to become a world-champion fighter. I thought it was my one true path to happiness.

Oh, how unbelievably mistaken I was.

I was training four to six hours a day at my house and at a boxing gym I went to at the time. I'd read multiple books on top professional boxers and adopted many of their training routines as closely as possible. That four to six hours was something all the greats did, and so it became a must for me.

I'd jump rope for a half hour straight, run about six miles every day, hit the heavy bag and speed bag for several hours, then finally cap it all off with some shadow-boxing for a half hour or so more.

Before I started sparring with other fighters at the gym, I practiced at home with my trusted heavy bag, just to make sure I could take a shot.

I'd swing the bag up as high as the swivel would allow, then let gravity take over as the brute beast would come soaring back down to earth, plowing into my young and naïve face. I'd repeat this process over and over, mimicking the hits that a real boxer might throw at me, doing my best to simulate an actual fight.

Sometimes I'd take a whole three-minute round of heavy bag work and just let the bag smash into various parts of my head: my nose, my chin, the side of my head, my eyes, my forehead. I'd let this son of a bitch whack me all over, in what I foolishly believed at the time to be a strengthening of my ability to take a punch. (In actuality, it weakened it.)

Yes that heavy bag and I had many moonlight dances, but unfortunately it never quite worked out the way I intended. By the end of our affair, I was left heartbroken and modestly brain damaged.

MY SELF HATRED

Looking back at those days now I feel saddened.

I don't regret them really (more accurately, I don't dwell on them), but I do wish I'd never done those things. Let's just say if I had a time machine, that punching bag and I would've never had such an intimate relationship. (Nor would boxing and me, for that matter.)

Pounding myself in the face repeatedly, multiple days out of the week, for months on end, is certainly one of the stupidest things I've ever done. But again, I can't dwell on the mistakes of the past and the excessively misguided ideations of a troubled young man. I can only focus on now and on improving the future, which is what I do. And thankfully I've been pretty good at that.

But thinking about this moment now does make me wonder.

Why would I hit myself over and over again in the face with an 80-pound object?

Why would I continue to do it, even after I'd get headaches and go to sleep with a pounding head?

Why did I even have the desire to want to be a fighter in the first place and put myself through all that pain and damage, even when I knew deep down it wasn't for me?

The answer to all of these questions comes down to one thing and one thing only: I hated myself.

I hated who I was.

I hated the way I looked. I hated how short I was. I hated that I couldn't get a date. I hated that I didn't have any friends. I hated that I was too skinny, and smaller than other guys my age. I hated my weird hairline. I hated my crooked teeth. I hated that I wasn't going to any good college. I hated that I wasn't naturally tough. I hated that I couldn't relate or connect with anyone. I hated the fact I couldn't sleep good at night. I hated the fact I had no money. I hated that I was insecure. I hated that I was not confident. I hated that I was lonely. I hated that I was depressed. I hated everything about me at that point in life. And I hated myself even more for hating myself.

And because of all the hatred I held so deeply in my core, I punished myself for it. I punished myself without even knowing I was punishing myself. But I did, as I came to find out years later.

MY SELF-HARM

Looking back at my actions, it's so obvious now. I was practicing self-harm.

Self-harm is the act of physically hurting yourself, through a multitude of potential means, in an effort to cope with mental anguish. The anguish may stem from depression, anxiety, borderline personality disorder, PTSD, or another condition associated with mental health issues.[1]

Loving Yourself

Self-harmers partake in burning, hitting, scratching, picking or piercing skin, hair pulling, and most notoriously, cutting themselves. They do so mainly as an escape from their pain (I know, it's quite horrifically ironic).

You see, by causing a "real" pain like cutting one's wrist in a non-lethal way, or say, I don't know, swinging an 80-pound punching bag into one's face, the self-harming individual causes a self-induced and "controlled" pain. One that they can moderate and actually have power over. In their minds, it's a way to take back some semblance of control in their life, when they feel like they've lost it everywhere else.[2]

They feel like because their life is so shitty and because they have problems with depression or anxiety or whatever else, they've lost control over their minds. By harming themselves, they can temporarily induce the belief that they're in charge again.[3] It's a bizarre philosophy, trust me I know, but to them it seems like a good one. And to my 16-year-old self it did too.

Of course most of the time this isn't consciously thought out.

It's not like a severely depressed person analyzes his thoughts and says, "Let me burn my hand in an attempt to momentarily feel in control of my mental state, as a coping mechanism for the mental issues I'm currently facing," and then meticulously carries out a predetermined dose of agony.

No, it's not that sophisticated.

It's more like an unconscious urge to hurt yourself that you one day act upon, just because, and then when you realize you kind of felt good while doing it, you keep doing it periodically thereafter. A totally fucked up system for healing pain that in the long-term only causes more of it.

Trust me, I can attest to this.

The one-sided ass beatings in my garage, administered to myself and by myself, lasted on and off for about a year. Some weeks I'd go superfluously hard and give myself a really good thrashing, only letting up when my head started throbbing to the point of feeling like it would explode; other weeks I'd just give myself a blow or two, focusing more on the actual doling out of punishment, albeit to an inanimate object.

But the entire act of self-harm, which I'll extend to the infatuation with becoming a professional boxer, as it encompasses (at least for me) the same type of fucked up psychological pathways as the smashing of my heavy bag into my face, lasted about two years. What I mean by this, is that I truly believe my desire, and then my actions which followed, to box and fight others for about two full years was in and of itself a form of self-harm. I was regularly sparring guys three or four times a week, allowing my head to get smashed in all the while.

By *spar*, I don't mean like going through the motions, and dancing around each other practicing your form. Spar is such a placid word, and masks the true brutality of the act. By spar, I mean like getting in there for 20-30 minutes with someone at your gym and pounding the fuck out of each other nonstop, until one or both of you is gushing out blood or becomes mildly concussed. Yeah, in my delusionally misplaced mind, this sadistic venture was a brilliant idea.

One tough, future pro-boxer who took a liking to me and was actually a really cool guy and someone I looked up to, gave me big props one day when he said, "Justin, you're a real tough kid, man. You could be a world champ one day. You know how I know?"

"No," I responded back, both surprised and honored.

"I know, because when most people get hit they back up and they get afraid, he explained. "I see you sparring all these dudes in here and when you get hit, you just keep coming forward."

Now, at the time, I was fucking thrilled to hear this. Getting this type of praise from such a talented and tough older fighter was the height of triumph for a young up-and-comer back then. I was truly flattered by his words. And I gave myself the proverbial pat on the back, and let this further fuel my hunger for boxing glory.

But looking back now, that older, seasoned vet was wrong. I was never going to be a boxing champ, no matter how much I wanted to be back then. And the truth is, I only came forward after being hit because I was unconsciously intent on self-harm, not because I was some sort of fisticuff protege.

After about the two-year mark, while working on the techniques for beating anxiety and depression I've talked about earlier, I gave up boxing. In doing so I gave up my self-harm and self-hate, choosing self-care and self-love instead.

And I've never been happier.

LOVING YOURSELF

Loving yourself comes down to accepting who you are.

I know it's easier said than done, but choosing to accept who you are is truly the best way to get over feelings of inferiority, self-worthlessness, self-hate, and of course depression.

There will always be things you don't like about yourself. But I've got ground-breaking fucking news for you: *Get over it!*

Everyone has these issues. Everyone wishes they were a little more this, or a little more that, and everyone wishes they could improve some faults or imperfections they shoulder. You're not unique in aspiring to be better. That's normal.

But letting these thoughts get to you and letting them take over your happiness is a problem. Instead of marinating on things you can't control, accept that that's who you are, and instead focus on the things you can control.

That's the key.

Who doesn't wish from time to time that they looked like Brad Pitt, or were as tall as Michael Jordan, or had the body of Arnold Schwarzenegger (in his prime of course, not the old, saggy figure he boasts now)? Even Jordan probably wishes he looked more ripped like Arnold, and I'm sure Arnold wishes he had Pitt's face, and Pitt probably wishes he was taller. It's a vicious, ego-driven cycle, but one you've got to look past to truly be happy.

It really comes back to gratitude, the very first topic we covered in your fight against depression. Stop focusing on the negative and focus on the positive.

Focus on all you do have, not what you don't.

Love yourself every day more and more and love the imperfections that make you unique. The idiosyncrasies of everything that make up who you truly are, both inside and out, are to be cherished, not resented.

In one of my favorite all-time movies, *Good Will Hunting*, Robin Williams' (rest in peace) character, Sean Maguire, talks about how his wife used to fart in her sleep habitually during their marriage. Sometimes she'd even let one off so loud she'd wake herself up, to which Sean would silently giggle to himself. She had later died from a losing battle with cancer, and upon reflecting on her life and their marriage together, Sean said it wasn't her stunning beauty or her amazing personality that anyone could immediately pick up on from her that he missed the most, it was the idiosyncrasies and the little quirks that made him truly love her, and wish she were still with him. It was the farts-in-her-sleep type of things that made her unique and made her truly special to him.

This is what it's all about. Love yourself as a whole, all your seemingly negative characteristics, and all your positive ones too. Embrace your essence fully and love yourself like you've never loved anything else. Consequently, others will fall in love with your entire essence as well, just as Sean did with his flatulent wife.

MY SELF-LOVE

I'm a short man.

I'm about 5'7 on a good day, and most guys I come across tower over me. I'm usually about the same size as the women I meet, or microscopically taller.

It used to eat me up inside. It used to be one of the things I hated about myself. But I've learned to get past it over the years.

Would I like to be six-foot-fucking-six and possess the ability to dunk a basketball like Air Jordan? Abso-fucking-lutely! Who wouldn't want to slam one home from time to time?

But realistically, it's just not something I dwell on anymore, or honestly care much about.

Instead I focus my attention on other things.

I've focused on improving different areas of my life, on learning new skills, on enjoying different moments, and embarking on new adventures. I've long gotten past this and other insecurities I used to have (my weird hairline, my skinny frame, my crooked teeth, to name but a few), and have accepted these things as part of the entire package.

They're the necessary evils, if you will, that go into creating the overall badass and totally fucking awesome quintessence that is me, Justin Erik Stenstrom, First of His Name, Conqueror of Anxiety and Depression, and Helper to Many.

And goddammit I do love who I've become and love where I'm headed. After all these years I finally and truly love myself.

And you should too. It's the secret to happiness.

PART IV
Confidence

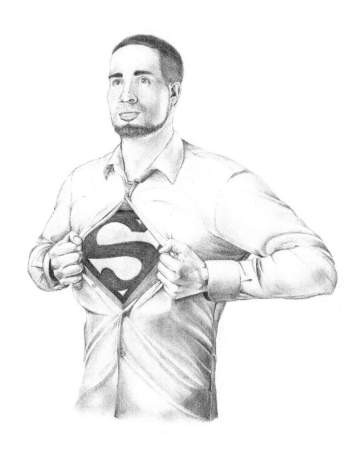

Chapter Twenty-Five
Your Untapped Confidence

By now, I've given you the clear-cut tools to conquer your anxiety and depression. Epic fucking cognitive instruments that will have you mastering your mental woes in no time, with the epiphany-like clarity of an enlightened monk. Yeah, I know, it's pretty fantastic.

But now we must traverse into our next cerebral obstacle. That of gaining true confidence.

This is, in my view, the last step to being psychologically complete. When you get a hold of your depression and anxiety you come back to a baseline of being a healthy human being. This is great and all, but it still leaves more to be desired. After all, life is about pushing your limits and growing in all areas. But to do this, you must first possess earth-shattering and mind-blowingly magnificent self-confidence.

And that's what I'm now going to teach you how to get.

EVERYONE'S GOT IT

I want you to picture for a moment the prototypical video game nerd. You know, the 22-year-old college graduate who sits at home for the better part of each day in his mother's basement, sniping out virtual Afghani terrorists or blowing the shit out of alien armies from a nearby galaxy. His thrill in life is duking it out against other nerds (with equally titillating personality traits as his) and imposing his artificial dominance over them.

This young man, whose sole sustenance consists of cheese puffs and ramen noodles, is quite clearly lacking in several crucial life areas, the least of which would have to be his deprivation of a real social life, or even just a *life* for that matter. But without picking on the misguided *Call-Of-Duty*-obsessed youngen too much, I do want to point something out. If this guy (or any of his dorky friends) was to actually step outside his basement while the sun was still shining, and try to have some type of social interaction with a normal human being, he'd be absolutely fucking lost. God forbid he came across a decent-looking woman too. He'd be more out of place than Peter Griffin at a Mensa meeting.

It'd be like a blind man trying to ride a motorcycle. This poor gamer would be fucked.

Why? Because he'd be completely out of his element. He'd be like a fish who'd just got his ass scooped out of water by a grizzly-looking, Captain-Ahabesque seaman. He wouldn't know what the fuck to do next, and yeah, he'd probably flop around lifelessly in a strange attempt to eradicate his social awkwardness.

But, without crushing the video game guy's existence too badly, as much as I do like to laugh, believe it or not, all is not lost. You see, I've worked with these guys frequently over the years. And truth be told, I have a soft spot in my heart for them. As much as I may like to crack jokes on them and make light of the fucked up and weird behaviors they routinely demonstrate, I actually really do like these gamer guys, and like to help them find the light.

The one recurring theme with guys like this (as with all guys who severely lack confidence, especially in extreme social settings like parties, bars, nightclubs, weddings, work get-togethers, classes, and more) is that they all think they have *zero* confidence. Across the board, they truly believe they're the most uncertain and insecure people on the face of the Earth, and that confidence is simply a mystical skill for which they were not endowed nor are ever destined to obtain. But I tell them right away that they're wrong, on two accounts.

The first, is obvious, and that's that by working with me, I will absolutely instill a stronger sense of confidence in them, almost immediately. The second, less apparent but more important blunder to their suppositions, is that they don't already possess confidence. They unequivocally do.

Let me explain.

Everyone has confidence in them already. It's a fact. No matter how insecure, unconfident, dejected, or otherwise anxious people may be in any given domain, they still possess self-confidence somewhere else, even if they don't realize it.

Take video game dude for example. As we mentioned, he's going to stick out like a sore thumb in social situations because he's unfamiliar with them. He's not confident in these areas as he hasn't spent much time in them. But if you take gamer boy and throw him into a roomful of other gaming lads, what happens? Gold dust.

This young man will thrive. He'll have the right body language, he'll be laughing, he'll be joking around, he'll be shit-talking his buddies, he'll be talking strategy, he'll be loving life, and he'll be one confident motherfucker. Why? Because it's what he knows. It's what he's familiar with. It's his environment and his game (both literally and figuratively) he's playing.

Yes, it's probably an excruciatingly painful sight to see this young man struggle through social get-togethers with peers who don't live in their parents' basements and survive off nutritional dogshit like he does. But stick this same youngster in a group full of Jedi-loving supernerds, and all of a sudden, he's the fucking man.

So what's going on here?

How can this guy jump from one extreme to the other without even thinking about it?

He does it because he naturally has confidence in him already. It's a part of his and everyone else's DNA. We're born to be confident, and to have the self-belief that we can succeed in life. But over the years we seem to forget this, and lose that confidence with time.

Maybe someone laughed at us when we were younger. Maybe someone picked on us at school. Maybe the girl we really liked turned us down and then told the rest of the class. Maybe we just sort of took the back seat and let some of the louder, more outgoing peers take the spotlight, allowing them to soak up all the glory and confidence, leaving us to doubt ourselves and feel second-rate.

Whatever the case, I'm telling you now, you have it in you already. It's time to bring it back up and let it shine. Awaken the sleeping giant of your confidence and step the fuck up in your life. No more back seat, sideline-standing bullshit allowed. Get in the game, and take back your confidence.

Decoded Neurofeedback

Scientists have recently demonstrated just how easy it can be for you to regulate your emotions. Using a technique called multivoxel pattern neurofeedback, or decoded neurofeedback, they've been able to track the neuronal activity of participants' brains and see more clearly than ever what's going on when specific emotions like confidence get activated.

But more importantly, through their work with decoded neurofeedback, they've demonstrated the ability to regulate this powerful sentiment and facilitate its presence using a stimulus.

That stimulus in this case was money, which always seems to work well for motivating people.

By rewarding the participants in the form of cold hard cash whenever they displayed a brain pattern associated with a high-confidence state, they were able to get their participants to display this brain pattern more regularly, and almost at will.[1]

It's quite impressive; simply by using an influential trigger, the scientists could generate a true and tangibly documented emotion in their volunteers.

Confidence, as science is proving, can in fact be frequently manipulated.

GETTING YOUR CONFIDENCE BACK

Think right now about your own life. Think of your day-to-day and week-to-week routine. In what areas of your life do you absolutely fucking shine? In what areas of your life do you lack confidence and take a back seat?

Take your time and really brainstorm here. Using your trusty notebook or journal is highly recommended.

After brainstorming both the confident and unconfident areas of your life, put a strong emphasis on the confident places and really detail what your confidence looks like in these settings.

I want you to write down all the facets that go into what your peak confidence state looks like. Just like our lovable video game dweeb example, focus on everything that goes into your confidence and how that appears: your tone of voice, your body language, your mannerisms, the words you use, the way you carry yourself, the attitude you have, everything.

Now remember this, because I'm going to come back to it later on when I dive into a specific technique for quickly boosting your confidence in any arena.

For now, however, I want you dwell on the fact that you, like everyone else on this planet, already possess an extraordinary amount of confidence inside you. But unlike so many others, you're now aware of it. This profound realization is the first, and perhaps most enlightening, step of all when it comes to obtaining confidence.

Keep this in mind as we dive into some of the upcoming chapters. And slowly start acting more and more like the way you do when you're at your confident pinnacle. Start implementing those mannerisms, body language, tone of voice, and everything else from your peak state, into the areas of your life where you want to have more confidence.

Begin to condition yourself for gaining unbelievable confidence in those areas where you've been struggling, and open the door to living life on your terms.

Confidence is already inside you, but I'm going to help you pry it the fuck out and put it on a silver platter, so you can showcase it to the world, in any situation.

I hope you're ready.

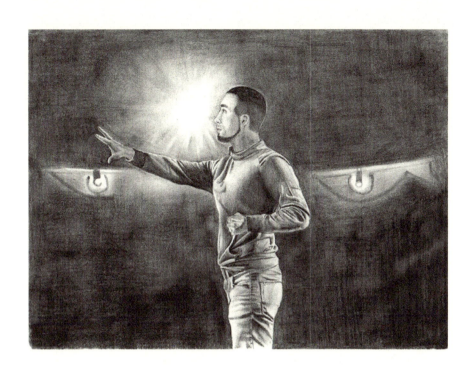

Chapter Twenty-Six
Pretend to Be Great

My palms were sweating as I waited in the murky hall, anticipating my call at any moment.

I wiped them both on the legs of my recently-tailored dress pants. Then I pulled out the paper towel I'd just nabbed from the men's bathroom minutes before, and wiped down my brow. The sweat was unmistakably accumulating on there as well. *What the fuck.* I said to myself. *I hope this goes well.*

"You ready, bro?" my friend and impending partner Phil asked, interrupting my internal doubt.

"Yup, I'm fucking pumped. Can't wait dude!" I lied to him.

"Fuck yeah, man!" he excitedly replied back.

I hid it as best as I could, but inside I was terrified. I'd have been more than happy to postpone and wait for forever, before having to do what I knew was only seconds away now. My nerves were taking over and I was starting to sweat profusely.

This was going to be one hell of an experience.

A few months back, I'd signed up for an acting class, when I was feeling bold and adventurous. I'd enjoyed it. No, actually, I'd loved it ever since then, but it wasn't until today that I'd had to really be tested. Sure we'd done the various exercises, and delved into the fabric of our emotions, pulling out pieces of ourselves we hadn't even known existed, and sure we'd challenged ourselves in immeasurable ways of fortitude, testing both our mental and emotional limits. But we hadn't done anything like this yet, and I was scared.

Phil wasn't, though. That guy was as cool as a cucumber. (Or at least he played the role well enough to fool me.)

I looked at him, and wondered if he was bullshitting me just as much as I was bullshitting him. *Goddammit, I can't tell*, I thought to myself. And I continued to freak out.

We were set to go up in front of the entire class and perform a scene out of a play called *The Pillowman*, an incredible, surprisingly awesome story about a man whose mentally-retarded and seemingly harmless brother ends up being a serial killer. It's such a clever plot, with multiple mysteries and hidden clues sprinkled throughout. Not to mention, it's a story which references multiple other short stories (made-up short stories by the first brother, who's a writer and not the serial killer), which themselves are clever as hell and exceptionally entertaining.

Pretend to Be Great

(As an aside, I recommend reading this little gem at some point in your life. It's that good.)

As my role, having been assigned this play to read and act out, I was playing the part of one of the detectives who interrogates the writer about his short stories, which seem to be the inspiration for all the murders that have been taking place, and seem to implicate him (rightly so). Phil was playing the writer I was interrogating.

"And now," a crisp, loud, female voice bellowed out, "we have Justin and Phil performing *The Pillowman*, by Martin McDonagh."

I heard the applause and immediately felt my heart drop.

Fuck, fuck, fuck, I thought to myself. *What if I bomb? Fuck, there's so many people here. There's gotta' be twice as many as usual. Shit, what the hell did I get myself into?*

And then a thought popped into my mind, just as we were getting ourselves situated with a couple of stage props. I'm not sure where it came from, but it came. I guess I can chalk it up now to karma or perhaps just sheer dumb-luck. But in that moment I just decided, *Fuck it, I'm going to keep pretending that I'm good. If Phil is doing it, he's fooling me, so it must work, and if he's not, well fuck it, he's fooling me anyway, so what's the difference?*

I decided to just pretend to be fucking confident, even though I was scared shitless and ready to yack at any moment.

Not only was I going to act out a scene and pretend to play a part in this short story, but I was also going to pretend to be fucking great at it. I was going to pretend to be a tough-guy detective like the role entailed. I was going to step inside my character and assume the role of the take-no-shit, confident cop. I was going to pretend to be like one of my favorite self-assured and always cool actors, Robert De

Niro. *No, fuck that, I'm not going to pretend to be him, I'm gonna' be him.* I thought to myself.

And then I crumpled up my forehead and put a scowl on my face. The bold, confrontational, and domineering expression of Jimmy Conway from *Goodfellas* took the form of this accusatory detective I was personifying for the audience.

"I bet you're all adrenaline now, aren't you," I began, "all 'Ooh just shouted at a policeman,' . . . all 'Ooh probably shouldn't've but ooh got really angry.' Ooh. Calm the fuck down!" I yelled at Phil, in my authoritarian, De-Niro-like voice.

And Phil collapsed back down in defeat, imitating the writer's defeated demeanor to a tee.

He and I then carried on for about five minutes, going back and forth, rattling off our rehearsed lines like one might recite their favorite song in a car. We were crushing it.

When our time came to a climactic finale, we faced the audience, smiled, and took a long, soul-radiating bow.

They loved us.

MY REALIZATION

Something dawned on me soon after my performance that day. By pretending to step into that role of being Robert De Niro's iconic wiseguy character, I'd been able to get past my fears in that moment of stress. But even better, I'd summoned up a level of confidence that I'd previously not embodied.

It was almost as if in those five minutes, on stage in front of all my classmates and some friends, I really *was* De Niro. It had felt so real. The self-doubt and worry I'd held about messing up had been instantly replaced with this feeling of being fucking cool and unbelievably assertive.

That role-playing I did, to give myself confidence in those final few seconds before we began, came through in a last ditch, Hail Mary sort of way. But I knew I was on to something, even if it had been just pure luck that I'd stumbled upon it (In hindsight, this strategy certainly echoes the approach I'd used to beat my fear of riding roller coasters, which might explain where I'd hatched the idea.).

I began applying this concept to everything in my life where I needed to feel more confidence, when I couldn't naturally conjure it up.

When I first started going up and talking to women, I'd pretend to be a great seducer, or one of the dating coaches I'd seen online approaching women. When I went out to the bar at night and waltzed over to the dance floor to frolic with some hotties, I'd pretend I was Usher or Chris Brown as I moved my torso about.

And soon later, when I'd go to give my first speech in front of a decent-sized crowd, I temporarily assumed the role of Tony Robbins. I may not have been nearly as good as Tony, but it didn't matter. I was far better than I would have been, because of the confidence it allowed me to exude.

WHY PRETENDING WORKS

This practice of stepping into the role of someone who has unbelievable confidence works because it allows you for the first time to feel what it's like to have confidence in a specific environment you're unfamiliar with. You can sense it, experience it, and most importantly, get feedback from others, which allows you to have even more confidence, as it reassures you and reiterates to your subconscious mind that you can in fact, really be confident in that area.

If you are lost in the beginning, and unsure of how to get started in gaining confidence fast, try this approach. Rather than solely attempting to steadily build up your confidence over time, which does work but obviously takes much longer, this acting method dramatically allows you to experience confidence immediately and begin setting a new standard of self-belief in any walk of life.

It's essentially the old "fake it 'til you make it" method. But it actually works. In his book *Liar's Poker*, author Michael Lewis talks about how he mimicked the master salesman above him when he first began selling bonds and was an inexperienced trainee. But after a while of using the techniques that the master was using, he soon became a master too.[1]

One study, conducted by psychological scientists Tara Kraft and Sarah Pressman of the University of Kansas, investigated whether faking a smile when you're feeling down, can actually improve your mood. They examined 170 volunteers and by the end of their experiment demonstrated that everyone who smiled, even if it was a forced smile, improved their response to stress and lowered their heart rates, indicating the physiological and psychological benefits for maintaining positive facial expressions during stress.[2]

Another study, published in the *Quarterly Journal of Experimental Psychology* in 2013, examined the placebo-like effects of confidence in the performance of test takers divided into two groups. After pretending to give one group of the study's participants the answers to a forthcoming test and making these students believe they'd been exposed to the answers prior to taking the test, this group outperformed the second group which hadn't been primed to believe this. Both of the groups actually had *zero* insight into the test, and absolutely no tangible advantage for taking the test, but the group who thought they'd been given a benefit significantly outperformed

Pretend to Be Great

the other group, simply because of the confidence-boosting belief that they'd been privy to the answers already.[3]

Yes, the power of your mind cannot be denied. Making it truly believe something can dramatically affect your performance in any area.

When stepping into a confident role, like I did the day I acted out that play, you're working on both your conscious and subconscious mind at the same time. You're consciously feeling and experiencing the sensations and emotions of a high-status, confident person, and for someone who's never felt this way in a social setting, this can be incredibly powerful. But you're also subconsciously getting the feedback from those around you (who are completely unaware of your role-playing game), who act, speak, and treat you more favorably, as they treat all confident individuals more favorably than those who are not. This positive reaffirming to the most powerful part of your mind, starts to condition it (immediately and then gradually) into actually believing in this confidence.

Not only do you feel better and feel more confident when you assume this new confident persona, but you actually start to become truly confident. This game, this feigned confidence if you will, after a certain period of time, no longer becomes a performance, it becomes a reality. Soon enough, you don't even have to act out any role, you *are* that role.

STEPPING INTO YOUR ROLE

About four or five months after I performed *The Pillowman* in front of my acting classmates and teacher, I was procrastinating on YouTube in my college library between classes. I'd taken a break from doing some schoolwork, and was aimlessly surfing around between old *Judge Judy* clips, MMA knockouts, and cats doing goofy shit, when I stumbled across an old interview with the legendary Marlon Brando. I clicked on the video and was immediately drawn in by something that caught my attention.

It was Larry King, or one of those old talk-show zombies, and they were asking Marlon about acting and how he was able to be so good at it. How he'd been able to step into some of the most iconic roles in cinematic history with what appeared to be such ease.

Brando coolly went on to explain that it was easy. He'd just done what was natural to him and natural to everyone else. He was just assuming the role of whoever his character was and doing what we all do, every single moment of every single day: act.

Larry was initially perplexed and asked Brando to elaborate, so he went on to say something along the lines of this: We all act. In every moment. I'm acting right now. You're acting right now. We all have these roles that we play throughout the day. We change our roles as different situations require us to be a certain way. But we're always playing a role, I'm just playing roles on the big screen, but we all play a role in real life too, in fact many, many of them.

Brando was dead on, though I don't know if King ever fully grasped what he was saying. Perhaps he thought Marlon was just being wise and trying to one-up him on his own show. Or perhaps Larry was just too dilapidated to really comprehend the acumen of such a statement. Either way, I got it, and loved the message completely.

Brando was right. We do all have roles we play. We play the role of the husband when we wake up, the role of the loving parent when our kids get up, the role of the employee when we go to work, the role of a friend when we meet up with a buddy after work, and finally the role of a parent again when we come back home. Maybe our child acts up and we step into the role of a disciplinarian, but after 20 minutes we step into the role of consoler, telling our kids that we still love them, and just want them to behave next time. And then, *Boom!* We step into the role of excited family man, as we pop on our favorite family show and gather round for some laughs and entertainment.

You get the point.

We have many, many roles we play throughout the day, different ways of acting around different people and in different situations while with those people. It's an essential part of life.

My question, after knowing this, is why not choose to step into more favorable roles? If your go-to in different situations is to step into self-doubt or uncertainty, why not change this habit and step into the role of confidence? Choose to be confident and choose to be someone who plays this role all the time. Leave behind your old roles of unconfidence, self-doubt, even meekness, and adopt the new roles of self-assuredness, self-belief, and self-confidence.

It's something you already do, just do it more often.

THE CRITICS

Trust me, I can hear you already . . .

Every time I talk about this technique there's always someone who inevitably says, "Yeah, I get it Justin, but I don't think that pretending to be someone you're not is a good idea. It seems disingenuous."

Well, you can label it whatever you want if you feel that way, but the fact of the matter is it works. If you want to think of stepping into various roles as being disingenuous, then I guess every human being on the planet is disingenuous, because as I mentioned before, and as Mr. Brando concurred with in his interview, we all play fucking roles! All the fucking time.

And for someone who has no idea what it feels like to feel confidence in a certain area, this role-assuming strategy is the fastest and easiest way for him to adopt this new feeling. It's not like you have to pretend to be someone you're not the rest of your life either. It's more of a temporary adoption of a new positive belief system to get your ass going in the right direction,[4] a jumpstart of confidence, that soon translates into a smooth and powerful ride.

HOW TO APPLY THIS CONCEPT

I want you for a moment to consider the area of your life where you want to have more confidence. Whether it's confidence delivering a speech, or talking to women, or being the center of attention at a party, or selling products to potential customers, take a moment and think of this area. (If it's nothing specific, that's okay too; this technique will still work just the same.)

After you come up with the aspect of your life where you want a boost in confidence, brainstorm and think of one to three highly confident people who've already had incredible amounts of success in that domain. Think of everything about them that makes them confident. Really do a mind rattle with this (journaling helps, as always) and consider all of their confidence-emanating characteristics: the way they talk to others, their body language, their tone of voice, the way they walk, the energy they have, the way others react to them . . . everything that makes them unbelievably fucking confident. Reflect on that.

I recommend watching them as well and studying them as much as possible until you get them down. Remember, you're doing research into a new role here, just like any great actor. Think Brando's Don Corleone, De Niro's Jake La Motta, even Ledger's Joker character . . . all of these actors spent countless hours of preparation studying the role they intended to play. Do the same.

Pretend to Be Great

If that means watching several movies of the confident actor you intend to mimic, or watching some interviews of the celebrity you'd like to imitate, or YouTube clips of the self-help coach you admire most (*ahem*, me), do it. Even if the role you intend to play is not that of a celebrity or someone you can pull up on video, still spend some energy studying as much as you can of that individual elsewhere.

It might be someone you see in person, who's got just the right amount of confidence you aspire to obtain. Start watching and listening to that person more intently. Pick up on everything they do and open your eyes to what makes them confident. When you feel like you fully understand a person's confidence and where it stems from, it's time to adopt it.

Go out in those situations where you want to have confidence, and step into the role of the person you've been studying. Assume the new role you want to play in life and make it your own. Remember, we're acting at all moments of the day already, just pick the role you want and enjoy the life you create with it.

Pretty soon you're going to be a real confident motherfucker and someone's going to copy you.

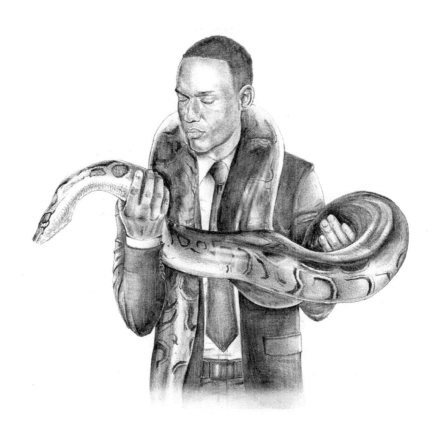

Chapter Twenty-Seven
A Powerful Confidence Tool

The six-foot-five-inch monster of a man had made a living striking fear into the hearts of other gigantic human beings. Among titans, he reigned supreme for 15 full years. Even now, his broad, chiseled frame still looked as tough and ready to kill as it had just a few years prior, during his illustrious career.

But this wasn't the gridiron, and Michael Strahan was in a wholly foreign predicament. The man who'd sacked, tackled, and devastated some of the most brutal men on the planet for a decade and a half was now in a world of hurt, the likes of which not even he could deliver on his best day.

But it wasn't another mountain-sized-man that was causing Michael pain like in his playing days, it was a snake. A massive, python-looking beast, with sharp deathly eyes and thick ridged scales that ran well past six feet in length. Michael for his entire life was used to being the most dominant and physically intimidating presence in any given room, but this cold-blooded reptile was clearly the alpha here.

For as long as he cared to remember, Michael had carried a crippling fear of these slithering creatures, its degree accumulating so much over time that it'd manifested into a true phobia over the years, and one that left Michael turning into a blithering school-girl every time one's presence was made.

But in this moment in time Michael, against all rationale, was being forced to confront his fears head on.

It was on a talk show he hosted a few years back, aptly titled *Live! With Kelly and Michael*, Kelly being Kelly Ripa and Michael being Michael Strahan, the petrified ex-football star turned snake bitch. Both Kelly and Michael had been talking about his fear of snakes in the days leading up to this particular episode, and Michael had agreed, with great reluctance, to try to overcome his fear of snakes during one of their upcoming shows.

And so the show's producers had called on a man who's been recognized as perhaps the world's greatest healer of phobias and fears (and many other emotional and psychological issues) and asked him to come help. A man who's literally helped hundreds of thousands of people overcome their emotional struggles, all with astonishingly quick and seemingly effortless grace.

Enter Dr. Richard Bandler.

A Powerful Confidence Tool

Richard Bandler is a self-help legend. A charismatic if not quirky old man who co-invented his revolutionary psychological system known as Neuro-Linguistic Programming, or NLP, as it's more commonly referred.

Bandler, whose original background was in mathematics and gestalt therapy,[1] teamed up with the other co-creator of NLP, his friend John Grinder, whose background was in linguistics. Together they studied some of the smartest minds in the psychology world, including trailblazers like Milton Erickson, Fritz Perls, and Virginia Satir. From there they formulated a system combining several of the psychological principles they found most effective, giving birth to NLP, an innovatively effective method for solving the most difficult mental problems.

Using linguistics, visualization, mental patterns, hypnosis, and various other forms of psychological principles, NLP essentially retrains the mind to look at mental and emotional challenges differently, by removing the negative emotions typically attached to them and replacing them with positive ones. Within this broad spectrum there are many techniques and approaches to getting desirable results. And, naturally, there are many applications for NLP-like therapies, including counseling, psychotherapy, law, dating, relationships, sales, leadership training, and parenting, to name but a few.

Everyone from world-class athletes, to Fortune 500 CEOs, to household-name celebrities, to highly successful entrepreneurs, to handsome motherfuckers like myself, have used NLP to improve their lives in some way, shape, or form. (I'll happily elaborate on the last group in a moment, and yes, I did just call myself a handsome motherfucker.) But I digress . . .

Let me first finish the story of Strahan and Bandler's twirl with the python of doom.

STRAHAN VS. SNAKE

Bandler walks onto the set to great applause as Michael Strahan's sitting uncomfortably in an otherwise cozy chair. He's anxious as hell and it's written all over his face. He's smiling and trying to keep up appearances, but he's scared shitless, because he knows in just a few minutes he's going to have to face the vicious six-plus-foot nightmare head on.

Bandler, a few decades past his prime but sharp as ever, cracks a few dry but witty jokes to both Strahan and Ripa, and the eagerly tuned-in audience just feet away. He talks for a couple of moments with Michael about his fear of snakes; how long he's had it for, why he should want to get over it, and how it's taking up an unnecessary amount of his time. Then he walks him through the process of actually being able to overcome it.

The old psychological master walks the former gridiron stud through a series of steps which look something like this:

First he has Strahan visualize the fear he has of snakes. He has him think of the time (several episodes prior) where a guest brought onto the show a small, but real-life snake and threw it at Strahan in a playful attempt of on-air tomfoolery. Bandler continues to press, and has Strahan visualize his reaction (which was to both simultaneously jump out of his seat, and screech like a five-year-old Girl Scout). Bandler makes Strahan really focus on this picture for a minute and take it in.

Next, he has Strahan recall how big the picture he just visualized was, and whether it had any type of movements or motions in it.

A Powerful Confidence Tool

Strahan recounts that his picture was very large and that he could sense the snakes coming right at him in his visualization.

Finally, Bandler tells Strahan to take that massive and terrifying picture, and visually shrink it down to the size of a quarter. Not only that, but to turn the picture (almost always very colorful and vivid) into a black and white snapshot.

And just to solidify this process, he makes Strahan do it again: Visualize the first, scary, colorful, massive picture of the snake jumping into your lap, then shrink this picture down to the size of a quarter, then quickly turn it into an opaque, black and white image.

Strahan does it all again.

Afterward, Bandler asks Strahan how he feels about snakes, and how he feels about the original image of the snake soaring right at him. The football great just kind of shrugs and says, "I'm good."

To Ripa's surprise and to the surprise of all others watching, it appears like Strahan is nonchalant about his formerly heart-pounding phobia surrounding these dangerous reptiles. It seems like the kooky, old sage has once again eliminated a major mental block in another patient.

But to really put his method to the test, Bandler has Kelly bring out the python.

The titanic serpent is coiled around Ripa's arms and looks ready to strike death into any one of the unfortunate human beings on set who might happen to look at it the wrong way. Strahan, who previously would've been curled under a table off camera by now, instead confidently walks over to the snake and proceeds to pat this slimy and savage creature with the elegance one might use to pat a cute little tabby cat. But not only this, a moment or so after his loving caresses of affection, Strahan then decides to pick up the snake, out of Kelly's arms, and rest the beast onto his own arms and chest, allowing it to snuggle its scales onto the NFL-Hall-of-Famer's torso.

It's downright stunning to watch.

Here's a guy who just moments ago had been petrified at just the thought of seeing a snake, a man who'd lived his entire life with an incredible anxiety surrounding these creatures. And now he was smiling and laughing and wrapping the slimy and slithery fucking viper around his whole body! It was quite amazing to see. And it illustrates the magic that Bandler possesses to a tee.

But more importantly, it demonstrates the power of NLP.

NLP FOR CONFIDENCE

As I mentioned before, NLP has a number of practical functions, including its famous ability to quickly eliminate fears and phobias. I, myself, have used NLP in this regard, to help stifle a claustrophobic fear I was developing surrounding enclosed spaces a few years back.

Hyperbaric Oxygen Therapy

As the solid steel door slammed shut behind me, I realized just how real this solitary confinement would be. In a past life, I'd have already been freaking the fuck out, with sweat pouring down my cheeks and my heart pounding through my chest, urging me to take some kind of life-or-death action to save myself from imminent doom. As it were, however, I smiled, and perhaps even audibly chuckled, at the reflection of how silly I most certainly would have reacted years back.

I wasn't in a jail cell, but rather a hyperbaric oxygen chamber. And I wasn't being forced against my will, but voluntarily locking myself inside this constrainment for biohacking purposes.

A Powerful Confidence Tool

Hyperbaric oxygen therapy, or HBOT, is the process of using 100% oxygen at higher atmospheric pressures than normal breathing air to get inside your body and reach the deepest parts of your tissues and cells for the purpose of enacting healing. It's typically done inside a steel chamber (or other comparable container) that's filled up with pressurized pure oxygen. It's been used for a myriad of conditions including brain injury, autism, cancer, cerebral palsy, decompression sickness, stroke, and wound healing, to name but a few,[2] and has been popularized in the past few decades by Dr. Paul Harch,[3] considered by many to be the top HBOT doctor in the world.

In the right dosages pure oxygen can help just about any condition and is one of the most overlooked and effective treatments for a number of diseases. (As a reference, the air we breathe typically only has about 21% oxygen, while about 78% is made up of nitrogen, and 1% is made up of argon, carbon dioxide, and other smaller gases.)

In his book *Flood Your Body With Oxygen*, health advocate and bestselling author Ed McCabe talks about the countless benefits of getting more oxygen into your body on a daily basis, including its powerful ability to combat parasites, bacteria, fungus, cancer cells, viruses, and more.

And one of the most effective ways to flood your body with the vitality-boosting properties of clean oxygen? Yup, you guessed it, using HBOT.

So there I sat. Admittedly I've been calmer in my life, but honestly, there really wasn't a trace of fear to be had in this otherwise terrifyingly claustrophobic dilemma. With nothing but metal surrounding me on all sides of this tight concrete tank, I took a deep breath in and relaxed, thinking of the preparation I'd completed in the two weeks leading up to this moment.

I'd used both hypnosis, which by now, you know I'm a massive proponent of, and NLP, which you'll quickly see I'm an equal fan of. The hypnosis sessions were fairly straightforward and easy to implement every day for the 14 days leading up to my first session in the chamber. I'd just pop in a claustrophobia hypnosis track I'd found, and sit back and enjoy the 20-or-so minute experience, letting my subconscious soak in all the suggestions.

For the NLP, it too was simple and undemanding, but instead of letting my subconscious mind take over, I actively used my conscious mind to program my new emotions surrounding closed spaces. I actually used a process very similar to the one Michael Strahan used to get over his fear of snakes.

Just about every day leading up to the first hyperbaric day, I would imagine my fear of being in that closed-off chamber. I'd visualize it as vividly as possible and think of all the terror and anxiety that would be running through my mind and how alone and helpless I would be, while the steel door was sealed shut beside me. But then, I would shrink this terrifying, and naturally large image, down to the size of a penny. From here I would turn its bright colors into a dull black and white picture, and see it fading away in front of me. I'd even visualize myself picking the penny-sized depiction up with one hand and tossing it miles and miles away, into another universe, to symbolize its disappearance from my emotional repertoire.

Lastly, I'd replace this old picture with a new and improved, color-laden portrait of success. In my new vision, I'd be happily sitting in the chamber alone, smiling, and enjoying this time-induced seclusion as a much-desired, albeit transient, oasis from the madness of everyday society. And of course, I'd be turning innumerable amounts of pages in the books I'd be reading to break up my meditationesque retreat.

I'd make this visual as vibrant and realistic as possible, and bask in the feelings of happiness, contentment, and confidence, until it engulfed my being fully. And this became my new outlook every time I thought about sitting in that solitary chamber. The more I practiced this little visualization technique, the less and less clear that first image seemed to be, and the more and more alive that second, favorable picture became.

So when I finally did get in that chamber in real life, it was nothing to me.

I walked in, sat down, observed the space I had, laughed a little at my old, anxious self, and meditated for a few minutes on how far I'd come over the past few years. I ruminated about all the things I was grateful for at that moment in time, and then kicked my feet up onto a little platform across from me and whipped out a self-help book I'd been dying to check out.

When that first session ended after 60 minutes of being in there alone, I honestly was a little disappointed. Not because of the experience of being locked up in there all alone for the better part of an hour, but because I'd just hit a really interesting page in one of the book's best chapters. I'd have to

A Powerful Confidence Tool

> wait about 45 minutes until I got back home before I'd be able to pick the book up again.
>
> I repeated the chamber visits for the next month, without so much as a hiccup to my mental state whilst in the steel hollow. I have to give a big thanks to hypnosis for playing an integral role in this phobic win, and also my friend NLP for the massive boost in self-confidence it lent me during these visits. I truly couldn't have done it without these two fine companions.

But aside from fears and phobias, I've also used NLP in another manner, and that's what I want to share with you now. You see, NLP can be just as powerful and effective at producing confidence as it can be for eliminating fears. Rather than simply using it as a way to get past an anxiety (which is great and highly recommended), you can also use it as a way to cultivate incredible confidence . . . and basically at will.

Let me explain.

There's a technique in NLP called anchoring, the practice of associating an internal emotion with some type of external trigger. This anchoring concept is exactly what I'm going to show you how to do in just a moment with regard to precipitating confidence. But first let me give you a few examples of natural anchoring that occur in everyday life, so you have a better idea of what it really means.

Think of your favorite meal for a second. For me, I'm a pretty basic dude, so it would simply be a fresh and juicy cheeseburger, hot off the grill, with lettuce and tomatoes sandwiched between two nice buns. When I see this in person, and I smell the delicious aroma of that hamburger-steamed meat hitting my nostrils, my mouth instantly starts to salivate with pure lust.

What's happening here is the perfect example of what an anchor and a trigger is. The trigger is the luscious burger I so often love to mow down, that causes me to feel all licentious inside. The anchor is the entire act of this procedure happening: the thought of the burger, causing me to salivate and yearn to have it immediately.

For you it could just as easily be pizza, or chicken, or steak or whatever else you like, but you get the point. You're anchored by a specific food you love, so that when you see, touch, smell, feel, or taste it (obviously), or simply even think of it, it causes you to emotionally desire it and possibly even foam at the mouth like one of Pavlov's dogs.[4]

Another time-tested case of anchoring is what happens when you hear a baby cry. Just about every adult human being on the planet gets a jolt of cortisol when a baby starts crying, and their instant reaction is to begin worrying about what's wrong with the infant and how they can help. The trigger here is obviously the baby's cry, and the anchor is the whole process of the baby's crying, leading to your natural emotional response.

And lastly, for good measure, as sad as it is, a ubiquitous anchor across the globe is the surge of excitement and happiness (despite being fleeting) we get when we see notifications of some sort on our social media pages. Whether it be little red-squared numbers that pop up on the corners of our Facebook pages, signifying some sort of virtual recognition, or whether it be the red dots that pop up underneath our heart icons on Instagram, indicating somebody showed us some digital love, the anchoring effect is once again at play. The triggers are those notification signals, and the anchor is this entire sorry-ass display of us getting an emotional burst of excitement from a fucking virtual notification. (Yeah, our futures are all pretty fucked.)

A Powerful Confidence Tool

HOW TO APPLY ANCHORING

Now that you understand what anchoring is, it's time to learn how to apply this powerful NLP tool in your life.

Remember a couple of chapters back when I told you about the video game nerd who, like every other person on this planet, actually already possesses a certain degree of confidence? Of course you remember. How could you forget our lovable friend?

Do you also remember how I told you to think about an area of your life where you already possess unbelievable confidence? Remember how I told you to focus on everything that goes into your confidence and recall precisely what it looks, feels, and sounds like? Hopefully you do, if not, make sure you do that right now.

Either bring back that memory now by cuing up the inner workings of your hippocampus, or take a second, and actually do the exercise now.

EASILY ANCHOR YOUR CONFIDENCE

Now that you've pulled up these thoughts of your tremendous confidence, it's time to step into that confidence.

So take a long deep breath in, then a long deep breath out, and relax. Now, for the next minute or so, step into that time and place where you held unbelievable confidence. Take a mental trip through space and assume that role once again. Think of everything that's going into that moment. Make this picture as bright, vivid, colorful, and real as possible.

Focus entirely on everything that goes into your confidence: your body language, your tone of voice, your feeling of being on top of the world, your feeling of knowing what to say and when to say it, your feeling like you can literally do anything you want in that moment, no matter how challenging. Add in your charisma, your positive and happy facial expressions, your self-assured mannerisms, the way others treat you with respect, the way they engage with you, their excitement, their energy, and their clinging to your every word with celebrity-like infatuation. All of it.

Take this all in and feel these feelings and emotions fully and completely. Smile as you experience this incredible moment once again, and let all of the wonderfulness of this memory sift through the entirety of your body and being. And after a moment of this, take one more deep breath in and then out, while simultaneously pressing together, on one of your hands, your index finger and your thumb. Hold that thumb and forefinger together for the duration of this breath.

And that's it.

What you've just effectively done is create an anchor for confidence, one you can use in any moment where a confidence boost is needed. The anchor is this positive feeling of remarkable confidence you've associated with taking in a deep breath and pressing your thumb and index finger together. The trigger is clearly the deep breath combined with the digit press.

Any time you do this little move, you'll get a surge of the feelings you just got a moment ago when visualizing and stepping into that confident memory you had.

I've used this exact anchor for many years: before going on a date, before stepping on stage, before taking a test, before just about everything I do where having more confidence behooves my performance. It's a secret little weapon I carry at all times.

A Powerful Confidence Tool

You can strengthen this association by walking through the aforementioned exercise every so often and stepping into that confident memory. Feel all those incredible feelings and visualize that picture of you having the utmost confidence, and then take the action: breathing in and pressing your thumb and index finger together to make the trigger more powerful. It takes literally a minute or two to do, and trains your brain to keep the association alive and potent.

NLP's been developed and used by some of the most successful individuals in the world, including guys like Tony Robbins and Paul McKenna, two pioneers in the personal development space. They, along with celebrities like the aforementioned Strahan, comedian Russell Brand, and even talk-show titan Oprah Winfrey, have all reaped the many benefits of this innovative practice. Yup, NLP is exceptionally powerful and extraordinarily easy to start using. Add it to your bag of tricks today.

Hmm, using the power of your mind to overcome mental and emotional problems? How diabolically clever. Hats off to you, Bandler, you clever old warlock. You've conjured up quite the confidence contraption indeed.

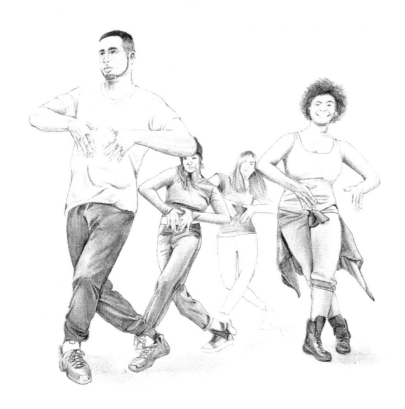

Chapter Twenty-Eight
Shattering Your Comfort Zone

I looked around at the auditorium's occupants and thought, "Holy fuck! This is gonna' be fun."

It was September and the fall semester had just started at Massasoit Community College. I'd just entered my second year and was hoping to finish in the spring (ended up doing another year, but that's neither here nor there). I'd decided to switch things up in my second year and pick some courses I'd never done before, thus the basis for this next tale of immeasurable courage, which of course begins with unfathomable self-doubt.

As the crowd slowly trickled in, I was growing more ecstatic by the minute. I felt like the first 49er when he took his pickaxe and struck gold in Coloma, California way back in the mid-1800s. This was like winning the lottery, only better.

Smoking-hot woman after smoking-hot woman walked through the auditorium doors and gathered around a table being leaned on by an equally-smoking-hot but older woman at the center of this forum, whom one could easily surmise as the leader of this room's assembly.

A number of chairs had been ceremoniously placed around the table and I happened to be joyously sitting back and occupying one of them. I honestly (God's truth) felt like the fucking Bachelor on that stupid TV show as I watched each new classmate enter the room. In my head I kept thinking, *Yes! Fuck yeah!* and *Wow!* as each one approached. I'd be floored by some new female classmate's beauty, and have to quickly regain my composure, only to be floored even further a moment later when the next one came in and outdid the first. It was never-ending.

It was like playing one of those casino games where you finally hit the ultimate jackpot. You know those ones you've seen in movies, where the lights go off and start flashing, and this celebratory music starts playing, and the coins just seem to pour the fuck out of the machine from every mechanical orifice imaginable, dousing you with enough gilded metal to make Blackbeard himself jealous. And the best part is . . . it just keeps coming, and coming, and fucking coming some more!

That's how I felt. This unrelenting conglomerate of beautiful women was multiplying around me like a houseful of gorgeous Gremlins, and I was loving every second of it.

Shattering Your Comfort Zone

Finally, after what seemed like years of pure happiness in my life (excuse me as I wipe off a few tears of nostalgic joy that have just trickled down my cheek in this moment of warm reminiscence), the coins, I mean women, finally slowed to a halt. And I was surrounded with the best prize any young man could dream up in his wildest fantasy: 30 super-model-attractive women, all sitting next to and around me, eagerly waiting to get started on our new class together. (There actually, in full disclosure, was one other male in this class. He was okay at dancing, and was actually a pretty cool dude, but he's really not significant in this story, so I'll probably omit him from this point forward. I didn't notice him that day and I really didn't notice him any other day thereafter. Again, good dude, but there was far more to behold, especially in my sex-charged and confidence-seeking mind. Also, I'd fully expect to be forgotten from any of said dude's future interpretations of this same class, if and when he ever decides to pine over the past and rehash this epic period in time with his future grandchildren. No hard feelings bro, I get it . . .)

Anyway, as I'm naturally lusting over the bonanza surrounding me, the teacher, who extracts even more yearning from my already dwindling supply, begins to address the class.

"Hi everyone, I'm really happy to meet you all. My name is (I forget), but you can call me (I also forget, so let's call her Jane)," the really attractive teacher announces.

"Do any of you have any prior experience taking classes like this?" Jane continues.

Every single person's hand but mine shoots up.

"Oh, that's great. I'm happy to see just about everyone has some experience in dance," she enthusiastically adds, and then glances over at me, one hand tucked in my pocket, the other awkwardly resting on my lap as it searches for a new comfortable home amidst the gaze of this stunning beauty, who will be my dancing instructor for the next four months.

She smiles slightly, and I can't tell if it's a smile of delight or pity, but I smile back anyway, hoping it's the former.

As she continues, I come to the realization that I'm the only one in here who has absolutely no fucking experience in dancing. Up until that point I've seemingly possessed two tied-up left feet every time I tried to move my body around, in what one could only assume was a horrific attempt at rhythmic movement. My dancing spectrum has consisted of a head nod and a foot tap; anything more than that and I was flirting with disaster. If you or anyone else witnessed me going beyond this self-imposed limit, you were liable to take out a restraining order, or simply call the police to end my indecent crimes against humanity.

But putting my ego aside (and perhaps my freedom if someone did feel the urge to get the authorities involved at any given point in this class), I'd decided to take the plunge and sign up for this dance course anyway. I knew I sucked. But I figured, "Fuck it, I might as well try to get better."

CHALLENGING MYSELF

It was during this time that I was taking on all challenges in my life. I was on the cusp of pushing past all of my biggest fears, and I wanted to continue. Armed with the courage of a man who'd beaten depression and anxiety, and who'd woken a sleeping giant within, I started to bang on, and knock down, all the doors of things I'd previously been terrified of. I felt like a kid who'd been bullied all his life, but suddenly hits puberty and gets jacked, and goes back and beats the shit out of all the assholes who picked on him.

I was picking a fight with all of my bullies and winning.

Shattering Your Comfort Zone

Aside from signing up for the dance class, I'd been riding roller coasters, taking acting classes, doing speech classes, taking improv lessons, singing karaoke every couple of weeks (sober), and walking up to and striking up a conversation with just about every attractive woman I'd come across. One incredible fear after another I was picking out and mastering. These were all things I was terrified of doing, but just by pushing myself into doing them, and making sure I stuck through it and didn't quit, I always gained more confidence by the end of it.

It felt so good too. Living life without fear, and with the belief that you can do anything, no matter how terrifying it may appear, is just an incredible sensation.

Don't get me wrong, I was scared shitless every time I pushed myself out of my comfort zone. I'd always immediately feel like I'd finally gone too far, in whatever I was trying to overcome, but I'd promised myself not to give in. As much as I was afraid, as much as it didn't come naturally to me, and as much as I was totally out of my element, I doggedly stuck with each and every challenge. From acting, to improv, to speech class, and dance, I persistently showed up and broke past my self-beliefs.

But of all the steps I took out of my comfort zone, taking that dance class was the most nerve-racking of them all. But it also turned out to be the most rewarding.

DANCING TOWARDS CONFIDENCE

For the first few weeks, I'd drag my feet before every single class, concocting an infinite number of excuses for why I should sit that day out and maybe try the next class in a few days instead: *I've got a lot of homework to catch up on. I'm feeling a little under the weather today. Ah, if*

ELITE MIND

I just reset my alarm clock, I can sleep in for another two hours and catch up on my sleep and be refreshed for the rest of my classes today.

Excuse after excuse would spring to mind every morning as I'd get up for the day's courses. But I never succumbed to them. Not once.

I knew if I did, I'd get in the habit of skipping all the time, and my goal was to conquer this fear, just like all the others before it.

Refreshingly, though, I'd feel on top of the world by the end of every class. The beginnings were always a little tense, but once I got going and we'd start to move around and learn some new dance moves, it became a blast. I actually truly enjoyed the class and loved moving around, slowly getting less and less awkward with my bodily flow.

As the semester progressed I started looking forward to the classes, and couldn't wait to get in there. I actually enjoyed learning how to dance, and learning how to be more confident in my own skin. It's one thing to dance at a bar when it's dark as hell and loud as fuck and everyone is half-in-the-bag or completely shitfaced, and can't discern whether or not you're a good dancer because they've had ten-too-many Fireball shots and they're sloppy as sin. It's pretty easy when your only potential audience can't hold an additional thought because their sole focus and life's purpose in that moment is consuming more alcohol and becoming bombastically inebriated. No, the rummies in your local dive bar aren't as critical, or meaningful, as a class full of sober and super-sexy babes.

So learning this skill was something I welcomed with open arms. Even if I still wasn't turning into Michael Jackson anytime soon, I was slowly (incredibly slowly) but surely, getting better.

At the end of the year we had one final dance routine to perform in front of the class. We'd learned a number of others throughout the semester—everything from contemporary dance, to salsa, to hip-hop and more, taking the guidance of Jane and her hypnotically attractive method of teaching (which needless to say I loved and grew more and more fond of by the day). But for our final performance, we were paired off into groups of twos or threes, and told to create our own dance routines based on the arbitrary genre of music we'd ritualistically plucked out of a hat earlier in the year to determine precisely this.

I got hip-hop, which wasn't too bad, I guess. I also got paired off with a couple of smoke-shows, which was even better.

After a few weeks of hard practice and even hanging out with my partners outside of school to go over our routines (among other things), we were set to perform. Now, before I continue, anyone who knows anything about dancing, like even the tiniest fucking minuscule bit of it, knows that it takes a long, long time to get good at it. Like *years* in fact for most people, or if you spend ten hours a day with a personal dancing coach and a world-class partner on something like *Dancing With The Stars*, you might hack the proverbial learning curve and cut your time down dramatically. But that doesn't come without nearly complete dedication for weeks or months on end, spending the better parts of your days practicing over and over again. And even then, mastery of dance is probably still not truly within grasp. So for the common man, like you or I, we're almost certainly on the *yearly* plan.

With that said, let me just cut to the chase and end your hope for the cliché, movie-ending climactic moment of glory, where I come out with my two head-turning partners and work the crowd like Patrick Swayze in *Dirty Dancing*. It doesn't quite play out like that. In reality, to be fully transparent here, I actually kind of sucked.

I had a ton of confidence going in, using some of the concepts I've mentioned already, and felt great throughout, but I just didn't have the necessary skill needed to be that good. My partners were good, and they looked sexy doing their number, but I just sort of danced around with a big smile on my face, one step and one beat behind them, skipping ahead at times to keep up with the quicker-than-desired pace.

I fucking bombed. It was like watching a fish flail around in the Sahara.

Okay, maybe I'm being a little too harsh on myself here. Perhaps I didn't really bomb as badly as I think, but I do know I wasn't nearly as good as I'd hoped or thought I was going to be. I was a little behind in some parts of the song and I did mess up a couple of times, but all in all, it wasn't that bad. For instance, it wasn't like I'd been thrown into a pit full of snakes and everyone in the audience was just painfully watching me get bitten and choked to death, which would've been the case in my pre-confidence era. Actually, I had fun, and I could tell the audience was having fun watching us.

About midway through the routine, I realized I wasn't doing as well as I'd wanted to, and that maybe, given a few more weeks of practice, I'd have done a lot better, but that the couple of weeks we'd had just wasn't nearly enough time. But I also recall not really caring about whether I sucked or not, and allowing myself to have fun, despite being in front of an ordinarily horrifying audience of people watching my every move.

I'd thought to myself before I went up there, and then re-thought this again midway through, that this whole thing was just for fun anyways. It wasn't like I really had anything to lose or anyone to actually impress. And so, prior to and during the routine, I stopped myself from getting negative about how I was doing and instead focused on enjoying myself.

Shattering Your Comfort Zone

As badly as I may have actually done, I probably had more fun than anyone who performed that day. And when our three-minute act came to its conclusion, the whole class erupted in applause. It was the loudest and most energetic applause I'd heard that entire semester. At the time I thought it had been because my two partners had carried my ass to the promised land and actually salvaged our performance. But looking back now, I honestly believe they were clapping because I'd stuck with it.

They were clapping because I was visibly so far below everyone else in that class in terms of talent, but so proficient at being confident in myself and being able to face my fears. They could see someone breaking down his walls and displaying ample amounts of incredible confidence right before their very eyes. And they could appreciate the beauty in that, despite the lack of beauty in my performance.

(Either that, or they were just going batshit crazy with applause because they were so pumped my rhythmically-challenged ass was finally ending its morbidly offensive assault on their optic faculties. I like to think it's the former sentiment though.)

THE DERIVATIVE OF MY CONFIDENCE

As bad as I was at dancing, I had so much fun doing it. When people see you doing something and enjoying yourself, it often supersedes the level of skill you display in that area. Confidence isn't quite everything, but it sure is a lot.[1]

With this new level of confidence, derived from pushing myself out of my comfort zone and regularly challenging myself in all aspects of life, I felt like a new man. I felt like a person who finally knew how to enjoy himself and live life as it was meant to be lived.

There was no stopping me. My confidence was at an all-time high and continuing to grow. With just a few more steps I'd be unbelievably fucking confident and mentally elite.

HOW TO APPLY THIS

If you're serious about gaining confidence you have to take this step.

To gain the ability to feel like you can do anything in any situation successfully, you have to do things that scare the fuck out of you. Things like dancing in front of a bunch of women, or singing to a crowd full of people (must be done without the aid of alcohol or drugs), or giving a speech to a roomful of guests, or riding on roller coasters that scare the shit out of you, and so many other things that scare the hell out of you. If you want to gain true confidence, it's imperative to push past those self-imposed limits you've had for so many years.

When you do this, you realize that there's truly nothing you can't do. You are the only person restricting your own success in anything. We all are our own biggest critic and our own worst enemy. When we buck up and take on the challenge of facing the things we most fear, when we survive them, we realize our true power. We realize how much untapped potential dwells inside of us and how much willpower we truly possess to take on anything life throws our way.

Go out today and sign up for something that scares the hell out of you. Whatever it may be. Maybe it's something I've listed already or maybe it's something you fear that's been terrorizing you for so long. A social challenge, a mental class, an emotional test, a physical pursuit, whatever you've been holding back from taking because it's too far outside of your comfort zone . . . sign your ass up for it today and take the plunge.

Shattering Your Comfort Zone

Look, I'm not advocating doing anything beyond reason here. Just to be clear, I don't recommend doing anything ridiculous or down-right dangerous, like jumping off a bridge or running across three lanes of highway traffic. Don't do anything stupid that may put your life at risk, seriously. What I am advocating, however, is taking on those fears you've been holding off for years and going all-in on beating them. Why? Because at the heart of your deepest fears lies the soul of your truest confidence.

Take action today and see how much you can do. My guess is you'll amaze yourself with just how much you can accomplish. And, my other guess, is that your confidence will shoot through the fucking roof.

ONE LAST THING

Taking the approach of facing my fears, stepping out of my comfort zone, and doing shit that scared the absolute hell out of me might have been the smartest thing I ever did in my life. It's perhaps the most powerful confidence-building tool in this entire book.

If there's one thing you absolutely must do out of this confidence section, it's this step here. So make sure you don't take this advice lightly and put it off until never. The time is now.

By the way, as much as I love going out and starting up a dance party, whether at the bar, a nightclub, a wedding (I'll literally be the first one out on the dance floor most of the time), that doesn't mean I'm any good at it. Even now, many years after taking that dance class of super-babes, I still honestly suck.

But that doesn't stop me from getting out there and tearing up the dance floor like a fucking *Footloose* champ. And in reality, it doesn't matter, as long as you're confident you could move around like Pee-Wee Herman doing his *Tequila* dance and still get women. As long as you can laugh, have fun, and be confident while doing this, you'll excel.

Confidence can often override skill and make you look like you know what you're doing, even if you have no fucking clue. If you're confident in yourself, you'll be successful in *almost* anything you do (there are certainly limits; this isn't magic!). Overall, it's a hell of a tool for success.

Remember, confidence isn't everything, but it's huge, and oftentimes more than enough to get you by.

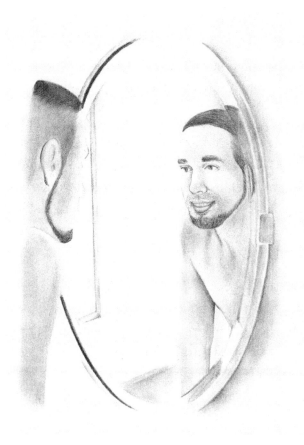

Chapter Twenty-Nine
Improving Your Self-Image

"Goddammit, I look fucking sexy!" I boldly exclaimed, with a slight snicker forming from the corners of my mouth, to one of my best friends Chris, as we stood in front of a life-sized mirror in the hallway of one of the coolest clubs in Boston.

I was beaming with satisfaction as I looked down at my wingtipped light brown shoes and dark blue fitted jeans (with a sprinkling of just enough light blue in the middle to match the tan wingtip Oxfords to a tee). I then glanced up at my slick, slim-fitted, light blue Calvin Klein button shirt that accentuated the best parts of my Adonis-like figure, and a shit-eating grin of satisfaction swept across my face. (Okay, *Adonis* is totally stretching it here, but I felt great!)

I loved my outfit. And I said, "I look fucking sexy," in the humblest way possible. Really. I did look good, and I love dressing up, but by no means do I mean to imply that I'm conceited about my looks. I'm quite simply not. Do I love being confident and showing off the hard work I put in at the gym? Absolutely. Do I truly think I'm unworldly handsome, and that women get all hot and heavy every time I enter a room? Fuck no.

In fact, it took me years to get over my insecurities surrounding my self-image, so I know just how important it is to not get carried away with the influence it garners over my contentment. I'm happy with my self-image and work hard at optimizing it every day, but I'm not attached to it; at least I try my best to not be.

I learned a long time ago that it doesn't matter so much that you're where you wish to be in terms of your self-image; far more important is how you're working your way toward getting there. In other words, you gain your confidence from the fact that you know you're striving to be your best, not necessarily that you've arrived at that place.

For years my height bothered me. For years my weight bothered me. For years my hairline bothered me. For years my eyes bothered me. But after adapting many of the principles found in this book, I let that shit go and started focusing on what really mattered.

I mentioned before that I'd love to be taller if it were possible. I wouldn't mind one bit being a giant, towering over most of the denizens in my city and invoking immediate respect from all who gazed upon my magnificence. I'd be fucking thrilled in fact if some

Improving Your Self-Image

Robin-Williams-looking genie popped up from the depths of the earth and magically made me like 6'6 or something. That'd be pretty sweet.

But I'm not delusional, as much as I may have thought I was way back when I smoked that laced marijuana. I know this will never happen and so I've come to terms with my modest stature and am totally cool with it now.

And the same goes for my hair, my eyes, my skinnier-than-average frame (though unlike the others this can be somewhat manipulated), and every other insecurity I've harbored over the years. If I can't work on improving something, I do something unbelievably fucking radical and astoundingly bizarre: I accept it.

We're all blessed with different gifts.

This isn't just some nice Kumbaya sentiment, it's fucking true. Some people were born to be physical specimens and make a living beating up other men, whilst others were born to launch rockets into outer space for the greater good of humanity. And still others have a mixture of inborn strengths and weaknesses, and are not innately destined to master any particular field but to test out and enjoy many, using a multitude of skillsets to traverse through life tackling various challenges.

We all have our things we love about ourselves, like our creativity, our ingenuity, our independence, or maybe our looks. But on that same token, we also all have things we hate about ourselves and wish that we could change—our height, our looks, our voice, our intelligence, or whatever else.

The point here is that there are two sides to the token: one cultivates happiness and gratitude for what we have, and the other promotes insecurity and inferiority. What I'm suggesting is that you put the token down and keep the side up with all the things that make you feel good about yourself.

Accept what you cannot change, embrace your strengths with open arms, and focus on that which you can improve. By taking this approach your day-to-day happiness will augment, and your confidence too will follow suit.

So step number one is dropping the negative feelings surrounding your personal dislikes. Drop them now like a bad habit.

Step number two is focusing on your strengths and all that you were blessed with in life. (Love yourself for Christ's sake, will ya'?)

Step number three is working on that which you can improve, and more specifically, working on your self-image. And this is what I want to focus on most in this section.

YOUR SELF-IMAGE

Your self-image is the way you view yourself. That's it. It takes into account your looks, your physical health, your feelings, your emotions, your strengths, and yes, your weaknesses. It's the way you feel about who you are as a human being. And when it comes to confidence, this is obviously extremely important. As a matter of fact, true confidence is derived from your self-image.

Let me repeat that once more to nail it home and for dramatic effect: *True confidence is derived from your self-image.*

As far as improving your feelings and emotions, we pretty much annihilated that issue in the depression and anxiety chapters, so I'll refrain from beating that dead horse any further for the moment. And as for the strengths and weaknesses bit, I'll repeat this once

Improving Your Self-Image

more: quit dwelling on shit you can't change and embrace the shit you've been endowed with!

So that said, we're left with your physical health and your looks, which can both be improved, and even hacked to a certain degree.

Here's a fairly comprehensive list of things you can and should immediately start optimizing to enhance your physical health and looks, and thus your self-image and confidence.

Diet

We talked at length about the power of your diet in the previous section of this book. The biggest takeaway from that segment is quite simple: You are what you eat, so eat like a champ.

Sleep

Sleep, too, we covered extensively in the anxiety portion of this book, so I'll hold off on reiterating all the specifics for improving it. Just know that not only is sleep important for anxiety reduction, as well as depression, but it's also critical for your confidence level.

Exercise

Once more, we've covered exercise at length, so I won't dive into great detail here, but just remember, your self-image is often derived from how you look. If you look like shit, and you think (and know) you look like shit, you're going to have shit for confidence. Therefore, it only makes sense to optimize how you look, and perhaps the finest way to do this is through hitting up the gym and regularly working out.

It doesn't matter that you're at your ideal body physique in order to receive the confidence-boosting benefits of exercise, only that you're moving toward your personal goal.

Clothing

There's an old quote attributed to two of history's most distinguished authors, Mark Twain, and William Shakespeare. Who really uttered it first, or at all, is debatable, but nonetheless it reads, "Clothes make the man." And well, it's true.[1] Wearing the right clothes is one of the most powerful techniques to feeling amazing about yourself. It's also one of the easiest things you can do right away, and with little to no effort, instantly feel better about the way you look and feel.

Look, I'm no fashion aficionado by any means, but I do know that dressing up a little can go a long way. Get rid of your old baggy, beat-up, faded clothes that effectively make you look like a homeless bum, and buy some nice, new, fitted and stylish shit that looks good on you. For guys, that means fitted shirts, fitted pants, and nice pairs of shoes. For women, it could be a well-fitting and stylish dress, fitted blouse or top, fitted pants, and nice heels or shoes to add some sexiness or class, depending on the occasion.

In general, fitted works best for both sexes. But you always want to accentuate your body type and skin tone with the outfits you choose.

Some people look great in red, while others look better in blue. Some look fantastic in white, while others look transparently weird wearing this same color. Find what naturally highlights your skin complexion and stick mostly with those colors.

For body type, play around with different styles of clothes, as some will make your shoulders look big, your biceps look cut, and your waist look skinny, and therefore make you look more attractive as a man. Others, although fitting well on other men, may not ideally conform to your figure. As for women, the same applies. Some outfits make your waist look skinnier, your breasts firmer, your arms more toned, and your butt more Jennifer-Lopez-like. Whilst these same garments might make someone else look more like Rosie O'Donnell. Go for J-Lo whenever possible.

Hairstyle

When I was depressed and younger I used to have a very plain haircut, not because I thoughtfully tried to display my depression to the world by choosing a boring haircut, but because it sort of mimicked my inward feelings in a subtle way. It was kind of like my subconscious mind expressing itself, basically mumbling to the world, "I'm boring and insecure."

My haircut was as basic as haircuts came: straight down, blunted bangs, with I think a number 2 clipper for the sides. That was it. Don't get me wrong, this hairstyle of simplicity can look great on some guys, but for me, it just muttered *blah*. Looking back, I absolutely rocked this do because I wanted to blend into the crowd and not be noticed by anyone. And that's exactly what happened.

As I got older though, and my confidence grew, I started styling my hair up, and back. The undercut hairstyle and faux hawk became my go-to looks respectively, and they both screamed nothing but confidence.

Now occasionally, I switch things up and cut my hair really short, but I never go back to putting it just down. For me at least, it's too depressing, and boring.

The biggest takeaway when it comes to finding a good hairstyle is to choose something that fits you, and perhaps challenges you to stand out a bit. If you've had the same boring do for years, it's time to switch things up. Get a little more edgy and perhaps a little more fashionable, and try something new. In fact, try a few different looks and play around with a few styles, until you find one that really resonates and makes you look and feel sexier. No more blah and boring, we want new, exciting, and attractive.

Your hairstyle may not seem like a big deal, but trust me, when you know you look good, and better than you did before with your old haircut, you're going to automatically feel more confident.

Oh, and if you're losing your hair, like a ton of it, don't be afraid to shave the rest off. The bald look can work great for some men. Just make sure you're one of those men first. Try using one of those bald apps or something to see how you'd look with a shiny top. If you think you'd look better, take the plunge; if not, find a style you can work around and that still looks fairly natural. And then *own* it.

Grooming

Facial hair, clear skin, trimmed nails, trimmed body hair, even hygiene of various sorts, can all be lumped into the grooming category. These each play a factor in the way you maintain your looks and ergo your confidence level.

If you're a man, either keep the clean-shaven look clean and shaven, or grow a nicely trimmed beard. If you're a woman, remove all facial hair from your face, aside from your eyebrows and eyelashes. There shouldn't be any little whiskers creeping out of your facial structure—no excuses, especially in this day and age with all of the phenomenal technological advances in razor blades.

Clear skin is also important, though for some it's a lot tougher than others. Usually if you have bad skin, there's an underlying dietary or allergenic issue that needs to be addressed. This can be fixed through getting yourself tested for various toxins, allergens, and food sensitivities. Knowing what foods you're highly sensitive to can be very helpful in providing you a map for which ones to eliminate from your diet. Typically, cases of acne can be healed entirely by getting rid of these bad foods and allowing the body to run more cleanly.

Also, lowering your glycemic load appears to improve acne,[2] as does removing dairy from your diet. Consuming nutritional compounds like antioxidants, omega-3 fatty acids, zinc, vitamin A, and dietary fiber can further assist as well.

Additionally, the more obvious, but equally important aspect here, is to take care of your skin. Shower regularly, and don't use harmful, chemically-laced rinses, creams, or lotions (Think Dirty is a great app for helping you identify the insidiously dangerous ingredients in your products). Moreover, don't overuse soap, which can dry out your face or skin, don't take extra long showers (same drying-out effect), and use a "healthy" acne cream, if you choose to use one at all.

Most of the acne creams are not good for your skin with long-term use, as they're loaded with unfavorable ingredients. But for acute situations of clearing up your skin (especially pimples on the face, which I know can be devastating to many), go for it. Keep your confidence high by keeping your skin nice and clean.

Trimming your nails. This one's easy: Trim your fucking nails. That is all.

The same goes for body hair. Looking like the Abominable Snowman is so 1970s porn. Having a bushful of pubic hair and a shaggy Austin-Powers chest is unacceptable these days. Get a $15 set of Wahl clippers on Amazon, put the clipper setting on 1 or 2 (or 0 if you're like me), and go to town on your pubes, and on your chest if applicable. Your romantic partners will appreciate this move, trust me.

If you're a woman, armpit hair is a sin. Your job is to take the same clippers we men use, remove all the numbered attachments, and go to town on your armpit hairs, every couple of days (or just a regular razor will do). And the same goes for your legs, and of course for your vaginal area. No pubic hairs, and no unwomanly hairs at all for that matter, should be visible to the naked eye. Not on your face, not on your legs, and not on your ass. (Sorry, the short-lived feminist movement of growing out hairs in unwanted places just didn't quite catch on. It hit the sex-appeal roadblock head on.)

Quit being lazy and grab a razor, unless of course you're content being utterly unattractive to those you desire. It may sound harsh but it's true. (Men can get away with a little more hair in a few places.)

It may take a couple extra minutes for women to shave than for men; you're right, that's not fair. But we guys have held open thousands of doors over the course of our lives to make up for this evolutionary discrepancy. So there, we're equal. Not to mention, we have fucking beards we must either shave off or attend to every day for fuck's sake (plus hairy balls, hairy ears, hairier noses, hairier unibrows, and back hair that on some men completely stakes claim over their spinal columns and sprouts dense shrubbery comparable to the thicket found only in the jungles of the Amazon). Give us a break.

Lastly, as far as hygiene goes, brush your teeth, wash your hands, take showers as mentioned before, get the boogers out of your nose, and smell like roses as much as possible. Basically, be a clean and sanitary person on all fronts, not a smelly, disgusting one.

Putting all of this together, grooming can certainly make or break someone's confidence level. When you've got these fairly simple steps nailed down you know you're operating at your best. You feel good about yourself and how you look, and naturally, confidence grows.

Don't overlook grooming, it takes only a few minutes to do each day, but it's essential for maintaining and producing your optimum level of confidence.

<u>Body Language</u>

Body language could probably be its own confidence chapter, but because it's so intimately tied into your self-image, I felt inclined to add it to this section. Having great body language is perhaps the quickest and easiest way to boost your self-image.

So without further ado, here are my best body language tips.

BODY LANGUAGE MASTERY

<u>Head Up, Shoulders Back, Standing Tall</u>

Always keep your head up when attempting to display confidence. Those who have their heads down immediately lose value in the eyes of others, and hence feel less confident. This is probably the most basic of all confident body language tips. Just keep your chin slightly up and out at all times, the opposite of if you were in a boxing ring or fighting someone. By having your chin stick out, you display that you have nothing to fear and are very relaxed and comfortable.

You also want to make sure you keep your shoulders back, which prevents you from slouching over and puffs out your chest in a subtly cool way. Don't take this overboard and start strutting around like that toolbag at your gym who thinks he looks like a juiced-up Ronnie Coleman. (You know, the guy who walks around with his shoulders aberrantly pulled back and his chest obnoxiously puffed up; that'll just make you look like a cocky dumbass, not a confident cool person.)

But yes, a slight shoulders-back look and a minor puffing up of the chest is a good way to exhibit confidence. It prevents you from having any bit of a questionably meek-looking appearance. We're going for confidence here, not compliance.

Standing tall is the last part of this little trio of bodily expressions. It goes hand in hand with the other two examples, in that your whole goal here is to showcase your body as much as possible, to essentially say, "Hey, look at me," to the world. You're making yourself, in a subtle but effective way, stand out more, simply by erecting your body to its fullest capacity. Confident people do this time and again. They naturally position themselves to the utmost limits of their body and have absolutely no shame in sticking out in the right way.

Stop lowering your head, stop rounding down your shoulders, and stop slouching. Stand up straight, puff that chest out a little, and keep your head up high.

Eye Contact

Make solid eye contact with everyone you come in contact with. It immediately displays your confidence and shows that you have a strong sense of character. People who can't look someone else in the eye often act this way because they feel like they are inadequate, inferior, or have done something wrong; they do this as a way to "cover up" their actions and not be discovered.

As a confident person, look every motherfucker in the eye and hide nothing. Show people you're the one with value, the one with a strong backbone. Looking down, looking away, looking around at something else . . . all of these actions should be completely eliminated from your repertoire.

But don't overdo it. Sometimes, men and women who want to feel more confident will stare too long into someone else's eyes in an attempt to display their confidence. It's like the asshole who wants to have a good handshake so he squeezes your palm with the death-grip from hell, crunching your fingers and leaving you wondering, "What the fuck is wrong with him?"

Those who stare into your eyes for far too long have the same insulting effect. Don't be that person who fucks up good eye contact. Instead, look someone in the eyes for a few seconds, then look away naturally during a break in conversation, and then look back again, and then rinse and repeat indefinitely.

Taking Up Space

Taking up space has the same psychological effect as popping your chin and head up (confident), as opposed to looking down or tucking in your chin (no confidence). When we are confident we naturally let our guard down as we don't fear a threat to our well-being. This takes the shape of moving our hands and legs away from our vital organs—heart, liver, kidneys, genitalia—and freeing them up to show others how sure of ourselves we are. (Kind of like a peacock who spreads his feathers.)

The more capacity you take up, the more confident you're going to appear. So feel free to open those arms up, stand a little wider (or put your feet up if you're sitting down), and own the fuck out of the space around you.

After all, it is *your* space. Take it.

Tone Of Voice

"It's not what you say, it's how you say it."

I'm sure you've heard that gem before.

How about this one?

"Go fuck yourself, ya' fucking asshole."

This said to your best friend in a serious, pissed-off manner could mean the end of your friendship, as it would most likely be very hurtful in that context. But the exact same words uttered in a sarcastic, playful tone of voice, would mean a completely different thing. Actually, you and your friend would probably both start giggling over the reason for you sarcastically calling him out in this manner.

Identical phraseology, but in two drastically different tones, and therefore two radically different outcomes. Tone is almost everything when it comes to your verbal expression. How you say something far outweighs what you say. That's why it's so important to mind your tone of voice. If you want to be more confident, you need a confident tone of voice.

This can come down to several different things, but the common theme is that you have a self-assured inflection in your voice: you're not ambiguous or unsure; you're not hesitant, and certainly not meek; and you're absolutely not fucking timid. Instead, you're bold, assertive, unwavering, certain, and most definitely self-confident in whatever you say.

This confident pitch in your voice can take many forms: a playful vibe, a dominant attitude, a fun energy, a leadership approach, a sarcastic tone, and so many other displays of self-assuredness. The options are virtually unlimited here.

Voice Projection

Right along with your tone of voice, comes projecting your voice. The projection of your voice is critical in demonstrating your level of confidence to those around you. You can have the right confident tone all day long, but if nobody can hear you, they'll never be able to

Improving Your Self-Image

see the confidence you actually have. You must speak louder, especially in our ever-growing noisier world. Your voice will be lost amongst the crowd if you don't consciously speak up.

I know firsthand.

Trust me, I don't inherently have a booming voice, and it took me a while to come out of my naturally-introverted shell, once I realized how important it was for others to hear me in order for my confidence to grow. If you're like me and don't have an intrinsically loud volume of speech, start consciously enunciating your words a few levels higher than you normally would. It may be a little uncomfortable to have others hear you and perhaps become the center of attention at times, but that's part of the price you pay for getting more confidence. (This goes really well with stepping out of your comfort zone.)

Be loud and be proud.

<u>Movements</u>

Every move, from your arms and hands to your legs and feet, should be relaxed and controlled. A confident person doesn't have nervous tics, they don't fidget, they don't have weird jerks, they don't touch things unnecessarily, and they don't adjust or try to "fix" jewelry, hair, or articles of clothing merely from unconscious habit.

No, when confident people move, it's because there's a reason to. Spreading your arms across the table (if you're sitting down) and leaning back, now that's a solid movement. It shows you're relaxed and owning your space. Tapping your foot on the floor, then adjusting your watch for the third time in five minutes? That's an unnecessary pair of movements that reveal you're most likely anxious and looking to leave as soon as possible.

Remain calm unless making a confident motion. That's pretty much the simplest approach to mastering your movements. Of course you can scratch an itch if you get one, or check your watch if you need to know the time, or fix a collar if it wasn't folded over correctly, or whatever else. But incessantly making movements out of a feeling of unease is a no-go.

Do not, for the mother of all things big and small, do this. Ever.

<u>Walking</u>

You may have up to this point never really thought much about the way you walk, but you should. It's a huge part of your non-verbal communication. Just like all your other movements, a walk should be relaxed, controlled, and comfortable. Don't walk too fast or you'll come across as nervous. Don't walk too slow or you'll appear unsure of what you want to do. Instead, find the right balance of cool, controlled movement, one that demonstrates you're confident enough to take your time, but also shows you know where you're heading.

A little bit of swagger in your step can go a long way here. (Just a bit of it though; too much can make you look like you're trying way too hard.)

Also, make sure you keep your head up, shoulders back, and stand tall, as mentioned earlier. Gaze forward at where you're going and don't look down. You can glance around if you'd like, but only briefly. Keep your focus on where you're headed; don't get caught up in worrying about what others are doing around you. Confident individuals keep the focus on themselves and what they want to do, not on others.

Improving Your Self-Image

<u>Smiling and Laughing</u>

Smile regularly. Those who are confident in themselves are almost always people who are incredibly happy. So show the world this: smile when you say things; smile when you meet someone new; smile when you enter a room; smile when you see someone you know; smile . . . as much as you possibly can. It's not only good for your confidence, but good for your health. Studies have actually found that smiling can directly lead to happier mood changes.[3]

Try not to fake a smile either, but rather actually smile and enjoy life more. Start to take life less seriously and more playfully. View different situations and different people as ways for you to further enjoy life and share more meaningful experiences.

That said, if you do have to occasionally fake a smile or two, to pull off a more confident demeanor, make sure you smile with your teeth. This is how people smile when they're really happy, and it's much harder for someone to discern if you're faking a smile when you smile fully and expose your pearly whites, as opposed to a sort of half-smile that doesn't display teeth. These half-smiles are easy for people to pick up on as being disingenuous.

Laughing, as I mentioned in the beginning of this book, is probably the greatest gift to mankind. It's the breaker of tension and liberator of souls. It connects two people like nothing else (aside from perhaps sex, and even then sometimes more so). It lifts the mood of the most dejected individual and brings happiness to all who experience it. Laugh, and laugh often. This is perhaps the best medicine for your health currently in existence, and it also does wonders as far as revealing your level of confidence to the world.

He who laughs most is most happy. And he who laughs most has the most confidence.

Handshakes

Having a good, solid handshake can reveal a lot about your self-belief.

You ever shake someone's hand and think, "This is fucking gross!" as you covertly make a disgusting face and reflect to yourself, "I can't wait to wash the hell out of my hands!"?

I have. Many times. So many people don't even consider this, but it's very important. Going up and shaking someone's hand with a sweaty, clammy, weak-gripped shake is probably one of the dumbest things you can do if making a good impression is on your mind. It immediately ruins all chances of you coming across as someone who garners respect and possesses confidence.

Instead of being a clammy-hand handshaker, make sure you rub off the sweat (preferably when no one's looking), wipe off any dirt or other crap that might be on your fingers, and have a firm and strong extension of your hand as you embrace the person in question.

When you interlock hands, give it a solid up and down for a full second, maybe a second and a half at most, and then release. Do not, and I mean DO NOT, try to give a death-grip handshake in an attempt to impose your masculine dominance. The only thing this will effectively do is convey what a complete douchebagged-asshole you are. It's completely ineffective for trying to do whatever you think it's supposed to do.

Not too hard like you have a stick up your ass, and not too soft and clammy. Strong but flexible will do.

Your Words

I mentioned earlier that your tone of voice is a lot more important than the actual words you utter. But that doesn't mean the words

Improving Your Self-Image

themselves still aren't a critical component. They are. Your words don't need to be the specific things you say. I'm not going to tell you to recite a bunch of paragraphs and then repeat them verbatim in public. Not only would that not work, that would just be ridiculously tedious for you, and more importantly, me.

What I mean by optimizing your words is, think about the words you use in conversation, and make them more favorable to cultivating your confidence.

For instance, think about saying things that are more positive. Try putting a positive spin on things, even if you're having a shitty day or if something isn't going your way. Use positivity to switch negative things into beneficial things, and to display your confidence to others. Everybody hates that guy who's always complaining about how horrible his life is. Don't be that guy. Be the guy who sees things in an optimistic light, and who makes good shit happen, even when circumstances aren't going his way.

You can also say things that are self-entertaining, to telegraph your confidence to those around you. It's counter-intuitive but people who couldn't care less about what others think are people who others end up caring more about. These are the ones who hold massive amounts of confidence, and to whom society in general is most attracted.

These people often say things only intended to amuse or entertain themselves, without so much as a single fuck given to the opinions of those around them. But what magically happens is, others are more enthralled by them. People get drawn to these types of people because they're so few and far between.

Most people are scared to say a lot of things. Scared to say controversial shit. Scared to voice an unpopular opinion. Scared to stand up for a belief. Scared to say jokes that may offend a few. Scared to be politically incorrect. Scared to say something that's really on their mind . . . Some people are even scared to breathe because they fear taking too much of their fair share of oxygen.

Don't be someone like this. Be someone who steps up and puts himself out there from time to time. Take the heat, be a lightning rod, offend a few people; in the end, your confidence will skyrocket and most people will love you for standing up and doing what they can't. By losing a few fake friends you gain an infinite number of real ones.

PRACTICE IN FRONT OF A MIRROR

Practice your body language, your tone of voice, and yes, even some of your speech in front of a mirror. Seriously. I know it sounds fucking stupid, but it really works. If you want to really get good at stepping into the role of your new confident self, you've got to perfect the way your new confident self looks.

Spend 10 minutes a day for the next 10 days, going over everything I mentioned above, especially the areas you really want to focus on. This isn't a big commitment or a big time-suck on your part, so you should easily be able to do it. No excuses.

Practice your body language forms, and get it down. Talk to yourself, move your body around, project your voice louder, do it all. And then rinse and repeat, every day for the next 10 days. I want you to own the fuck out of that confident new image.

You're a confident person inside, now act like it.

LOVE WHAT YOU SEE IN THE MIRROR

When it comes to putting everything together and shaping your self-image, I say this:

At the end of the day, fuck it all.

Improving Your Self-Image

Fuck having six-pack shredded abs like Cristiano Ronaldo. Fuck having luscious golden locks like Charlie Hunnam. Fuck dressing to the tee like David Beckham.

You don't need any of these things to be confident. What you really need is to be working toward reaching your own goals, whatever they may be. As I mentioned earlier in this chapter, the most important thing to having confidence, derived from your self-image, is not that you have that perfect body you've always wanted, but that you are working toward getting it. Looking like a modern day Hercules can be cool, but it's not a prerequisite to being confident.

The most important thing to remember when it comes to having confidence is loving what you see when you look in the mirror. Having your ideal body is a process, but taking care of smaller, easier things (grooming habits, haircut, wardrobe, body language), is the perfect way to get the ball rolling. And in the meantime, tackling your diet, mastering your sleep, and working out most days out of the week will be more than enough to remind you you're giving it your all when you look yourself in the mirror.

This reassurance that you're putting in your best effort to maximize your self-image and maximize your happiness, that's where your true confidence is bred.

Put in the effort, get the confidence.

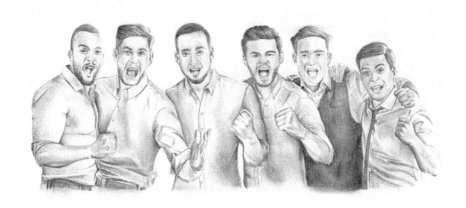

Chapter Thirty
Averaging Your Way to Greatness

"You are the average of the five people you spend the most time with."

Just about every human being on the face of the Earth has heard this quote at some point in their lives. It's attributed to the late great Jim Rohn, but like all quotes, I'm sure some sort of derivative of this has been used for hundreds, if not thousands, of years before Rohn's time. In any case, it's true.

Human beings are social creatures. We pick up on the social cues of those around us, whether good[1] or bad.[2] We're hereditarily inclined to live in tribes, where we must communicate, congregate, and work together in order to survive. Without the pack we'd be all alone, and almost certainly doomed to imminent death.

Just think about it from a practicality standpoint for a moment, to fully grasp the importance of this tribal concept and why living amongst others is so important. Let's journey back for a minute to about 40,000 B.C., and let's briefly pretend you're a hairy-balled caveman, who bangs rocks together to make music and rubs sticks together to make fire. (Yeah, we can even call you Mr. Flintstone if you'd like.)

Now Fred, imagine for a moment trying to hunt a deer by yourself with a crude weapon like a glorified sharpened tree branch. How fucking bad would it suck to have to run around, unsuccessfully throwing this rudimentary spear at an animal twice as fast and twice as athletic as you? Pretty fucking bad, I would imagine.

Now, envision having eight or so other guys with sharpened sticks and knives, and maybe a few with cool and innovative technologies like maces, throwing axes, and prototypical bows with arrows, also hunting the soon-to-be-roasted buck. How much better do you surmise your chances of having venison for dinner that night (and then getting lucky with Wilma) become?

The correct answer, Freddie my boy, is *infinitely*.

That's why groups matter, even today.

Arbitrary Neanderthal metaphors aside, we're wired to be like others. It's in our DNA to socialize, communicate, and to think like those we surround ourselves with. We've learned, we've grown, we've evolved, by sharing our ideas and living amongst those with whom we spend our time.

So with that in mind, it only makes sense to spend your time with those who have the things you want.

Would you want to spend your time with someone who brings you down, or someone who has things in life you don't want in yours? Someone who would quite literally slow your growth as a human being? Of course you wouldn't.

And jumping back to our Bedrock analogy for a moment, would spear-wielding Fred Flintstone want to spend his time hunting with cavemen whose best weapons were hurling *rocks* in their attempt to bring down a deer? Of course he wouldn't. Rock throwing cavemen would've been considered the dumbest of the dumb, the bottom of the class, no-brained morons, and so 41st millennia B.C. No, Fred would've been intelligent about who he surrounded himself with. He'd go hunting with the smart fucks who'd invented the bows that could shoot arrows, so he could rise to their level, eat more food, and get kinky with Wilma more often.

And that's precisely what you want to do too.

You want to find those five or so people, more or less, who can elevate you and make you rise to their level. In terms of confidence, you want to find five confident motherfuckers who can rub their self-belief off onto you.

It's exactly what I did.

MY CONFIDENT FIVE

<u>Bobby</u>

I mentioned Bobby earlier on in the anxiety section. You remember him, the guy who convinced me, against every fiber of my being, to go riding on that death-trap of a monstrosity known as Bizarro, way back when. The guy who inadvertently showed me the antidote to conquering my greatest fears with that one fateful roller coaster ride. Yup that Bobby, or "The Natural," as history's come to refer to him as.

I reintroduce The Natural once again because of all the men I surrounded myself with who bestowed upon me their sense of self-confidence, Bobby gave me the most.

He wasn't tall, he wasn't big, he wasn't remarkably handsome or otherwise physically gifted to where you'd look at him and think, "That's just not even fair."

No, Bobby was a pretty average-looking guy, who just so happened to possess an exorbitant amount of self-worth, not in a narcissistic way, but in an I-believe-in-myself-completely kind of way. And it showed.

Women loved him, guys loved him, old people loved him, kids loved him; everywhere he went, with his colossal self-belief pioneering his interactions, he immediately endeared himself to all he came across. He'd make girls fall for him in minutes. He'd have random guys shooting the shit and laughing with him in seconds. He'd get old folks to smile and have moments of inspirational small talk that would undoubtedly be the best couple of minutes of their day. And as for kids, every child he ever came across instantly thought he was the coolest adult they'd ever met.

Seriously, his social acuity was astounding. I've yet to meet anyone as good with people in my life. And by now, I've met quite a number of social masters, but even they couldn't hold a candle to The Natural.

The Natural's gifts to me were twofold. For one, he gave me the mindset to master the art of attracting women. Which as you know by now was a focal point in my life at this period of time. In fact, it had been my sole purpose back then: to get good with women after failing miserably with them for so many years. And Bobby, like a blessing from above, was my crash-course instructor for showing me just how it was done; even though he was completely oblivious to the fact. Simply through watching his genius at work, I learned substantially more than any book, course, or coach could possibly have taught.

The other contribution Bobby made to my self-belief system was the profound notion of not giving so much of a fuck about what other people think. Mark Manson, a great dude and a former guest on my podcast, talks about the concept of not giving a fuck in his bestselling book, aptly titled *The Subtle Art of Not Giving A Fuck* (which honestly I've still yet to read as of this moment, but from what I've heard it's really good). But long before Mark was writing hot-cake-selling bestsellers on this concept, The Natural was embodying this sentiment unconditionally.

When we'd go to a bar or club, Bobby was always the first one out on the dance floor (soon after my dance class I'd be right there with him, if not racing him to be the first). He'd grab a beer, and after a few laughs and regaling of stories, he'd hop right on over to the dance floor and work his charm.

Bobby, like me, completely sucked ass when it came to dancing. He had one real move and he used it often, no matter what was playing. It could be hip-hop, or house music, or R&B, or even fucking salsa, and he'd still figure out a way to incorporate his little move (distastefully of course) into the dance. It's kind of hard to describe the move, as uncanny as it was, but it involved both hands raised in the air, a slight bending of the knees, a head-sliding motion along with a matching shoulder sway, and a shit-eating and confident-as-fuck grin plastered across his face.

To this day I'm not entirely sure whether Bobby knew that he was absolutely terrible and just totally didn't give a fuck, or whether he was so self-assuredly delusional that he'd actually convinced himself he was good. But I can fairly accurately predict, knowing how blatantly obvious his dancing skills sucked balls, it's the former. Either way, it didn't matter. He was incredibly effective. It would only take a couple of minutes of dancing around before women would come up and make him look like a stud.

ELITE MIND

Whether it was dancing or the way he talked, The Natural's confidence was unwavering. He said things that came to mind. He talked about things he wanted to talk about. He made jokes that just about nobody else could get away with saying, some of the funniest fucking lines of any given night. He led the way dominantly but respectfully when it came to women, and they absolutely loved that masculine resolve. Every so often when he did fuck up and maybe crossed a social line or offended a girl in some way (and yes Bobby was incredibly great but he wasn't perfect), he just played it off like it wasn't a big deal. And it never became a big deal.

The most significant thing I took from my time with Bobby was how he believed in himself more than anyone else, and therefore didn't really give a fuck about what others thought. And the funny thing is, people loved him even more because of this.

The less he gave a fuck the more they loved him.

There's a difference between not caring at all about other people—you know, like sociopaths and shit—and caring too much about what others think, as insecure people do. Bobby had the perfect balance of these two opposites. He cared about his close friends, his family, and himself, and loved talking and laughing and hanging out with others, wishing them nothing but good fortune. But he never let the opinions of the masses ever affect his mindset. And that to me was a powerful realization. I've lived my life with this outlook ever since I discovered it in him.

Simon

Simon was not your prototypical stoner. Yes, he smoked weed numerous times throughout the day, and probably hadn't skipped a day in years, but he was different. One quick glance at his tall skinny frame, shoulder-length greasy hair, and backward snapback, and you'd immediately assume he was some video-game-addicted, mama's-basement-dwelling, Ramen-noodle-eating pothead who couldn't get laid in a houseful of hookers. But you'd be wrong.

Simon's social game was second only to The Natural's, and that's saying quite a lot. As much as Bobby was social and people naturally loved his presence, Simon was actually more inclined to be the center-of-attention kind of guy, at least most days of the week. He loved the role, and thrived in it. Bobby was, and is, the master of all social situations, and would totally turn on his charm whenever he wanted to, but really excelled more in the one-on-one role, or with just a couple of people.

Simon on the other hand, loved crowds, and crowds of people often loved Simon. He was loud, he was funny, he was high energy (I know, one of the only potheads I've ever met with high energy), and he was great at making everyone around him have a good time.

Like Bobby, he had an unwavering conviction of who he was, and impressed upon others this belief. And like Bobby, people loved him for it.

We used to go to a lot of parties back in the day. Sometimes they were in Boston, sometimes Fall River or Taunton or Plymouth. (All are cities in the Eastern part of Massachusetts, but none are connected or even all that close to one another.) But no matter where we went, if we were with Simon, you knew two things would happen by night's end: One, just about (if not literally) *everyone* at the party would know who Simon was by the end of the night. And two, just about every one of them (again, if not literally *every . . . single . . . person*) would *like* Simon. He was just that kind of guy, a really fun, outgoing, and confident dude.

As a natural introvert, being the center of attention is not my normal go-to state of being. But watching guys like Simon have so much success working a room, I certainly picked up more than my fair share of what worked, and used it often.

I owe a lot of my life-of-the-party talent now to my observations of Simon many years back. This potheaded lanky dude could work a crowd like no other, and I learned a hell of a lot just from being around him.

Peter

Peter was a really short, skinny guy, who I liked immediately, not because he was shorter and skinnier than me, which is typically hard to come by, but because he was just so incredibly likeable. He was from out west but had moved to my state for a period of time.

He'd gone up to me one day at the gym in between sets and started talking to me about . . . God knows what. The next thing I know, we're shooting the shit for like the next 20 minutes, and we became instant friends.

You might think it odd for someone to go up to someone else at the gym and start chatting away, as naturally I wouldn't do this either, but Peter made it look so normal. Never once in our first interaction, or any interaction ever for that matter, did he give off any weird or awkward vibe. He was just one of those very rare people you love to talk to. And he was damn good at it.

I've never seen someone spend so much time chatting with other people. The man was impressive. He'd go into the gym for a workout, just about every day, and would probably leave about five or six hours later. Not because he was some iron-man, pushing his body to the extreme, but because he'd go around and have conversations with fucking everyone in the gym—the entire fucking lineup of people. In fact, of all the hours he'd spend their, I honestly don't think he ever worked out for more than 20 minutes.

He was the definition of a social butterfly. And he was also a funny fucking bastard. Every time I'd see him he was in some sort of deep and elaborate conversation with one of the members. People I'd walked past for years without so much as a head nod would be spilling their guts to Peter and opening up about their deepest and most intimate confessions.

It was really quite amazing. I'd walk in and see him and he'd just sort of smile at me in recognition, and then continue on with his gripping exchange. Then, at some point after, he'd head over to me and pull me into an entertaining chat, where I'd remain for the next 20 minutes or so. But I never minded. I actually quite enjoyed our banters, even though they always fucked up my workouts. They were funny and entertaining, and they always put me in a good mood. Peter always had some sort of funny story to share about something that'd happened in his life. They were all worth listening to and the tradeoff of a slightly diminished training session was well worth their cost.

Peter had sort of an effeminate manner about him. He was not gay, as I knew of multiple women from the gym he'd seduced, but if you didn't know him you might think he was. He had kind of a girly voice that ended with a very slight lisp, sort of a womanly walk, and body and hand gestures that didn't do him any favors in terms of masculinity: He would put his hand on his hips, cross his legs oddly from time to time, and wear very questionable clothing, like sandals with socks and extra-tight skinny jeans, even before skinny jeans became popular. (Not like it mattered if he was gay, I truly could give a fuck less and liked him either way, but taking into account all of the clues, I honestly don't think he was.)

In fact, I kind of liked that he had this sort of feminine style about him. He was different, but in his own way tremendously confident. Juxtaposing his character to that of The Natural's was like night and day. One man was tough and masculine, while the other was soft and feminine. But each man was wildly successful in his own approach. And I learned significantly from both.

Looking back, I think I modeled a lot of my social game from Peter. Remember when I'd walk around my old supermarket job and talk to everyone from the meat guy to the produce lady to the guys stocking the shelves, and everyone else in between? Guess whose book that page came out of? Yup, Peter gets the nod for that one.

He also showed me that confidence doesn't have to look a certain way. Again, you don't have to be extra manly or super dominant to have confidence. You can be more relaxed, more calm, and—yes, even more effeminate to a certain degree—and still be confident in yourself. It was almost like a passive confidence that he had, so strong that he didn't mind sitting back and letting you take the spotlight. He knew who he was and didn't mind letting you shine, kind of like what many great leaders do. They lead from behind the scenes and often let others think they're in charge, even when they're really pulling all the strings.

Caleb

Caleb was the archetypal cool guy. In all the years I've known Caleb I don't think I've ever seen him rattled. Come to think of it, I don't think I've ever even seen him mad. He was just always as confident and cool as a cucumber.

Another social genius, Caleb was also known to be the life of most parties. He too, was funny, sociable, endearing, and incredibly likeable. Like Simon, he had an incredible knack for winning over crowds and getting nearly everyone to both remember and like him by the end of any given night.

Caleb had more friends than anybody I've ever met. And not just Facebook friends, like the thousands of people we barely know who get mindlessly added to our friend count on there. I'm talking about real people. Caleb was (and is) friends with literally thousands if not tens-of-thousands of real, actual people.

People went out of their way all the time in public to say "Hi" to Caleb. Just about everywhere we ever went with the guy, he knew at least a couple of people on a personal level. Where Simon would be great at going to new places and making friends with a ton of new people, with Caleb when we went to new places, he'd already know a ton of people. He was like an undercover celebrity.

People liked him so much mainly because of his confidence. He wasn't brash or bold, he wasn't overly friendly or super nice, he was just a cool motherfucker with a lot of self-confidence, and people were attracted to it. Caleb was sort of a trendsetter as well. He always dressed a little different than the guys around him. He acted a little more mature, maybe a few years older than he really was. And he never followed others and the popular opinion of the group. If he wanted to do something he did it. Whether it was with you, with the group, or totally by himself, he didn't care. He thought about things and saw life through his own lens, and wouldn't waver in his decision once he committed to it.

I'm sure Caleb's contribution to my confidence is multi-faceted, but the biggest role I think it had in terms of my own self-belief was the confidence he demonstrated in being yourself. I watched him time and time again, going against the grain and coolly doing what was best for him. He never got mad, never got rattled, never tried to be someone he wasn't, he just kept his contented, chilled attitude and did whatever he wanted in the end.

He kind of reminds me of that famous Robert Downey Jr. quote, "Listen, smile, agree, and then do whatever the fuck you were gonna' do anyway." That's Caleb. I think Iron Man stole that line from my buddy.

Chase

Chase, unlike the others on this list, didn't seemingly possess an unbelievable amount of natural confidence. He wasn't good with women like Bobby. He was certainly not the life of any parties I can think of like Simon. He wasn't naturally great, or even good, at striking up conversations with people throughout the day like Peter. And he didn't possess the social reputation and cool resolve that Caleb did. But Chase did have something all the others really didn't have: a confidence and happiness in being alone.

It wasn't something that came naturally either, but something he'd gotten used to over time.

You see Chase had a much tougher life than most. He was born with the looks of . . . well, let's just say he's not going to be winning People Magazine's Sexiest Man Alive award any time soon, or ever. He's a few inches shorter than me, he's got glasses, he's been balding since midway through high school, and he's got acne scars on both sides of his cheeks from years of erroneous oil buildup. He's not ugly, but he's certainly not the most attractive man you'll ever meet.

Not to mention his father has unfortunately passed away, his mother has been out of the picture for years, his older brother is addicted to drugs and nowhere to be found last I checked, and his sister is much older than him, lives many miles away, and sees him about as often as the Earth sees a solar eclipse.

His parents never had much of any money; they were both immigrants who couldn't really speak English, and Chase was essentially an only child, oftentimes left to fend for himself. Having lived virtually on his own for years, he officially moved out at 18 and has lived by himself ever since.

Naturally, depression, loneliness, anxiety, and a host of other issues have crept into his life over the years; after all, life can be incredibly tough, especially when you have to survive it all by yourself. But Chase never gives in. And he never will.

He may not be socially confident and he might waver in his self-belief to do things from time to time, but at the end of the day there's a toughness that few others I've ever come across possess. He's got a confidence in himself to keep going, no matter how shitty life gets.

I've mentioned just a few of his issues, and out of respect for his privacy I'll refrain from delving into anything specific, but let's just say if you're reading this, I can almost certainly guarantee if you stacked up your life stresses against those of Chase, you'd be thanking God for aligning your lucky stars. With all the shit I've gone through in my life, I know that Chase has gone through much, much more.

And I'm constantly reminded of how incredible this man's determination to succeed is. His confidence, though not as apparent to others, is omnipresent. He believes, against some of the worst odds for people who've been dealt comparably fucked-up playing cards in the game of life, that he will find peace, happiness, and success in his life. And this hope and belief in himself is what constantly drives him. And quite honestly, it drives me.

I've learned a ton about true confidence from Chase, but his biggest gift to me has been his remarkable ability to remain confident and optimistic, even when life seems to strike a crippling knockout blow. I'll always have a confidence that I can pull myself out of anything that comes my way, and a lot of that belief comes from the fact that Chase has already done it, time and time again.

FINDING YOUR FRIENDS

The gentlemen I've listed above have all had a huge impact on my life. In one way or another they've helped shaped my level of confidence and who I am today. They, along with a few others to a lesser but tangible extent, have shown me what's possible with regard to my own self-confidence.

By surrounding myself with positive people and people with varying degrees of confidence, I was able to cherry pick the essentials for what I wanted in my own life. And I recommend categorically that you do the same.

Find five or so individuals who have what you want. Find the people who have the certainty and confidence you're looking for and the skills you'd like to possess, and then spend as much of your spare time hanging around them. You'll naturally pick up on what it is they do and how they operate, and their incredible traits and characteristics will unquestionably rub off on you.

Remember, as Jim Rohn said, "You are the average of the five people you spend the most time with." So choose your friends wisely and let their greatness rub off on you.

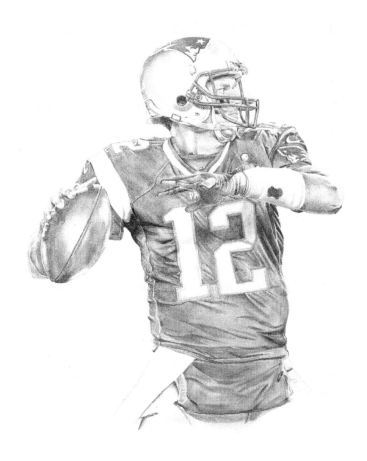

Chapter Thirty-One
It Takes Work

As the blur of the red-jerseyed man crossed the white, momentous line-marker stretching across the width of the entire field, all hope was lost. This was not just a dagger in the heart of all who lived in the northeast section of this country, more like a spear.

It was over. There was literally no chance now. Down 28-3 midway through the 3rd quarter in the 51st Super Bowl, our beloved Patriots were officially fucked.

Even I, a man who clings to even the slightest bit of hope, and who's been known by many of my peers to be delusionally optimistic, knew it was all but over.

"How the fuck could this happen?" I yelled out loud in utter frustration.

"What the fuck are they doing!?" I continued, as I pounded the sofa cushion with all my might.

"This game's fucking over! What a fuckin' shitty fucking game!!!" I bellowed out in a finality-like way, choosing to take my frustrations of their loss in the only way I could conceive, by yelling and cursing at the top of my lungs, like the true New Englander I was.

And then I fell silent, along with the rest of my houseful of family and friends, the shock of such a devastating performance not quite registering with any words that could articulate what we'd all just witnessed.

The dozen or so of us New England denizens huddled around my living room big screen (and the rest of the other Patriots fans watching from all over the globe) had painfully, by all intents and purposes, given up on our team.

Some of us even stopped watching at this point.

Others, like me, continued to watch this unmerciful beating more so because of the shock-induced comatose-like-state which rendered our bodies temporarily paralyzed and unable to pick our asses up and off the couch from the distress of it all, and less so because we thought they had any actual chance of turning things around. Yes, it was the ultimate ass-whoopping, of all ass-whooppings previously documented in history.

It Takes Work

It seemed like everyone knew the Pats were fucked. Except for one man: Tom Brady.

You may have heard of this guy; he's pretty good. He's won six Super Bowls, four Super Bowl MVP awards, three Regular Season MVPs, has the most wins by any quarterback in history, along with the best win percentage, and is right at the top for just about every passing record there is. He's unquestionably the greatest quarterback to ever step foot on the field, and I say that as someone who looks at all the numbers, not just someone who's rooting for the hometown favorite.

Although I can appreciate any questions surrounding potential bias here, there really is none. He's the best that ever fucking lived.

Back to our tale though.

Tom Brady, unlike any other person on the planet, knew there was still hope. He knew he was capable of pulling off the unthinkable and he knew he couldn't give in, no matter how dire it all looked. Brady had to keep his composure and had to get his team on board.

He went up and down his sideline after the Falcons' last touchdown, refusing to give in, and demanding that his team get their shit together and focus. He yelled to his team, "We gotta play tougher. Gotta play harder. Harder, tougher, everything. Everything we've got![1]" And he displayed his patented world-class confidence a moment later as he jogged back onto the field with his team, with his head up and nothing but unwavering determination in his eyes.

Tom Brady, against all odds, was still confident he could win, and why wouldn't he be? The man had spent his entire life overcoming the odds and proving people wrong. He prided himself on outworking everyone else and doing everything possible to succeed.

He wasn't about to let a 25-point deficit shake his self-belief, a self-belief that had been hardened from years of battle-tested labor.

THE WORK ETHIC OF A CHAMP

He wasn't the biggest. He wasn't the strongest. And he certainly wasn't the fastest. But what Tom Brady lacked in physical prowess, he more than made up for in work ethic. Given his lack of natural talent, he was always the underdog. But this chip on his shoulder fueled the motivation and discipline it took to train exceptionally harder than everyone else. The doubters were always there, but Brady used them to ignite the effort that would eventually lead to his greatness.

From high school, where his Junipero Serra team in San Mateo, California was just a mediocre 5-5 squad. To college, where he was literally the seventh-string quarterback on the Michigan Wolverines when he joined. To draft day, when he was passed over by every team but one and taken 199th overall. To his rookie season, where he was the fourth-string QB, barely even making the squad. To the next year, when he was finally given a chance to play only after Drew Bledsoe (thank the Lord) was injured by Boston's second-greatest sports hero of all time, New York Jet Mo Lewis (which directly led to Tom Brady's takeover and record-shattering career). To the successive years thereafter, where he was doubted over and over again and told that his "lucky" run wouldn't last. To the numerous playoff and championship games, where he was forced to come back from seemingly insuperable odds to achieve victory. Tom Brady is possibly the world's greatest underdog, and also its greatest overachiever.

Brady's work ethic is legendary. He's been known for years to always be the first one at practice and the last to leave. And while other guys go home and wrap things up when practice ends, Brady continues to study the game, watch film, and work on the things that can add to his performance.

He's obsessed with being the best and is driven to do everything he possibly can to outperform others. In an interview with WEEI, a local Boston radio station, Brady mentioned the following when asked about his early bedtime routine, "I do go to bed very early, because I'm up very early. I think that the decisions that I make always center around performance enhancement, if that makes sense. So whether that's what I eat or what decisions I make, or whether I drink or don't drink, it's always football-centric. I want to be the best I can be every day. I want to be the best I can be every week. I want to be the best I can be for my teammates. I love the game and I want to do it for a long time. But I also know that if I want to do it for a long time, I have to do things differently than the way guys have always done it.[2]"

Additionally, he takes all practices incredibly seriously—life-or-death-type serious. Brady knows that the skill and confidence gained from practicing the way you want to perform on game day is essential to success, and treats each practice as if it were a real game. He yells, he directs, he runs plays at full speed, he celebrates with his teammates when they do something right; to Brady, practice isn't just a means to getting better for the game, it's an extension of the game itself.

Rob Gronkowski, a superstar both on and off the field and an all-time great tight end, said of Brady regarding practice, "It's a lot of fun. It's every day, he comes out, he competes every single day. Everybody chirping at each other just makes the game fun and makes it special, too." And Patriots receiver Malcolm Mitchell added, "But practice here is like the game and I love every bit of it. Every time you come out here, it's game day. That's how I feel when I suit up and put on this uniform.[3]"

Yes, Brady's true secret to success has been his tireless work ethic and dedication to practice. It's been the catalyst for all he's been able to do, and is truly renowned.

What's also renowned is the level of confidence he's cultivated from this give-it-all-you-got attitude. Even way back when, when he first entered the league, there's a famous story of awkwardly built and not-quite-put-together-yet rookie, Tom Brady, introducing himself to Robert Kraft, the billionaire owner of the New England Patriots. Here's the brief but profound conversation the two had one day after Brady came over to Kraft following a training camp practice:

"I'm Tom Brady," Brady said to Kraft, introducing himself assertively.

"I know who you are," Kraft responded back. "You're our sixth-round pick."

And then Brady said something that stuck with Kraft, and rather than turn him off because of its bold nature which may have on the outside verged on arrogance, it resonated with the mogul.

Brady's famous response back was, "I'm the best decision this organization has ever made.[4]"

Kraft didn't know it then, but Brady was right. And he has proved it over and over again with each winning season and each championship trophy he brought home.

THE GREATEST GAME EVER PLAYED

Down 25 and running out of time fast, Brady wasted no more of it after jogging out with his fellow comrades. He marched right down the field and immediately threw a touchdown to his running back

It Takes Work

James White, making the score 28-9. Still dismal, but a step in the right direction.

After getting the ball back a few minutes later, Brady marched down the field again, and set up a Stephen Gostkowski field goal for 3 more points, again changing the score, this time to 28-12.

With the clock still ticking away and the Falcons controlling the ball, it still seemed like the Patriots were fucked, although now it would just hurt more because a little ounce of hope had been restored. At least if they'd gotten blown out, we'd all have seen it coming from a mile away, and wouldn't have to deal with the inevitable plummet from the roller coaster of emotions our beloved team was enacting on us. At least that's what I was thinking at the time.

But with just 10 minutes left in the fourth quarter, and the rest of the game, the Patriots defense finally made their mark on that Super Bowl, causing the Falcons to fumble the ball and turn it back over to Brady's offense. Brady, capitalizing on opportunity like no other, seized the moment and delivered a six-yard bullet into Danny Amendola's arms for a remarkable touchdown, bringing the New England tally up to 18, and then to 20 a minute later after getting a two-point conversion.

After another strong display by the Patriot defense, Brady was given the ball back once again, after the Falcons were forced to punt it away. With just 3:30 left on the Super Bowl clock and pinned down at their own nine-yard line, the Patriots still faced devastating odds. But Tom Brady, with the sheer determination that could only be found in someone who'd overcome years and years of insurmountable odds, and with the confidence obtained from his obsessive madmanesque practice routine fueling him, took the ball and promenaded downfield, throwing the football with laser-like precision to all his wide receivers and running backs.

His accuracy and poise that drive would've made the most successful Navy Seal snipers jealous. And just two minutes later, after getting his team all the way downfield, he handed the ball off to White, who ran it in for 6 more points, making the score 28-26. A minute later, however, with the help of one of his favorite receivers, Amendola, Brady threw another 2-point converting pass, evening up this game and setting the stage for the greatest comeback in Super Bowl history.

At this point, the momentum had completely shifted onto our side. All of us Patriots fans went from being the most dejected, spoiled, and miserable assholes on the planet half hour earlier, to being the most ecstatic, enthusiastic, and joyous bastards you'd ever find.

Overtime was essentially just a formality at that point. We'd won the coin toss, got the kickoff, and gave the ball back to Brady to do his thing. And he did.

Tom Brady led the overtime drive, leading his team with his time-tested self-belief and resolve. One dart after the next was fired on cue, as the Patriots marched down the field one last time. And just like he had before, Brady got the Pats right down to the goal line, just two yards out from the end zone, and handed the ball off to James White, who then took it and secured their game-winning score. With that, Brady and the Patriots capped-off the greatest comeback in Super Bowl history, and in the eyes of many, perhaps the greatest game ever played, in any sport, in any time.

It was mind-blowing to say the least.

But the most impressive part of that whole game was the poise and confidence that Brady showed. Really, the man never gave up or even got down on his team. He, and he alone, had the self-assurance that he could do it, and through his mindset and unshakeable presence he convinced the rest of his teammates to follow suit.

Long live TB12, a true legend, and a man who constantly defied all odds on his path to greatness. He's an inspiration on what you can achieve when you put in the hard work to achieve it.

LEARNING FROM TOM

Now before you go on thinking this was just a love-fest for Tom Brady and that I have an undeniable man-crush on number 12, let me just clear the air and say, "Yeah, I actually do. So fuck off."

I mean seriously how could you not love a story like Tom's? The man was a perpetual underdog and was constantly overlooked and prejudged his entire life. Nobody ever gave him a shot, but because of his will, he created his own destiny, a destiny that just so happened to make him one of the greatest sports stars in history (I say THE GREATEST, but I'll make the concession that this can be argued.).

Don't you see? His story is *our* story.

It's my story and it's your story. We all have the power to create the life we want and to shape what our destiny becomes. We just need to understand that we have this control, and then we have to take the steps needed to enact it.

Brady's work ethic is truly remarkable; it's what made him great. Not his arm, which was good, but not extraordinary by any means. Not his size, which again by quarterback standards was decent, but not really exceptional. And certainly not his innate athletic ability, which by all accounts was horrible. (He once held the dubious record of having run the slowest 40-yard dash in NFL Combine history.)

No, Brady relied on something that we all have: willpower. He wanted it more than anyone, and so he put in the time it took to get it. The biggest takeaway here is really that you can achieve whatever you want, but you have to do the work it takes to become great.

If you really want something, go after it with unrelenting resolve, and maybe, just maybe, you can one day lead your team through the greatest comeback in Super Bowl history . . . or something epically comparable.

BRADY'S CONFIDENCE

Tom Brady exudes confidence like no other athlete I've ever seen. He's not cocky, but he's tremendously self-assured on the gridiron, and it shows in every game he plays. I suppose it can be argued that he's not the number one greatest quarterback ever, though this probably comes from people who really hate the Pats. But what can't be argued is that he's somewhere at the very top of that list. And further, what can't be disputed is that, at last check, he holds the highest winning percentage of any quarterback to ever play in the NFL.

At the time of this writing, after playing 18 seasons, he holds a winning percentage of 77.4%, meaning that he wins the overwhelming majority of the time he steps on the field. Just for a reference, another sports legend, considered by many to be among the greatest athletes in history, Michael Jordan, held a career win percentage record of 65.8%.

Brady, using his driven desire to be the best, continues to shock fans again and again with incredible feats of football excellence and come-from-behind wins. He's not perfect, but he's fucking great. And his greatness is due in large part to the confidence he carries with him every time he throws on that Pats jersey. It's a confident belief that he can, and will, create his own destiny.

GAINING CONFIDENCE FROM PRACTICE

If you want to have confidence in something, there's no substitute for actually putting in the work and getting good at it. You can mentally perform as many techniques as you want, and they all help to a certain degree, but if you lack skill in something or completely suck, all the mind training in the world will mean jack shit at the end of the day.

Even if you get so adept at convincing yourself you're good, and can derive a feeling of superfluous confidence in a given area, that confidence is going to be absolutely useless when push comes to shove and you actually have to perform. As I've reiterated over and over, confidence is huge, and it can go a very long way in deciding your success, but it's not everything. Without actual skill, you really risk fucking up majorly and looking like a complete idiot in the process.

In some instances this is fine, but in situations where there's something meaningful at stake, do yourself a favor and put in the work to get good. It takes time, it takes work, and it takes many hours of practice in most cases, but if you want to succeed at something it's a necessity.

Like Tom Brady and his world-class confidence, adopt a mindset that favors a strong work ethic and a great routine for practice. Practice like you're performing something for real. Take it as seriously as number 12 on the Patriots takes his practices. This way you'll undoubtedly gain confidence from knowing you're putting in all that's necessary to succeed, and furthermore, you'll actually cultivate the skill required to succeed.

Gaining confidence from practicing is the most tried-and-true method for building your self-belief. It's not glamorous and it's definitely not flashy, but it works. Not only do you increase your actual skill when you practice, but you enhance your self-belief in performing that skill, and thus when it comes time to perform, you execute on an even greater level.

It's a win-win. Put in the work, develop your skill, and cultivate your confidence all the while.

P.S. Go Pats!

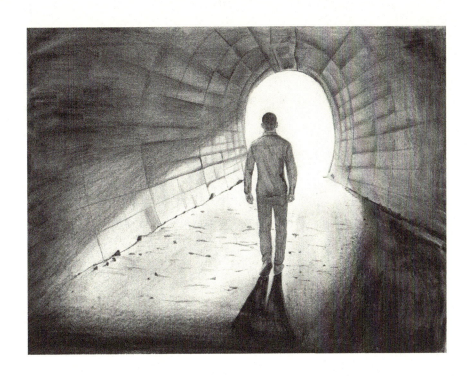

Last Words

There you have it.

I've laid everything on the table for you.

You now have the tools to master your mind and change your life for good. Within this book resides the playbook for overcoming anxiety, conquering depression, gaining confidence, and becoming a truly happy person again.

I wish I had this book way back when, but thankfully, with the help of some incredibly loving family members, a few exceptionally inspirational friends, and with the innate tenacity afforded to me by the good graces of God, I've somehow been able to traverse through the darkest of days and finally find the light.

It certainly wasn't easy. It definitely isn't something I'd like to do again. And it's not something I'd wish upon my worst enemy. Panic attacks can take over your life. Anxiety can make it unbearable. Depression, especially of the suicidal nature, can literally make you want to end it all.

But even more insidious, perhaps, might be the lack of true confidence so many have in themselves, a self-doubt that conditions the vast majority of individuals to live their lives on the sidelines— taking the easy route, doing what everyone else is doing, and letting the hours, days, and years unfold while they idly watch but a few others enjoy them.

This is the true evil.

Life is meant to be lived, not wasted away.

Too many people lack the true confidence needed, however, to step out from the norms of society and follow their dreams. They lack the desire, the motivation, the heart, and the self-belief to think they can do it.

Don't be one of these people.

If you have anxiety or depression, use this book to get over that. Take the steps and actions presented throughout these pages now and get your mental health back today.

But don't stop there.

That merely gets you to your baseline. Once you're back to your mental normalcy, take on the challenge of getting more out of life. Take on the challenge of being the best you can be and going after the things you want.

It will certainly be tough. And it will certainly be hard.

You will fall down.

You will fail.

You will suck for a while.

But if you keep your determination and your persistence through the struggle, I promise, you will eventually make it. Resiliency is the key. True self-confidence is attainable to all who seek it.

Know that.

And know this: Once you gain true confidence, the sky is the limit.

HOPE

Thinking back, during the days where suicide occupied the preponderance of my thoughts, there was one thing that was always missing, something I couldn't place at the time, but was surely the biggest driver of my insufferable depression: hope.

Hope eluded me back then. And it left me thinking there was no way I could ever get better, no way I could ever fix my problems. The depression was initially caused by a number of factors, but once I lost hope of ever pulling myself out of it, that depression exponentially increased. And it would've continued to get worse if I hadn't gotten lucky and stumbled upon a few good resources early on in my journey.

Even still, at times my hope would falter, and I'd slip back into my negatively dejected state.

But slowly, as I trenched through my pilgrimage and desperately clawed my mind away from the relentless grips of this mental disease, my hope grew more and more, until one day, it encompassed me. And with this ally fully in tow the battle became much easier.

Hope afforded me the ability to defeat the mental enemies that had lurked within and taken over my life for so long. It was the one thing that tipped the scales in my favor and allowed me to take my mind back.

My hope now, in writing this book, is that by reading it, you'll have the hope you need for taking your mind back too. Hope is an extraordinarily potent ally, and the moment you get it on your side, is the moment you begin to realize you can actually overcome whatever problem you're facing.

Sometimes I like to joke around and say funny or ridiculous shit. Other times I get a bit egotistical and think I'm the coolest thing since sliced bread. And still, every now and then I ponder to myself in the still of the night and reflect on all my greatness and worldly accomplishments, considering myself to have a truly gifted and special mind.

But it's during these times, especially those latter moments, when I'll be rudely thwarted from my narcissistic daydreams of self-delusion: by a smoke alarm going off because I forgot about the frozen chicken I was cooking in the oven; a phone-vibrating email alert from my bank for a bill I forgot to pay, a text message from a girl who thought I was an asshole, because my sarcastic attempts at being both witty and clever had in fact been neither witty nor clever, but instead just fucking lame and nonsensical.

The truth is, I'm a normal dude.

Sure I've got some special gifts, and I do think I'm pretty smart and fairly clever, but I also have my faults. Many in fact. I don't actually have a bizarre egotistical view of myself (at least I don't think so) because I know I'm not uniquely special. I have a desire to succeed and a dogged determination to achieve great things in life, but that's really it.

Everything else is pretty normal. My IQ is pretty average, my looks are pretty average, and my height is very average. The only thing that really separates me from others is my belief that I can do anything I set my mind to (hope) and my unrelenting pursuit in obtaining it thereafter.

But you can have this too.

Hope and a never-give-up attitude is simply a mindset shift. And a shift that by now I trust you understand.

If you take nothing else away from this book remember these subsequent words.

You can do anything you set your mind to. Every problem you face can be overcome; no matter how hard your life gets, there's always a solution to your problems—in fact, many, many, solutions. You just have to find them, and of course, take action on them once you do.

Your mind is an infinitely powerful instrument. You can try to play it blindly, though it will often sound chaotic, or you can learn to master it, and play the most beautiful songs imaginable. Personally, I've chosen to master this eternally complex device, and I love the music I'm able to create now that I know how it works.

TAKING RESPONSIBILITY FOR YOUR HEALTH

"The cavalry ain't coming," as my friend Gary John Bishop says.[1]

You are the cavalry. It's up to you to make a change. Nobody's going to come save your ass, you gotta' save yourself.

Stop relying on your doctors. Stop relying on your parents. Stop relying on your friends. These people may have the best intentions for you, but at the end of the day, your health is in your own hands. Only you can truly facilitate the change needed to be healthy and happy.

The sooner you realize this, the faster your life will transform.

Take responsibility now for your health, your happiness, and for the path you wish to travel for the rest of your life. Fuck what you've heard on TV. Fuck what you've seen on the internet. Fuck what you've read in self-help books. When it's all said and done, none of it matters. Only *you* matter. And nothing can happen until you decide to take action and make it happen.

You are responsible for everything that happens in your life. Embrace this fact now.

HAVING A SUPERPOWER

If you've made it this far, the chances are you've dealt with depression and anxiety in the past, or are even experiencing them now. The good news is you either have a superpower or will have one by the time you overcome these struggles.

If you haven't faced anxiety or depression, the likes of which I've talked about at length throughout this book, don't fret; as I've said before, I wouldn't wish it on my worst enemy.

But if you have faced these issues, the superpower you now possess is that of resiliency. If you've overcome anxiety, panic attacks, and depression, or any other related mental-anguish, you're a survivor. You're a fighter and someone who won't give in. Just like my dad told me way back when in the kitchen that day, you too have this never-give-up attitude and a natural tenacity to succeed. The years of pain and suffering in your life have sharpened this resolve and made you tougher. You may not be able to see the gift you have, but it's there. Trust me, you've got something so many other people lack. Use this to your advantage.

Outwork your contemporaries. Train harder. Study more. Face adversity head on and bounce right the fuck back up when you get knocked down. This is in your blood. You've done it already and you've overcome the worst life has to offer. Everything else is easy.

Everyone else who has to face adversity in life has an uphill battle and many of them won't make it. But you, with superpower in hand, will conquer any new challenge that comes your way.

You're a goddamn fighter, just like me.

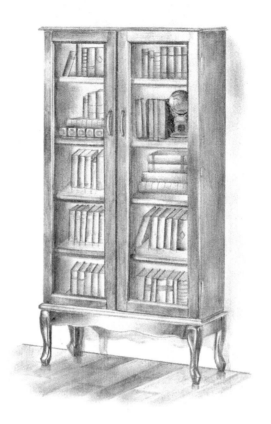

Epilogue

The bell rang out excitedly, three times in loud rapid succession, and Mary knew immediately what that meant. It was an old-school bell, installed many years back by her husband as a way to add a little nostalgia to the home's character, and to replace the regular doorbell previously affixed to their colonial. And she loved it. Especially in the last few years.

Every time the little chimer tolled out, it meant one thing, and one thing only: Her grandchildren had arrived.

ELITE MIND

It wasn't merely the fact that nobody else really used the old bell, as nearly all other guests would simply knock for sufficiency; it was also the enthusiasm that accompanied the chimes, an enthusiasm that could only be found in the essence of two very young children. Children who got a kick out of even the smallest things in life, and who found amusement where no others could. Children who brought out the best in her, and imparted their zest for life onto her spirit every time they came into her presence. She truly loved her grandkids and she smiled as she walked down the stairs to greet them.

"Grandma!" her two favorite rascals yelled out concurrently with equal ardor. "We missed you!"

"Oh, my two favorite munchkins! I missed you kids too!" Mary replied back, as a warm ear-to-ear smile crossed her face. "I just finished baking your favorite chocolate chip cookies too. You can have them after dinner!"

And after hugging her beautiful six-year-old granddaughter and her handsome four-year-old grandson, she embraced her son and her daughter-in-law, who'd created these little angels, and whom she loved just as much.

Just then her husband appeared out from the hallway, and the two lovable little rascals quickly ran over and leaped into his big arms. She smiled at the sight, and continued to affectionately greet her other two children.

Her son and her daughter-in-law looked great. Not just physically, but all over. They seemed genuinely exuberant, their mood was radiant, and their energy was incredible. She truly could not be happier for them.

Epilogue

She welcomed them inside and was really pleased to have made them such a good dinner. She'd spent the whole day preparing it, but didn't mind at all, as it filled up her heart to make others feel good. And Mary knew they were going to love her food. After all, her son had been eating it for years, and had told his mother numerous times that his now wife had always loved coming over, as she couldn't find this type of homemade brilliance anywhere else.

She smiled once more at the thought of bringing a little more joy into their lives.

A MEMORY

As the last specks of food were lifted off his plate and into his mouth, John felt great.

"Ma, I think you just outdid yourself with this one. Just when I didn't think you could make anything better than that bacon-infused meatloaf from last month, you go ahead and do this. I truly love ya'!"

His mother chuckled at his sarcasm and smiled at his appreciation. "I love you too, honey," she replied back.

And then John got up and picked up all the plates and utensils from his family members and brought them over to the sink. His old house never did have a dishwasher, but he didn't really care. He'd gotten used to doing dishes growing up here, and so could go right through them in just minutes. *Besides,* he thought, *that meal was probably one of the single greatest meals I've ever had in my life.*

"Speedy and spotless, that's how I do it," he remembered telling his mother as a kid. *Speedy and spotless,* he reiterated to himself, thinking back to his early days of scrubbing.

But John's skills weren't quite as sharp as they once were. Instead of whizzing through the plates, and the forks, and the knives, and the numerous pots and pans and bowls, John clambered through, at a fraction of the pace he'd taken in his youth.

But still he didn't mind.

He occasionally looked over at his wife and kids in the other room, and his mother and father who he loved so much, and every time he did so he smiled. He was truly a blessed man.

His wife was absolutely stunning. Many men say their wife or girlfriend is the most beautiful woman they've ever seen, but few actually mean it. John, however, was one of those few. She had long blonde hair, a thin waist, gorgeous legs, and the most attractive facial features he'd ever seen. It was literally love at first sight the day he met her. But as appealing as she was physically, mentally and emotionally she was even more attractive. Her personality would instantly endear anyone. She was caring, loyal, honest, sweet, funny, and smart all wrapped into one complete package. And she was his.

He turned over a bowl and poured on some more soap. *This bowl's probably older than me*, he thought, as he scrubbed the edges.

Then he looked back in the other room and smiled again, seeing his four-year-old son laughing and dancing to a song on TV, and then to his beautiful little daughter, a striking image of her mother, drawing some pictures with his own mother on scrap paper. Subsequently, he glanced over at his father, who too was watching his grandson sway to and fro like a mini James Brown, and laughing hysterically all the while.

John himself chuckled at this spectacle and continued to wash, polishing off a fork.

Epilogue

John was about halfway through when he thought about his work. Lately he'd been really busy, just before the Christmas break, but now he had a week off before he'd even have to think about his job. Not that he didn't love it, but it was certainly nice to take a little hiatus from time to time. Being a neuroscience researcher, he and his team were on the verge of making a major breakthrough in understanding the function of a very important mechanism in the brain, and he couldn't wait to publish his findings. But again, he did enjoy a good break from it all, even if it meant holding off a week on revolutionizing our comprehension of the most vital organ we have.

Putting work aside, he concentrated his attention back to the dishes, slowly but surely disappearing before him. All the forks and knives were gone, as well as the major pots and pans, and there remained only a few spoons and the plates used by each of his family members during the feast.

Continuing to wash and rub, John was pleased he was almost done. A few more minutes and he could join his family and kick back on the couch and crack some jokes with his dad. He looked back once more into the other room where his family was gathered, but was drawn to something else this time.

In the far corner of the room, far past his wife's blonde hair, stood a large brown bookcase. A bookcase that had been in the house for as long as John could remember, but one that was previously settled in the basement. As a kid, John had often gone downstairs to pick out a random book from that case, and then read on the basement couch for hours and hours, until one of his parents would snap him out of his trance and tell him dinner was ready, or one of his friends came over to hang out. He loved reading books and he loved drifting into the magical worlds of the stories he devoured.

It was funny to see the bookcase upstairs again, just feet away though. *Maybe dad was getting sick of walking up and down the stairs*, he thought. He was a big reader too and usually liked perusing through non-fiction and fiction alike after meals. *That must be it*, he decided. *Dad's knees are getting old, so he definitely moved this baby up here to relieve his achy joints.*

Just after he confirmed his theory, he noticed on the top shelf a book he hadn't seen in years. It stood out from the others, a book that he'd kept by his nightstand for many, many nights, many, many nights ago. It had been so long since those nights, but he still remembered them clearly. In fact it must've been about 20 years since he'd held that book, but he was struck by its presence because of the relationship he'd once had with it.

A BOOK

About 20 years ago, his life was completely different.

He had none of what he had today, and just about every horrible thing you could imagine. He was severely depressed, perpetually anxious and afraid, got heart-pounding panic attacks frequently, had no self-confidence and no self-esteem, and had lost all his friends from childhood. 20 years ago, John's life was a train wreck. And he'd wanted to end it.

After going to the doctors and taking prescription medications he'd thought things would get better for him. But they didn't. They only seemed to continue to get worse and worse, and his life seemed less and less like one he wanted to live. In fact, at one point he'd planned to commit suicide and end it all.

It would be so much easier to just put a rope around my neck and call it quits, he'd thought back then. *Move onto the next life, where everything isn't so fucked up and life's not so cruel.*

Epilogue

He'd walked through how he could do it and what instruments he might need to pull it off. He'd done a few searches on his computer too, and figured out what type of rope to get and how to tie the knot. It had taken him a few days, but soon enough he was certain he could pull it off.

He'd planned to do it on a Monday, sometime after school, as Mondays were always the worst days for him and he didn't want to go through another full school week.

On Sunday night, the day before he'd planned to hang himself, he'd remembered a book his father had gotten for him when he was a child. It was a human anatomy book with all sorts of pictures, charts, diagrams, and useful information on the human body. He'd felt like it would be a good idea to take a quick look through it, as it might offer more insight on the neck and the breathing process, and where the best location for the noose attachment should be.

He remembered walking down his basement stairs and coming to the massive brown bookcase.

He'd looked for that anatomy book but hadn't been able to find it. He'd fingered through the top shelf, the middle shelf, and the bottom shelf, but for some reason he could not locate its whereabouts. And then he did this again; searching high and low, he'd scanned every book on every shelf, but still could not unearth it. He knew it was in that bookcase somewhere, but for some reason his eyes were failing him.

He grew frustrated at his visual blunder, and knew his eyes were deceiving him. *That book is definitely in this bookcase, but for some reason I can't find the damn thing*, he thought to himself.

After another minute of this unsuccessful inspection, his eyes came upon another book, one he couldn't recall ever seeing before. A book that looked quite plain and rather ordinary but a book whose title caught his attention.

It caught his attention because its title boldly claimed to help people overcome their mental problems. And back then he had many.

Feeling curious, he remembered opening up the book and reading the chapter titles, to get a feel for what it was really about. And as soon as he did, he felt something strange: a feeling he hadn't experienced in what seemed like eternity. An odd sentiment he couldn't recognize at first, but that he knew had once existed within him.

As he read off the chapters the book covered, he felt, for the first time in years . . . the feeling of *hope*.

He had no idea where the book had come from, but he sat down on his basement's couch and began reading through it incessantly. Like the days when he was younger, and would get carried away for hours reading about knights, and wizards, and magical tales of mystery and suspense, John was completely enthralled by this book and the information it contained in overcoming mental woes.

Up until that point he'd found absolutely nothing to help alleviate his psychological condition; and all of it seemed to center around taking large doses of medication, something he innately knew was not good.[1] But this book, for the first time in his life, offered something different.

It provided a number of options and many ways for beating his depressive and anxious struggles, and judging by their methodologies, they all appeared to be very safe.

John spent about six straight hours reading that book from cover to cover, and by the end of it, he was a new young man. He didn't

Epilogue

actually conquer all his problems in those six hours, but he was given the resources to help him go about doing so. And just as importantly, he'd been rendered the hope he needed to defeat them. John was granted the opportunity he needed to keep fighting.

And he did.

He skipped his suicide plan the next day and instead embarked on his quest to take back his mind.

And soon after, he did.

John smiled to himself now, at the thought of how it all had changed, because of one book. At how it could have ended so drastically different, but how it didn't, and how he was able to turn it all around and create such an amazing life.

"Honey, are you okay?" his wife asked, as she touched his shoulder.

"Wha-what?" John replied, snapping out of his time-lapsed daydream.

"Are you alright, babe?" his beautiful wife reiterated. "You've been washing these dishes for like 30 minutes. Do you need a hand?" And she smiled, the smile he loved most in life.

"No, I'm just wrapping up now," John said, smiling back and rinsing off the last few plates with his old youthful prowess.

"And yes, hun, to answer your question, I'm not only okay, I've never been better." And John smiled and kissed his wife and turned off the faucet.

JOHN'S LIFE

John is me. John is you. John is your brother. John is your son. John is your friend. John is each of us and all of us. As I alluded to at the very beginning of this book, John is a fictional character based on the very real individuals I've known in my own life, and based on my own life experience.

But unlike poor Jonathan, who didn't happen to stumble upon a resource that offered up even the slightest bit of counsel or hope, John thankfully did. And it completely changed the direction of his life.

It's not that the book contained all the answers, or that its chapters were all-knowing and ubiquitously applicable to John's situation. It's that the book was enough to set him on a new course and steer him into a new path in life, one that encouraged further learning, knowledge, and understanding of his struggles, and more importantly, showed him how he could truly overcome them.

He didn't need a magic bullet to beat his depression, his anxiety, his panic attacks, his confidence issues, or his social and self-esteem troubles. He simply needed some guidance, and he needed to know that it was very possible, and very common in fact, for many people to win this mental war.

ALTERNATE ENDING

This is the ending I prefer.

The happy ending where John discovers there are many solutions—safe, natural, and healthy solutions for his psychological plight. And he realizes all is not lost and that he can, and will win the battle.

Epilogue

This is what happens, not just in tales of metaphoric prose, but in real life. When we're given even the smallest amount of hope, when we don't give up, and when we fight like hell to overcome our struggles, there isn't a single problem that can't be defeated.

Not a single fucking one.

The truth is there are many, many solutions out there, many right answers to your problems, so don't give up. Whether you find them in this book or whether you find them in someone else's, they exist. The only thing you have to do is seek them out and take action on them. Don't throw in the towel like the other Jonathan did. Fight like hell and change the course of your life, like this Jonathan.

At the end of the day, if you take nothing else away from this book, take away the hope that it gives you. The hope that countless individuals have already beaten their mental struggles with depression and anxiety and everything that goes along with these afflictions, and so can you.

Let this book bring you hope like the hope that the second Jonathan got and the hope that I got way back when.

The answers are out there, and many are in here, it's time now to take action, change your destiny, and write your own happy ending.

REFERENCES

Prelude

1. Kessler, R. and Bromet, E. (2013). The Epidemiology of Depression Across Cultures. *Annual Review of Public Health*, 34(1), pp.119-138.

How to Read This Book

1. Stenstrom, J. (2017). *Elite Man Magazine*. [online] Elite Man Magazine. Available at: https://elitemanmagazine.com/ [Accessed 7 Oct. 2017].

Chapter One

1. Lexico Dictionaries | English. (2017). *Masshole | Definition of Masshole by Lexico*. [online] Available at: https://en.oxforddictionaries.com/definition/us/masshole [Accessed 7 Oct. 2017].

Chapter Two

1. Stenstrom, J. (2017). *Elite Man Podcast on Apple Podcasts*. [online] Apple Podcasts. Available at: https://podcasts.apple.com/us/podcast/elite-man-podcast-lifestyle/id954083494?mt=2 [Accessed 7 Dec. 2017].

Chapter Three

1. Matthews, T., Danese, A., Wertz, J., Odgers, C., Ambler, A., Moffitt, T. and Arseneault, L. (2016). Social isolation, loneliness and depression in young adulthood: a behavioural genetic analysis. *Social Psychiatry and Psychiatric Epidemiology*, 51(3), pp.339-348.

Chapter Four

1. Citizens Commission on Human Rights, CCHR. (2019). *PCP Laced Marijuana: Creating Psychosis and Psychiatric Commitment – Citizens Commission on Human Rights, CCHR*. [online] Available at: http://www.cchrflorida.org/pcp-laced-marijuana-creating-psychosis-and-psychiatric-commitment/ [Accessed 8 Oct. 2017].

2. Hallucinogens.com. (2017). *PCP Effects on the Brain*. [online] Available at: http://hallucinogens.com/pcp/pcp-effects-on-the-brain/ [Accessed 7 Oct. 2017].

Chapter Five

1. Drugs.com. (2017). *How long does PCP stay in your system?*. [online] Available at: https://www.drugs.com/answers/how-long-does-pcp-stay-in-your-system-359519.html [Accessed 7 Oct. 2017].

Chapter Six

1. Wong, J., Motulsky, A., Eguale, T., Buckeridge, D., Abrahamowicz, M. and Tamblyn, R. (2016). Treatment Indications for Antidepressants Prescribed in Primary Care in Quebec, Canada, 2006-2015. *JAMA*, 315(20), p.2230.

Chapter Seven

1. Uzun, S., Kozumplik, O., Jakovljević, M. and Sedić, B. (2010). Side effects of treatment with benzodiazepines. *Psychiatria Danubina*, 22(1), pp.90-3.

2. Drugs.com. (2017). *Klonopin Side Effects: Common, Severe, Long Term - Drugs.com*. [online] Available at: https://www.drugs.com/sfx/klonopin-side-effects.html [Accessed 28 Oct. 2017].

Chapter Eight

REFERENCES

1. Nepon, J., Belik, S., Bolton, J. and Sareen, J. (2010). The relationship between anxiety disorders and suicide attempts: findings from the National Epidemiologic Survey on Alcohol and Related Conditions. *Depression and Anxiety*, 27(9), pp.791-798.

Chapter Nine

1. Adaa.org. (2017). *Facts & Statistics | Anxiety and Depression Association of America, ADAA*. [online] Available at: https://adaa.org/about-adaa/press-room/facts-statistics [Accessed 17 Oct. 2017].

2. Who.int. (2017). *Depression*. [online] Available at: http://www.who.int/mediacentre/factsheets/fs369/en/ [Accessed 25 Oct. 2017].

3. Michael Craig Miller, M. (2017). *1 in 10 Americans Depressed - Harvard Health Blog*. [online] Harvard Health Blog. Available at: https://www.health.harvard.edu/blog/1-in-10-americans-depressed-20101002478 [Accessed 7 Nov. 2017].

4. Cdc.gov. (2017). *FastStats*. [online] Available at: https://www.cdc.gov/nchs/fastats/depression.htm [Accessed 28 Oct. 2017].

5. Mojtabai, R., Olfson, M. and Han, B. (2016). National Trends in the Prevalence and Treatment of Depression in Adolescents and Young Adults. *PEDIATRICS*, 138(6), pp.e20161878-e20161878.

6. Martin, L., Neighbors, H. and Griffith, D. (2013). The Experience of Symptoms of Depression in Men vs Women. *JAMA Psychiatry*, 70(10), p.1100.

Chapter Ten

1. Goyal, M., Singh, S., Sibinga, E., Gould, N., Rowland-Seymour, A., Sharma, R., Berger, Z., Sleicher, D., Maron, D., Shihab, H., Ranasinghe, P., Linn, S., Saha, S., Bass, E., Haythornthwaite, J. and Cramer, H. (2014). Meditation Programs for Psychological Stress and Well-being: A Systematic Review and Meta-analysis. *Deutsche Zeitschrift für Akupunktur*, 57(3), pp.26-27.

2. Arias, A., Steinberg, K., Banga, A. and Trestman, R. (2006). Systematic Review of the Efficacy of Meditation Techniques as Treatments for Medical Illness. *The Journal of Alternative and Complementary Medicine*, 12(8), pp.817-832.

3. Gallant, S. (2016). Mindfulness meditation practice and executive functioning: Breaking down the benefit. *Consciousness and Cognition*, 40, pp.116-130.

4. Sharma, H. (2015). Meditation: Process and effects. *AYU (An International Quarterly Journal of Research in Ayurveda)*, 36(3), p.233.

5. Weil, M.D., A. (2017). *Breathing Exercises: Three To Try | 4-7-8 Breath | Andrew Weil, M.D.*. [online] DrWeil.com. Available at: https://www.drweil.com/health-wellness/body-mind-spirit/stress-anxiety/breathing-three-exercises/ [Accessed 8 Oct. 2017].

Chapter Eleven

1. Brody, S. and Costa, R. (2012). Sexual Satisfaction and Health Are Positively Associated With Penile-Vaginal Intercourse but Not Other Sexual Activities. *American Journal of Public Health*, 102(1), pp.6-7.

Chapter Twelve

1. Thomas, D. (2007). The Mineral Depletion of Foods Available to US as A Nation (1940–2002) – A Review of the 6th Edition of McCance and Widdowson. *Nutrition and Health*, 19(1-2), pp.21-55.

REFERENCES

2. Mercola.com. (2017). *Magnesium: The Missing Link to Better Health.* [online] Available at: https://articles.mercola.com/sites/articles/archive/2013/12/08/magnesium-health-benefits.aspx [Accessed 9 Nov. 2017].

3. Tarasov, E., Blinov, D., Zimovina, U. and Sandakova, E. (2015). Magnesium deficiency and stress: Issues of their relationship, diagnostic tests, and approaches to therapy. *Terapevticheskii arkhiv*, 87(9), p.114.

4. Cohen, M. (2007). Environmental toxins and health--the health impact of pesticides. *Australian Family Physician*, 36(12), pp.1002-4.

5. Saul, A. (2017). *Vitamin Deaths: Where Are the Bodies?.* [online] Doctoryourself.com. Available at: http://www.doctoryourself.com/vitsafety.html [Accessed 9 Nov. 2017].

6. Starfield, MD, B. (2010). *Is US Health Really the Best in the World?.* [online] Jhsph.edu. Available at: https://www.jhsph.edu/research/centers-and-institutes/johns-hopkins-primary-care-policy-center/Publications_PDFs/A154.pdf [Accessed 11 Nov. 2017].

7. Bollinger, Ty, *The Truth About Cancer* (Hay House, 2016), p. 23.

8. Adams, K., Lindell, K., Kohlmeier, M. and Zeisel, S. (2006). Status of nutrition education in medical schools. *The American Journal of Clinical Nutrition*, 83(4), pp.941S-944S.

9. Institute of Medicine (US) Committee on Conflict of Interest in Medical Research, Education, and Practice; Lo B, Field MJ, editors. Conflict of Interest in Medical Research, Education, and Practice. Washington (DC): National Academies Press (US); 2009. 5, Conflicts of Interest in Medical Education.

10. Möykkynen, T., Uusi-Oukari, M., Heikkilä, J., Lovinger, D., Lüddens, H. and Korpi, E. (2001). Magnesium potentiation of the function of native and recombinant GABAA receptors. *Neuroreport*, 12(10), pp.2175-2179.

11. Lewis, J., Tiozzo, E., Melillo, A., Leonard, S., Chen, L., Mendez, A., Woolger, J. and Konefal, J. (2013). The Effect of Methylated Vitamin B Complex on Depressive and Anxiety Symptoms and Quality of Life in Adults with Depression. *ISRN Psychiatry*, 2013, pp.1-7.

12. Rosenthal, H. (2017). *Alcoholics Anonymous, Bill W, and Niacin Therapy*. [online] Psychotherapy.net. Available at: https://www.psychotherapy.net/blog/title/alcoholics-anonymous-founder-bill-wilson-s-long-lost-treatment-paradigm [Accessed 9 Nov. 2017].

13. Tomen, D. (2017). *Vitamin B3 (Niacin) – Nootropics Expert*. [online] Nootropicsexpert.com. Available at: https://nootropicsexpert.com/vitamin-b3-niacin/ [Accessed 16 Nov. 2017].

14. Pratte, M., Nanavati, K., Young, V. and Morley, C. (2014). An Alternative Treatment for Anxiety: A Systematic Review of Human Trial Results Reported for the Ayurvedic Herb Ashwagandha (Withania somnifera). *The Journal of Alternative and Complementary Medicine*, 20(12), pp.901-908.

15. Andrade, C., Aswath, A., Chaturvedi, S., Srinivasa, M. and Raguram, R. (2000). A double-blind, placebo-controlled evaluation of the anxiolytic efficacy of an ethanolic extract of withania somnifera. *Indian Journal of Psychiatry*, 42(3), pp.295-301.

16. Bhattacharya, S., Bhattacharya, A., Sairam, K. and Ghosal, S. (2000). Anxiolytic-antidepressant activity of Withania somnifera

REFERENCES

glycowithanolides: an experimental study. *Phytomedicine*, 7(6), pp.463-469.

17. Kimura, K., Ozeki, M., Juneja, L. and Ohira, H. (2007). l-Theanine reduces psychological and physiological stress responses. *Biological Psychology*, 74(1), pp.39-45.

18. Lu, K., Gray, M., Oliver, C., Liley, D., Harrison, B., Bartholomeusz, C., Phan, K. and Nathan, P. (2004). The acute effects of L-theanine in comparison with alprazolam on anticipatory anxiety in humans. *Human Psychopharmacology: Clinical and Experimental*, 19(7), pp.457-465.

19. Zhang, C. and Kim, S. (2007). Taurine Induces Anti-Anxiety by Activating Strychnine-Sensitive Glycine Receptor in vivo. *Annals of Nutrition and Metabolism*, 51(4), pp.379-386.

20. Meldrum, B. (2000). Glutamate as a Neurotransmitter in the Brain: Review of Physiology and Pathology. *The Journal of Nutrition*, 130(4), pp.1007S-1015S.

21. Molchanova, S., Oja, S. and Saransaari, P. (2007). Effect of taurine on the concentrations of glutamate, GABA, glutamine and alanine in the rat striatum and hippocampus. *Proceedings of the Western Pharmacology Society*, 50(95), p.7.

22. Benke, D., Barberis, A., Kopp, S., Altmann, K., Schubiger, M., Vogt, K., Rudolph, U. and Möhler, H. (2009). GABAA receptors as in vivo substrate for the anxiolytic action of valerenic acid, a major constituent of valerian root extracts. *Neuropharmacology*, 56(1), pp.174-181.

23. Treiser, S., Cascio, C., O'Donohue, T., Thoa, N., Jacobowitz, D. and Kellar, K. (1981). Lithium increases serotonin release and decreases

serotonin receptors in the hippocampus. *Science*, 213(4515), pp.1529-1531.

24. Fernández-Ruiz, J., Sagredo, O., Pazos, M., García, C., Pertwee, R., Mechoulam, R. and Martínez-Orgado, J. (2013). Cannabidiol for neurodegenerative disorders: important new clinical applications for this phytocannabinoid?. *British Journal of Clinical Pharmacology*, 75(2), pp.323-333.

25. Stenstrom, J. (2017). *How To Truly Detoxify Your Body: Overcoming Lyme, Heavy Metals, Autism, Mold, And More – Dr. Chris Shade (Ep. 176) - Elite Man Magazine*. [online] Elite Man Magazine. Available at: http://elitemanmagazine.com/detoxify-your-body-lyme-heavy-metals-autism-mold-dr-chris-shade [Accessed 9 Nov. 2017].

26. Birdsall, T. (1998). 5-Hydroxytryptophan: a clinically-effective serotonin precursor. *Alternative Medicine Review*, 3(4), pp.271-80.

27. Calmclinic.com. (2018). *Rhodiola Rosea: a Risky Relief for Anxiety?*. [online] Available at: https://www.calmclinic.com/supplements-for-anxiety/rhodiola-rosea [Accessed 1 Nov. 2018].

28. Johnson, T. (2017). *Relief From Anxiety and Stress - page 1 | Life Extension Magazine*. [online] LifeExtension.com. Available at: http://www.lifeextension.com/magazine/2007/8/report_stress_anxiety [Accessed 19 Nov. 2017].

29. Elsas, S., Rossi, D., Raber, J., White, G., Seeley, C., Gregory, W., Mohr, C., Pfankuch, T. and Soumyanath, A. (2010). Passiflora incarnata L. (Passionflower) extracts elicit GABA currents in hippocampal neurons in vitro, and show anxiogenic and anticonvulsant effects in vivo, varying with extraction method. *Phytomedicine*, 17(12), pp.940-949.

REFERENCES

30. Palatnik, A., Frolov, K., Fux, M. and Benjamin, J. (2001). Double-Blind, Controlled, Crossover Trial of Inositol Versus Fluvoxamine for the Treatment of Panic Disorder. *Journal of Clinical Psychopharmacology*, 21(3), pp.335-339.

Chapter Thirteen

1. Cox, A. (2015). Sleep paralysis and folklore. *JRSM Open*, 6(7), p.205427041559809.

2. Takeuchi, T., Fukuda, K., Sasaki, Y., Inugami, M. and Murphy, T. (2002). Factors Related to the Occurrence of Isolated Sleep Paralysis Elicited During a Multi-Phasic Sleep-Wake Schedule. *Sleep*, 25(1), pp.89-96.

3. Kotorii, T., Kotorii, T., Uchimura, N., Hashizume, Y., Shirakawa, S., Satomura, T., Tanaka, J., Nakazawa, Y. and Maeda, H. (2001). Questionnaire relating to sleep paralysis. *Psychiatry and Clinical Neurosciences*, 55(3), pp.265-266.

4. Cheyne, J. (2002). Situational factors affecting sleep paralysis and associated hallucinations: position and timing effects. *Journal of Sleep Research*, 11(2), pp.169-177.

5. Otto, M., Simon, N., Powers, M., Hinton, D., Zalta, A. and Pollack, M. (2006). Rates of isolated sleep paralysis in outpatients with anxiety disorders. *Journal of Anxiety Disorders*, 20(5), pp.687-693.

6. Brooks, P. and Peever, J. (2012). Identification of the Transmitter and Receptor Mechanisms Responsible for REM Sleep Paralysis. *Journal of Neuroscience*, 32(29), pp.9785-9795.

7. Boeve, B. (2009). REM sleep behavior disorder. *Annals of the New York Academy of Sciences*, 1184(1), pp.15-54.

8. Sleepfoundation.org. (2017). *The Complex Relationship Between Sleep, Depression & Anxiety | National Sleep Foundation*. [online] Available at: https://sleepfoundation.org/excessivesleepiness/content/the-complex-relationship-between-sleep-depression-anxiety [Accessed 17 Nov. 2017].

9. Luojus, M., Lehto, S., Tolmunen, T., Elomaa, A. and Kauhanen, J. (2015). Serum copper, zinc and high-sensitivity C-reactive protein in short and long sleep duration in ageing men. *Journal of Trace Elements in Medicine and Biology*, 32, pp.177-182.

10. Miller, A. and Raison, C. (2015). The role of inflammation in depression: from evolutionary imperative to modern treatment target. *Nature Reviews Immunology*, 16(1), pp.22-34.

11. Leproult, R., Copinschi, G., Buxton, O. and Van Cauter, E. (1997). Sleep Loss Results in an Elevation of Cortisol Levels the Next Evening. *Sleep*, 20(10), pp.865-70.

12. Ranabir, S. and Reetu, K. (2011). Stress and Hormones. *Indian Journal of Endocrinology and Metabolism*, 15(1), pp.18–22.

13. Longordo, F., Kopp, C. and Lüthi, A. (2009). Consequences of sleep deprivation on neurotransmitter receptor expression and function. *European Journal of Neuroscience*, 29(9), pp.1810-1819.

14. Stenstrom, J. (2018). *The 6 Keys To A Happy And Healthy Life – Dr. Frank Lipman (Ep. 163) - Elite Man Magazine*. [online] Elite Man Magazine. Available at: http://elitemanmagazine.com/6-keys-to-a-happy-and-healthy-life-dr-frank-lipman [Accessed 4 Apr. 2018].

15. Düzgün, G. and Durmaz Akyol, A. (2017). Effect of Natural Sunlight on Sleep Problems and Sleep Quality of the Elderly Staying in the Nursing Home. *Holistic Nursing Practice*, 31(5), pp.295-302.

REFERENCES

16. Recommended Amount of Sleep for a Healthy Adult: A Joint Consensus Statement of the American Academy of Sleep Medicine and Sleep Research Society. (2015). *Journal of Clinical Sleep Medicine*, 38(6), pp.843–844.

17. Kang, J. and Chen, S. (2009). Effects of an irregular bedtime schedule on sleep quality, daytime sleepiness, and fatigue among university students in Taiwan. *BMC Public Health*, 9(1).

18. Vandewalle, G., Collignon, O., Hull, J., Daneault, V., Albouy, G., Lepore, F., Phillips, C., Doyon, J., Czeisler, C., Dumont, M., Lockley, S. and Carrier, J. (2013). Blue Light Stimulates Cognitive Brain Activity in Visually Blind Individuals. *Journal of Cognitive Neuroscience*, 25(12), pp.2072-2085.

19. Ribeiro, J. and Sebastião, A. (2010). Caffeine and adenosine. *Journal of Alzheimer's Disease*, 20(1), pp.3-15.

20. Okamoto-Mizuno, K. and Mizuno, K. (2012). Effects of thermal environment on sleep and circadian rhythm. *Journal of Physiological Anthropology*, 31(1).

21. Gooley, J., Chamberlain, K., Smith, K., Khalsa, S., Rajaratnam, S., Van Reen, E., Zeitzer, J., Czeisler, C. and Lockley, S. (2011). Exposure to Room Light before Bedtime Suppresses Melatonin Onset and Shortens Melatonin Duration in Humans. *Endocrinology*, 152(2), pp.742-742.

22. Uchida, S., Shioda, K., Morita, Y., Kubota, C., Ganeko, M. and Takeda, N. (2012). Exercise Effects on Sleep Physiology. *Frontiers in Neurology*, 3.

23. Park, B., Wilson, G., Berger, J., Christman, M., Reina, B., Bishop, F., Klam, W. and Doan, A. (2016). Is Internet Pornography Causing

Sexual Dysfunctions? A Review with Clinical Reports. *Behavioral Sciences*, 6(3), p.17.

24. Abbasi, B., Kimiagar, M., Sadeghniiat, K., Shirazi, M., Hedayati, M. and Rashidkhani, B. (2012). The effect of magnesium supplementation on primary insomnia in elderly: A double-blind placebo-controlled clinical trial. *Journal of Research in Medical Sciences*, 17(12), pp.1161-9.

25. Dubocovich, M. and Markowska, M. (2005). Functional MT1 and MT2 melatonin receptors in mammals. *Endocrine*, 27(2), pp.101-10.

26. Hadley, S. and Petry, J. (2003). *Valerian*. [online] Aafp.org. Available at: https://www.aafp.org/afp/2003/0415/p1755.html [Accessed 9 Feb. 2018].

27. Zhang, J., Sumich, A. and Wang, G. (2017). Acute effects of radiofrequency electromagnetic field emitted by mobile phone on brain function. *Bioelectromagnetics*, 38(5), pp.329-338.

28. Rupp, T., Acebo, C. and Carskadon, M. (2007). Evening Alcohol Suppresses Salivary Melatonin in Young Adults. *Chronobiology International*, 24(3), pp.463-470.

29. 10MinuteZen - The Evolution of You. (2019). *10 Minute Zen - Simple Breathing Exercises Better Than Meditation*. [online] Available at: https://10minutezen.com [Accessed 9 Feb. 2018].

30. Spencer, J., Moran, D., Lee, A. and Talbert, D. (1990). White noise and sleep induction. *Archives of Disease in Childhood*, 65(1), pp.135-137.

Chapter Fourteen

1. Denkova, E., Wong, G., Dolcos, S., Sung, K., Wang, L., Coupland, N. and Dolcos, F. (2010). The Impact of Anxiety-Inducing Distraction

REFERENCES

on Cognitive Performance: A Combined Brain Imaging and Personality Investigation. *PLoS ONE*, 5(11), p.e14150.

Chapter Fifteen

1. Jones, M. (1924). A Laboratory Study of Fear: The Case Of Peter. *The Pedagogical Seminary and Journal of Genetic Psychology*, 31(4), pp.308-315.

2. Rothbaum, B. and Schwartz, A. (2002). Exposure therapy for posttraumatic stress disorder. 56(1), pp.59-75.

3. ScienceDaily. (2018). *The neurons that rewrite traumatic memories*. [online] Available at: https://www.sciencedaily.com/releases/2018/06/180614213824.htm [Accessed 17 Jun. 2018].

Chapter Sixteen

1. Association for Psychological Science. "A Little Anxiety Is Sometimes A Good Thing, Study Shows." ScienceDaily. ScienceDaily, 5 April 2008. <www.sciencedaily.com/releases/2008/04/080403104350.htm>.

2. Mobbs, D., Hagan, C., Dalgleish, T., Silston, B. and Prevost, C. (2015). The ecology of human fear: survival optimization and the nervous system. *Frontiers in Neuroscience*, 9.

Chapter Seventeen

1. Lee, J. and Sung, Y. (2016). Hide-and-Seek: Narcissism and "Selfie"-Related Behavior. *Cyberpsychology, Behavior, and Social Networking*, 19(5), pp.347-351.

2. Sharma, M. and Khanna, A. (2017). Selfie use: The implications for psychopathology expression of body dysmorphic disorder. *Industrial Psychiatry Journal*, 26(1), p.106.

3. Raghunathan Ph.D., R. (2013). *How Negative is Your "Mental Chatter"?*. [online] Psychology Today. Available at: https://www.psychologytoday.com/us/blog/sapient-nature/201310/how-negative-is-your-mental-chatter [Accessed 16 Feb. 2018].

4. Cell Press. (2016, February 11). Why smiles (and frowns) are contagious. *ScienceDaily*. Retrieved October 29, 2017 from www.sciencedaily.com/releases/2016/02/160211140428.htm

5. Thompson, A. (2006). *Study: Laughter Really Is Contagious*. [online] livescience.com. Available at: https://www.livescience.com/9430-study-laughter-contagious.html [Accessed 19 Dec. 2017].

6. Boyd, R. and Richerson, P. (2009). Culture and the evolution of human cooperation. *Philosophical Transactions of the Royal Society B: Biological Sciences*, 364(1533), pp.3281-3288.

7. Yeung, J., Zhang, Z. and Kim, T. (2017). Volunteering and health benefits in general adults: cumulative effects and forms. *BMC Public Health*, 18(1).

Chapter Eighteen

1. Tracy, B. (2018). *The Power of Your Subconscious Mind | Brian Tracy*. [online] Briantracy.com. Available at: https://www.briantracy.com/blog/personal-success/understanding-your-subconscious-mind/ [Accessed 4 Mar. 2018].

2. Häuser, W., Hagl, M., Schmierer, A. and Hansen, E. (2016). The Efficacy, Safety and Applications of Medical Hypnosis: A Systematic Review of Meta-analyses. *Deutsches Aerzteblatt Online*, 113(17), pp.289–296.

3. Shih, M., Yang, Y. and Koo, M. (2009). A Meta-Analysis of Hypnosis in the Treatment of Depressive Symptoms: A Brief

REFERENCES

Communication. *International Journal of Clinical and Experimental Hypnosis*, 57(4), pp.431-442.

4. Ponton, MD, L. (2018). *All About Hypnosis and Hypnotherapy*. [online] Psych Central. Available at: https://psychcentral.com/lib/all-about-hypnosis-and-hypnotherapy [Accessed 18 Mar. 2018].

5. Hypnosisandsuggestion.org. (2018). *Measurement | Hypnosis And Suggestion*. [online] Available at: https://hypnosisandsuggestion.org//measurement-of-hypnosis.html [Accessed 4 Mar. 2018].

6. Untas, A., Chauveau, P., Dupré-Goudable, C., Kolko, A., Lakdja, F. and Cazenave, N. (2013). The Effects of Hypnosis on Anxiety, Depression, Fatigue, and Sleepiness in People Undergoing Hemodialysis: A Clinical Report. *International Journal of Clinical and Experimental Hypnosis*, 61(4), pp.475-483.

7. Cordi, M., Schlarb, A. and Rasch, B. (2014). Deepening Sleep by Hypnotic Suggestion. *Sleep*, 37(6), pp.1143-1152.

8. Stenstrom, J. (2018). *How To Double Your Life Span, Turn Back The Clock On Aging, And Reverse All Chronic Disease – Dr. Michael Fossel (Ep. 169) - Elite Man Magazine*. [online] Elite Man Magazine. Available at: http://elitemanmagazine.com/reverse-aging-and-all-chronic-disease-dr-michael-fossel [Accessed 2 May 2018].

Chapter Nineteen

1. Schuch, F., Vancampfort, D., Richards, J., Rosenbaum, S., Ward, P. and Stubbs, B. (2016). Exercise as a treatment for depression: A meta-analysis adjusting for publication bias. *Journal of Psychiatric Research*, 77, pp.42-51.

2. Blumenthal, J., Babyak, M., Moore, K., Craighead, W., Herman, S., Khatri, P., Waugh, R., Napolitano, M., Forman, L., Appelbaum, M.,

Doraiswamy, P. and Krishnan, K. (1999). Effects of Exercise Training on Older Patients With Major Depression. *Archives of Internal Medicine*, 159(19), pp.2349-2356.

3. Publishing, H. (2013). *Exercise is an all-natural treatment to fight depression - Harvard Health*. [online] Harvard Health. Available at: https://www.health.harvard.edu/mind-and-mood/exercise-is-an-all-natural-treatment-to-fight-depression [Accessed 15 Mar. 2018].

4. RANSFORD, C. (1982). A role for amines in the antidepressant effect of exercise. *Medicine & Science in Sports & Exercise*, 14(1), pp.1-10.

5. DiLorenzo, T., Bargman, E., Stucky-Ropp, R., Brassington, G., Frensch, P. and LaFontaine, T. (1999). Long-Term Effects of Aerobic Exercise on Psychological Outcomes. *Preventive Medicine*, 28(1), pp.75-85.

6. Sharma, A., Madaan, V. and Petty, F. (2006). Exercise for Mental Health. *Primary Care Companion to The Journal of Clinical Psychiatry*, 8(2), p.106.

7. Amen Clinics. (2018). *How To Walk Your Way to Better Brain Health | Amen Clinics*. [online] Available at: https://www.amenclinics.com/blog/walk-your-way-to-mental-health [Accessed 2 Apr. 2018].

8. Lincoln, A., Shepherd, A., Johnson, P. and Castaneda-Sceppa, C. (2011). The Impact of Resistance Exercise Training on the Mental Health of Older Puerto Rican Adults With Type 2 Diabetes. *The Journals of Gerontology Series B: Psychological Sciences and Social Sciences*, 66B(5), pp.567-570.

REFERENCES

9. Zhai, L., Zhang, Y. and Zhang, D. (2014). Sedentary behaviour and the risk of depression: a meta-analysis. *British Journal of Sports Medicine*, 49(11), pp.705-709.

10. CALLAGHAN, P. (2004). Exercise: a neglected intervention in mental health care?. *Journal of Psychiatric and Mental Health Nursing*, 11(4), pp.476-483.

Chapter Twenty

1. Eby, G. and Eby, K. (2006). Rapid recovery from major depression using magnesium treatment. *Medical Hypotheses*, 67(2), pp.362-370.

2. Lopresti, A., Maes, M., Maker, G., Hood, S. and Drummond, P. (2014). Curcumin for the treatment of major depression: A randomised, double-blind, placebo controlled study. *Journal of Affective Disorders*, 167, pp.368-375.

3. Al-Karawi, D., Al Mamoori, D. and Tayyar, Y. (2015). The Role of Curcumin Administration in Patients with Major Depressive Disorder: Mini Meta-Analysis of Clinical Trials. *Phytotherapy Research*, 30(2), pp.175-183.

4. McNamara, R., Jandacek, R., Rider, T., Tso, P., Chu, W., Weber, W., Welge, J., Strawn, J., Adler, C. and DelBello, M. (2016). Effects of fish oil supplementation on prefrontal metabolite concentrations in adolescents with major depressive disorder: A preliminary 1H MRS study. *Nutritional Neuroscience*, 19(4), pp.145-155.

5. Cui, X., Chopp, M., Zacharek, A., Roberts, C., Buller, B., Ion, M. and Chen, J. (2010). Niacin Treatment of Stroke Increases Synaptic Plasticity and Axon Growth in Rats. *Stroke*, 41(9), pp.2044-2049.

6. Jiang, G. and Xu, X. (2015). Niacin-respondent subset of schizophrenia – a therapeutic review. *European Review for Medical and Pharmacological Sciences*, 19(6), pp.988-97.

7. Saul, A. (2000). *DoctorYourself.com - Review of VITAMIN B-3 AND SCHIZOPHRENIA*. [online] Doctoryourself.com. Available at: http://www.doctoryourself.com/review_hoffer_B3.html [Accessed 10 Dec. 2017].

8. Orthomolecular.org. (1999). *The Adrenochrome Hypothesis and Psychiatry - A. Hoffer, M.D. Ph.D. and H. Osmond, M.D.*. [online] Available at: http://orthomolecular.org/library/jom/1999/articles/1999-v14n01-p049.shtml [Accessed 12 Dec. 2017].

9. Coppen, A. and Bolander-Gouaille, C. (2005). Treatment of depression: time to consider folic acid and vitamin B12. *Journal of Psychopharmacology*, 19(1), pp.59-65.

10. Lewis, J., Tiozzo, E., Melillo, A., Leonard, S., Chen, L., Mendez, A., Woolger, J. and Konefal, J. (2013). The Effect of Methylated Vitamin B Complex on Depressive and Anxiety Symptoms and Quality of Life in Adults with Depression. *ISRN Psychiatry*, 2013, pp.1-7.

11. MACHADO-VIEIRA, R., ZANETTI, M., DE SOUSA, R., SOEIRO-DE-SOUZA, M., MORENO, R., BUSATTO, G. and GATTAZ, W. (2014). Lithium efficacy in bipolar depression with flexible dosing: A six-week, open-label, proof-of-concept study. *Experimental and Therapeutic Medicine*, 8(4), pp.1205-1208.

12. Pinto-Sanchez, M., Hall, G., Ghajar, K., Nardelli, A., Bolino, C., Lau, J., Martin, F., Cominetti, O., Welsh, C., Rieder, A., Traynor, J., Gregory, C., De Palma, G., Pigrau, M., Ford, A., Macri, J., Berger, B., Bergonzelli, G., Surette, M., Collins, S., Moayyedi, P. and Bercik, P. (2017). Probiotic Bifidobacterium longum NCC3001 Reduces Depression Scores and Alters Brain Activity: A Pilot Study in Patients With Irritable Bowel Syndrome. *Gastroenterology*, 153(2), pp.448-459.e8.

REFERENCES

13. Bravo, J., Forsythe, P., Chew, M., Escaravage, E., Savignac, H., Dinan, T., Bienenstock, J. and Cryan, J. (2011). Ingestion of Lactobacillus strain regulates emotional behavior and central GABA receptor expression in a mouse via the vagus nerve. *Proceedings of the National Academy of Sciences*, 108(38), pp.16050-16055.

14. Desbonnet, L., Garrett, L., Clarke, G., Kiely, B., Cryan, J. and Dinan, T. (2010). Effects of the probiotic Bifidobacterium infantis in the maternal separation model of depression. *Neuroscience*, 170(4), pp.1179-1188.

15. Wallace, C. and Milev, R. (2017). The effects of probiotics on depressive symptoms in humans: a systematic review. *Annals of General Psychiatry*, 16(1).

16. Sciencedirect.com. (2012). *Chamomile - an overview | ScienceDirect Topics*. [online] Available at: https://www.sciencedirect.com/topics/agricultural-and-biological-sciences/chamomile [Accessed 6 Jan. 2018].

17. Amsterdam, J., Shults, J., Soeller, I., Mao, J., Rockwell, K. and Newberg, A. (2012). Chamomile (Matricaria recutita) May Have Antidepressant Activity in Anxious Depressed Humans - An Exploratory Study. *Alternative Therapies in Health and Medicine*, 18(5), pp.44–49.

18. Sarris, J., I. Papakostas, G., Vitolo, O., Fava, M. and Mischoulon, D. (2014). S-adenosyl methionine (SAMe) versus escitalopram and placebo in major depression RCT: Efficacy and effects of histamine and carnitine as moderators of response. *Journal of Affective Disorders*, 164, pp.76-81.

19. Hinz, M., Stein, A. and Hinz, M. (2012). 5-HTP efficacy and contraindications. *Neuropsychiatric Disease and Treatment*, pp.323-328.

20. Birdsall, T. (1998). 5-Hydroxytryptophan: a clinically-effective serotonin precursor. *Alternative Medicine Review*, 3(4), pp.271-80.

21. Butterweck, V., Böckers, T., Korte, B., Wittkowski, W. and Winterhoff, H. (2002). Long-term effects of St. John's wort and hypericin on monoamine levels in rat hypothalamus and hippocampus. *Brain Research*, 930(1-2), pp.21-29.

22. Wiley-Blackwell. (2008, October 13). St. John's Wort Relieves Symptoms Of Major Depression, Study Shows. *ScienceDaily*. Retrieved October 21, 2017 from www.sciencedaily.com/releases/2008/10/081007192435.htm

Chapter Twenty-One

1. University of Rochester Medical Center. (2018, February 2). Low levels of alcohol good for the brain, study shows. *ScienceDaily*. Retrieved February 10, 2018 from www.sciencedaily.com/releases/2018/02/180202085241.htm

2. Gershuni, V. (2018). Saturated Fat: Part of a Healthy Diet. *Current Nutrition Reports*, 7(3), pp.85-96.

3. de Punder, K. and Pruimboom, L. (2013). The Dietary Intake of Wheat and other Cereal Grains and Their Role in Inflammation. *Nutrients*, 5(3), pp.771-787.

4. MALEKINEJAD, H. and REZABAKHSH, A. (2015). Hormones in Dairy Foods and Their Impact on Public Health - A Narrative Review Article. *Iranian Journal of Public Health*, 44(6), pp.742–758.

Chapter Twenty-Two

1. Weeks, D., Michela, J., Peplau, L. and Bragg, M. (1980). Relation between loneliness and depression: A structural equation

REFERENCES

analysis. *Journal of Personality and Social Psychology*, 39(6), pp.1238-1244.

2. Matthews, T., Danese, A., Wertz, J., Odgers, C., Ambler, A., Moffitt, T. and Arseneault, L. (2016). Social isolation, loneliness and depression in young adulthood: a behavioural genetic analysis. *Social Psychiatry and Psychiatric Epidemiology*, 51(3), pp.339-348.

3. Stravynski, A. and Boyer, R. (2001). Loneliness in Relation to Suicide Ideation and Parasuicide: A Population-Wide Study. *Suicide and Life-Threatening Behavior*, 31(1), pp.32-40.

4. Stillman, T., Baumeister, R., Lambert, N., Crescioni, A., DeWall, C. and Fincham, F. (2009). Alone and without purpose: Life loses meaning following social exclusion. *Journal of Experimental Social Psychology*, 45(4), pp.686-694.

Chapter Twenty-Three

1. Błażek, M., Kaźmierczak, M. and Besta, T. (2014). Sense of Purpose in Life and Escape from Self as the Predictors of Quality of Life in Clinical Samples. *Journal of Religion and Health*, 54(2), pp.517-523.

2. Schaefer, S., Morozink Boylan, J., van Reekum, C., Lapate, R., Norris, C., Ryff, C. and Davidson, R. (2013). Purpose in Life Predicts Better Emotional Recovery from Negative Stimuli. *PLoS ONE*, 8(11), p.e80329.

Chapter Twenty-Four

1. Nami.org. (2017). *Self-harm | NAMI: National Alliance on Mental Illness*. [online] Available at: https://www.nami.org/Learn-More/Mental-Health-Conditions/Related-Conditions/Self-harm [Accessed 10 Dec. 2017].

2. Mayo Clinic. (2017). *Self-injury/cutting - Symptoms and causes.* [online] Available at: https://www.mayoclinic.org/diseases-conditions/self-injury/symptoms-causes/syc-20350950 [Accessed 4 Feb. 2018].

3. Peterson, J., Freedenthal, S., Sheldon, C., & Andersen, R. (2008). Nonsuicidal Self injury in Adolescents. *Psychiatry (Edgmont (Pa. : Township))*, 5(11), 20–26.

Chapter Twenty-Five

1. Cortese, A. *et al*. Multivoxel neurofeedback selectively modulates confidence without changing perceptual performance. *Nat. Commun.* **7**, 13669 doi: 10.1038/ncomms13669 (2016).

Chapter Twenty-Six

1. Ibarra, H. (2015). *You're Never Too Experienced to Fake It Till You Learn It.* [online] Harvard Business Review. Available at: https://hbr.org/2015/01/youre-never-too-experienced-to-fake-it-till-you-learn-it [Accessed 17 Jan. 2018].

2. Kraft, T. and Pressman, S. (2012). Grin and Bear It. *Psychological Science*, 23(11), pp.1372-1378.

3. Weger, U. and Loughnan, S. (2013). Rapid communication: Mobilizing unused resources: Using the placebo concept to enhance cognitive performance. *Quarterly Journal of Experimental Psychology*, 66(1), pp.23-28.

4. University of Melbourne. (2012, October 18). Self-confidence the secret to workplace advancement. *ScienceDaily*. Retrieved October 19, 2017 from www.sciencedaily.com/releases/2012/10/121018103214.htm

Chapter Twenty-Seven

REFERENCES

1. Jones, A. (1992). Gestalt therapy: theory and practice. *Nursing Standard*, 6(38), pp.31-34.

2. Thom, S. (2011). Hyperbaric Oxygen: Its Mechanisms and Efficacy. *Plastic and Reconstructive Surgery*, 127, pp.131S-141S.

3. Harch, P. (2017). *Harch HBOT*. [online] Hbot.com. Available at: http://www.hbot.com [Accessed 27 Dec. 2017].

4. Watanabe, H. and Mizunami, M. (2007). Pavlov's Cockroach: Classical Conditioning of Salivation in an Insect. *PLoS ONE*, 2(6), p.e529.

Chapter Twenty-Eight

1. Hays, K., Thomas, O., Maynard, I. and Bawden, M. (2009). The role of confidence in world-class sport performance. *Journal of Sports Sciences*, 27(11), pp.1185-1199.

Chapter Twenty-Nine

1. Townsend, J. M., & Levy, G. D. (1990). Effects of potential partners' costume and physical attractiveness on sexuality and partner selection. *The Journal of Psychology: Interdisciplinary and Applied*, 124(4), 371-389.

2. Kucharska, A., Szmurło, A. and Sińska, B. (2016). Significance of diet in treated and untreated acne vulgaris. *Advances in Dermatology and Allergology*, 33(2), pp.81-86.

3. Chang, J., Zhang, M., Hitchman, G., Qiu, J. and Liu, Y. (2014). When you smile, you become happy: Evidence from resting state task-based fMRI. *Biological Psychology*, 103, pp.100-106.

Chapter Thirty

1. Fowler, J. and Christakis, N. (2008). Dynamic spread of happiness in a large social network: longitudinal analysis over 20 years in the Framingham Heart Study. *BMJ*, 337(dec04 2), pp.a2338-a2338.

2. Cunningham, S., Vaquera, E., Maturo, C. and Venkat Narayan, K. (2012). Is there evidence that friends influence body weight? A systematic review of empirical research. *Social Science & Medicine*, 75(7), pp.1175-1183.

Chapter Thirty-One

1. McKenna, H. (2017). *Here's what Tom Brady told Patriots on sideline before mounting Super Bowl LI comeback.* [online] Patriots Wire. Available at: http://patriotswire.usatoday.com/2017/03/04/heres-what-tom-brady-told-patriots-on-sideline-before-mounting-super-bowl-li-comeback [Accessed 1 Mar. 2018].

2. Manfred, T. (2014). *Tom Brady Does Brain Exercises So He Can Go To Sleep At 9 PM And Wake Up Without An Alarm.* [online] Business Insider. Available at: http://www.businessinsider.com/tom-brady-sleep-plan-2014-12 [Accessed 3 Mar. 2018].

3. Puran, S. (2016). *Tom Brady's competitiveness is contagious.* [online] Sports.yahoo.com. Available at: https://sports.yahoo.com/news/tom-brady-competitiveness-contagious-182531850.html [Accessed 4 Mar. 2018].

4. Bishop, G. (2014). *The Other Side of Brady.* [online] SI.com. Available at: https://www.si.com/2014/12/12/tom-brady-off-field-former-teammates [Accessed 4 Mar. 2018].

Last Words

1. Stenstrom, J. (2017). *How To Unfuck Yourself And Create The Life You Want – Gary John Bishop - Elite Man.* [online] Elite Man Magazine.

REFERENCES

Available at: http://elitemanmagazine.com/unfuck-yourself-gary-john-bishop [Accessed 14 Mar. 2018].

Epilogue

1. Ferguson, J. (2001). SSRI Antidepressant Medications: Adverse Effects and Tolerability. *The Primary Care Companion to The Journal of Clinical Psychiatry,* 3(1), pp.22-27.

ACKNOWLEDGMENTS

I'd like to thank my family above all else for always supporting me even when they didn't quite get what I was trying to do. I didn't need them to fully grasp my plans, only to support me and have faith that they would work out. And they did, and so did some of those plans. Fufe, Javen, Dad, Mom, Jett, Janiyah, Jess, Joe, Junior, Old Man, love you guys.

I'd also like to thank everyone who contributed to this book, and in particular Steve T. and Marinda W., thank you for perfecting these lines and making them shine. I couldn't do it without your help. Also, thank you to Craig Ballantyne, Frank Miniter, Andrew Marr, Dr. Ted Achacoso, Ben Newman, Gary John Bishop, Dr. Pankaj Vij and many more for your support and friendship. I truly appreciate it.

Lastly, a special thanks to my friend and therapist Laura for helping me unpack a lot of crap over the years. You're truly a brilliant and kind soul and I sincerely appreciate everything you've done for me.

RESOURCES

For further learning and elite mind training go to:

EliteMindBook.com

For the best and most trusted nutritional supplements in the world go to:

EliteLifeNutrition.com

And for all-around exceptional content on mindset, success, and performance go to these links:

EliteManMagazine.com
EliteManMagazine.com/youtube
Instagram.com/JustinStenstrom

ABOUT THE AUTHOR

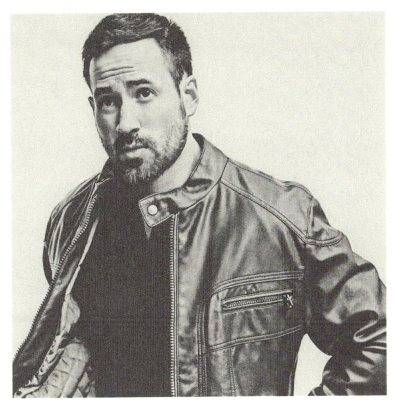

JUSTIN STENSTROM

Justin Stenstrom is a nationally-acclaimed life coach, bestselling author, and speaker. He is the Editor-in-Chief of EliteManMagazine.com, the founder of Elite Life Nutrition, and the host of the Elite Man Podcast, where he interviews some of the world's most successful entrepreneurs, authors, and high-achieving individuals, including guests like Robert Greene, Grant Cardone, Dr. John Gray, Bas Rutten, Wim Hof, Kevin Harrington, and many others. Once anxious, insecure, depressed, and unhappy, Justin's overcome many of life's greatest obstacles and loves nothing more than helping others do the same.

ELITE MIND